An Introduction to Generative Drug Discovery

This book focuses on the latest advances in computational *de novo* drug discovery methods, also known as generative drug discovery. This book describes the state-of-the-art methods and applications for de novo design of drug candidates using generative chemistry models as well as the ethical aspects of this technology. It will provide a foundation for those new to the field as well as those that may already have some experience of its utility. With contributions from scientists in both academia and industry 'An Introduction to Generative Drug Discovery' may represent one of the earliest, if not the first book, to focus on this topic.

DRUGS AND THE PHARMACEUTICAL SCIENCES
A Series of Textbooks and Monographs
Series Editor
Anthony J. Hickey
RTI International, Research Triangle Park, USA

The Drugs and Pharmaceutical Sciences series is designed to enable the pharmaceutical scientist to stay abreast of the changing trends, advances and innovations associated with therapeutic drugs and that area of expertise and interest that has come to be known as the pharmaceutical sciences. The body of knowledge that those working in the pharmaceutical environment have to work with, and master, has been, and continues, to expand at a rapid pace as new scientific approaches, technologies, instrumentations, clinical advances, economic factors and social needs arise and influence the discovery, development, manufacture, commercialization and clinical use of new agents and devices.
Recent Titles in Series

Emerging Drug Delivery and Biomedical Engineering Technologies: Transforming Therapy
Dimitrios Lamprou

RNA-seq in Drug Discovery and Development
Feng Cheng and Robert Morris

Patient Safety in Developing Countries: Education, Research, Case Studies
Yaser Al-Worafi

Industrial Hygiene in the Pharmaceutical and Consumer Healthcare Industries
Casey Cosner

Cancer Targeting Therapies: Conventional and Advanced Perspectives
Muhammad Yasir Ali and Shazia Bukhari

Molecular Recognition in Pharmacology
Mikhail Darkhovskiy

GMP Audits in Pharmaceutical and Biotechnology Industries
Mustafa EDİK

Purification of Biotechnological Products: A Focus on Industrial Applications
Adalberto Pessoa Jr, Beatriz Vahan Kilikian, and Paul Long

Principles of Research Methodology and Ethics in Pharmaceutical Sciences: An Application Guide for Students and Researchers
Vikas Anand Saharan, Hitesh Kulhari, and Hemant Jadhav

Good Clinical Practices in Pharmaceuticals
Graham P. Bunn

An Introduction to Generative Drug Discovery
Sean Ekins

For more information about this series, please visit: www.crcpress.com/Drugs-and-the-Pharmaceutical-Sciences/book-series/IHCDRUPHASCI

An Introduction to Generative Drug Discovery

Edited by

Sean Ekins, Ph.D., D.Sc.

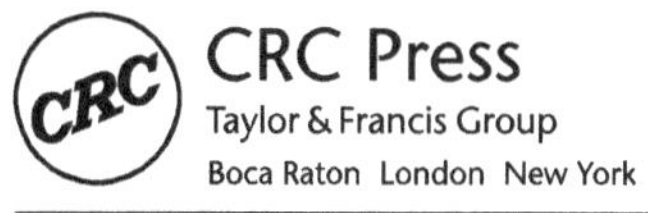

CRC Press is an imprint of the
Taylor & Francis Group, an informa business

Designed cover image: Sean Ekins, Joshua S. Harris, Fabio Urbina, Rıza Özçelik and Francesca Grisoni

First edition published 2025
by CRC Press
2385 NW Executive Center Drive, Suite 320, Boca Raton FL 33431

and by CRC Press
4 Park Square, Milton Park, Abingdon, Oxon, OX14 4RN

CRC Press is an imprint of Taylor & Francis Group, LLC

ISBN: 9781032506234 (hbk)
ISBN: 9781032506258 (pbk)
ISBN: 9781003399346 (ebk)

DOI: 10.1201/9781003399346

Typeset in Times
by codeMantra

I thought that it was time to expose my own research co-workers, to the power and limitations of knowledge engineering, otherwise known as "artificial intelligence".

Carl Djerassi, The Pill, Pygmy Chimps and Degas' Horse, 1992

For Dr. Steve Wrighton and Mr. Jim Wikel who let me explore computational approaches as a postdoc at Eli Lilly, which ultimately enabled this book nearly 30 years later!

Contents

Preface

Having spent nearly 30 years using software in drug discovery, one gets to see and apply many new technologies that are proposed to be 'game-changers'. The past few years have seen numerous rapid developments in hardware, software, and data such that artificial intelligence (AI) has become an everyday occurrence and is available in cars, phones, and other devices to help us with our everyday tasks. With the emergence of ChatGPT and the many similar generative tools, even the layperson has now heard of 'generative AI'. This book began just a few years ago as a rather ambitious idea to try to gather a number of the proponents of generative drug discovery in one place while the topic was in its early years. After observing the rapid progress and seeing increasing interest in the field, I saw there were no monographs on the subject up to that point. I thought the topic was rather 'hot' then, and it still seems to be having its moment so I hope this book will appear in time to feed the need for scientists to learn more about this topic.

The goals of this book are to simply describe the 'state of the art 'methods and applications for *de novo* design of drug candidates using generative chemistry models all the way through to the ethical aspects of this technology. I invited several leading authors from around the world who have published on this topic in the last few years to contribute their chapters. We are honored that these contributors agreed to participate and add their work to create this overview of the topic. Furthermore, to increase the practical appeal of this book to readers, we encouraged the authors to describe and make their respective software accessible. The mix of academic and industrial authors also provides for balance in the topics and also enables exploration of where the field could go in the future.

In the intervening time since starting on this project of course, considerably more publications on generative drug discovery have appeared, so this made it a little more difficult to capture everything. But still it should encapsulate a snapshot of where generative drug discovery has been, its potential (without overhyping), limitations, and the prediction of the overall direction it might go in future.

Ultimately, I look forward to hearing how this may lead to the next generation of generative drug discovery scientists and inspire the development of future drugs that will impact healthcare. Enjoy!

Sean Ekins,
Fuquay Varina, May 2024

Acknowledgments

What you have in your hands is the 'end result' and I have to sincerely thank those that took us up on the invitation to contribute chapters including Alex Aliper, Connor Coley, Wenhao Gao, Francesca Grisoni, Dragos Horvath, Gilles Marcou, Rıza Özçelik, Quentin Vanhaelen, Alexandre Varnek, and Alex Zhavoronkov. My colleagues Josh Harris, Thane Jones, Tom Lane, and Fabio Urbina are also kindly acknowledged for their assistance in helping me with this endeavor.

I am also grateful to the patience of the publishers Taylor and Francis, Hilary Lafoe and team who have been remarkably flexible as my 'day job' as a CEO has taken precedence. This is also a good opportunity to acknowledge colleagues for their willingness to provide advice and support along the way. A big thank you to Dr. Anthony J. Hickey for his sage advice and support, and to Dr. Alex Tropsha for earlier input on the proposal and help nudging a few authors.

My family (Maggie, Penny and Enzo) allowed frequent disappearances, time taken during vacations and holidays, and saw me hunched over the laptop writing and responding to emails. I hope it was all worth it. This is one of those few examples when you can still see a physical product of a specific effort at the end. Again, I thank the contributors and the many other scientists that inspired this book (and some that could not assist due to their workload but provided valuable suggestions of others to get involved).

About the Editor

Sean Ekins is founder and CEO of Collaborations Pharmaceuticals, Inc. (CPI) which is focused on using machine learning approaches for rare and neglected disease drug discovery. Sean graduated from Trent Polytechnic receiving a HND in Applied Biology then graduated from the University of Aberdeen, receiving his M.Sc., Ph.D. in Clinical Pharmacology, and D.Sc. in Science. He was a postdoctoral fellow at Eli Lilly before working as a senior scientist at Pfizer and then returning to Eli Lilly. He went on to join several startup companies at increasingly senior levels. Since 2005, he has been awarded numerous grants as PI for a wide array of start-up companies totaling over $12.2M as well as performing as a consultant on others. Since 2016, he has additionally won over 20 additional grants from NIH and DOD (STTR/SBIR grants, R21, UH2, and R01) totaling over $23.5M for CPI. He has a passion for advancing new technologies for drug discovery and is a prolific collaborator. He has authored or co-authored over 375 peer-reviewed papers and book chapters, edited 5 books on different aspects of drug discovery research and topics, and written 1 book on winning grants. Coverage of his recent research has also appeared in the *Economist*, *Financial Times*, *The Washington Post*, *Wired*, *Scientific American*, CNN, and Netflix, as well as several podcasts. When he is not writing he enjoys cycling and collecting vinyl.

Contributors List

Alex Aliper
Insilico Medicine Hong Kong Ltd and Insilico Medicine AI Ltd
Abu Dhabi, United Arab Emirates

Connor W. Coley
Department of Chemical Engineering
Massachusetts Institute of Technology
Cambridge, Massachusetts
and
Department of Electrical Engineering and Computer Science
Massachusetts Institute of Technology
Cambridge, Massachusetts

Wenhao Gao
Department of Chemical Engineering
Massachusetts Institute of Technology
Cambridge, Massachusetts

Francesca Grisoni
Department of Biomedical Engineering
Institute for Complex Molecular Systems
Eindhoven University of Technology
Eindhoven, The Netherlands

Joshua S. Harris
Collaborations Pharmaceuticals, Inc.
Raleigh, North Carolina

Dragos Horvath
Laboratory of Chemoinformatics
University of Strasbourg
Strasbourg, France

Thane Jones
Collaborations Pharmaceuticals, Inc.
Raleigh, North Carolina

Thomas R. Lane
Collaborations Pharmaceuticals, Inc.
Raleigh, North Carolina

Gilles Marcou
Laboratory of Chemoinformatics
University of Strasbourg
Strasbourg, France

Rıza Özçelik
Department of Biomedical Engineering
Institute for Complex Molecular Systems
Eindhoven University of Technology
Eindhoven, The Netherlands

Fabio Urbina
Collaborations Pharmaceuticals, Inc.
Raleigh, North Carolina

Quentin Vanhaelen
Pharma.AI
Insilico Medicine AI Ltd.
Abu Dhabi, United Arab Emirates

Alexandre Varnek
Laboratory of Chemoinformatics
University of Strasbourg
Strasbourg, France

Alex Zhavoronkov
Pharma.AI
Insilico Medicine AI Ltd
Abu Dhabi, United Arab Emirates

Part I

Introduction to Generative Chemical Design

1 Going beyond Serendipity
Generative Artificial Intelligence for Drug Discovery

Sean Ekins

1.1 INTRODUCTION

Discovery needs luck, invention, intellect- none can do without the other

Johann Wolfgang Goethe (1749–1832)

It is hard to imagine that humanity once almost entirely relied on serendipity to identify molecules with potential for therapeutic activity against diseases. Industrial pharmaceutical companies go back to the 17th century in the case of Merck, and many others are well over 100 years old (e.g. Pfizer and Eli Lilly) and have certainly capitalized on this. Historically, you do not have to go back that far to see this serendipity in action. Well-known examples are the discovery of penicillin by Alexander Fleming nearly 100 years ago, sildenafil (Viagra) in the 1990s[1] and the repurposing of GLP-1 agonists from diabetes to obesity.[2] Chance observation has likely led to many such discoveries that have been life-saving and impacted healthcare, subsequently creating massive economic value (or incredible costs, depending on the perspective). Rather than relying on just serendipity, the industry has also used trial and error experimentation often called the Edisonian approach. These twin approaches have long been the way how research and development was undertaken in the pharmaceutical industry. The cost of bringing a drug to market has however rocketed upward with estimates ranging quite widely from around \$1bn,[3] \$2.8bn[4] and beyond \$4bn.[5] This has necessitated the need to develop new approaches in an effort to 'industrialize' drug discovery and increase efficiency. Over the past 30 years alone drug discovery has been inundated with new technologies that have been heralded as going to revolutionize it, as the next big thing. These have included the likes of combinatorial chemistry,[6] high throughput screening (HTS),[7,8] phenotypic screening,[9] phage display,[10] fragment-based design,[11] structure-based design,[12] X-ray crystallography,[13] Cryo-EM,[14] docking and virtual screening,[15,16] organ-on-a-chip,[17] systems biology,[18–20] computer aided drug discovery,[21] DNA-encoded libraries[22] and drug repurposing.[23] While many of these widely used tools or approaches have

DOI: 10.1201/9781003399346-2

certainly contributed greatly to drug discovery, they have been mostly evolutionary in nature rather than revolutionary. This leads us to the most recent areas of interest that have followed in the last few years. It seems like we were no sooner caught up in the excitement around deep learning[24,25] than we were thrust into the field of generative artificial intelligence[26,27] and the flood gates were opened. While the general public perhaps only became aware of generative artificial intelligence (AI) once ChatGPT was launched in the fall of 2022, scientists in drug discovery have been applying these approaches for several years prior to this. What follows is a brief overview of generative approaches for *de novo* design and associated areas of interest to drug discovery such as methods to predict molecule synthesizabilty which may also be important before embarking upon the synthesis of molecules. We may be at the point where we can combine human and artificial intelligence to aid in pharmaceutical research and development.[28]

1.2 GENERATIVE AI FOR DRUG DISCOVERY

Normally, we would use a machine learning model to score an array of molecules to predict a property (e.g. bioactivity or absorption, distribution, metabolism, excretion and toxicity (ADME/Tox) properties, etc.). Now, if we start with a desired property value and imagine how we could get to molecules that fulfill these requirements (whether a single parameter or multiple parameter optimization), this is termed inverse design. One possible way to get to such molecules is to use a generative model. A generative model learns the probability of a chemical with the desired properties given the structure. This is an area that is increasingly being applied and also reviewed.[29] Of course, these approaches are not limited to drug discovery or even small molecule design as the method could also be used to explore chemical property space for materials design to develop molecules with other commercial applications, e.g. polymers.[28] There have been significant discoveries in the field of *de novo* drug design[30,31] which has renewed interest in generating new molecules using machine learning.[31] These have included several algorithms such as Recurrent Neural Networks (RNN),[31] Variational Autoencoder (VAE)[32,33] and Generative Adversarial Networks (GANs)[34] which can be used to design realistic molecules possessing physicochemical properties[35–38] that are in ranges that are desired. These approaches can also use different representations of molecules, whether 2D strings[39,40] or 3D graphs.[41] Many of the algorithms for RNNs and GANs, as well as graph-based algorithms such as junction tree variational autoencoders (JT-VAE),[40] are freely available as open-source python software. RNNs have been widely used in many areas, from generating libraries for HTS, hit to lead optimization, to fragment-based discovery.[27,38,41–44] Examples include training with molecules from ChEMBL, a two-layer long short-term memory (LSTM)-based RNN was used to generate libraries of SMILES followed by transfer learning to tune the model and generate a library of leads from a starting known active fragment[42] while another generated molecules using predicted properties.[43] These generative models can therefore enable the simultaneous optimization of multiple parameters like physicochemical properties or biological activity. However, most of the published examples have optimized against a single physicochemical activity or bioactivity, with one group using an RNN for multiple parameter optimization.[44]

Several groups have also focused on graph structures rather than SMILES such as Mol-CycleGAN,[41] which has the advantage of returning 100% valid structures. In some cases, the software was also open-sourced.[38,41] Recently, transformers and attention-based models were introduced and are *de facto* state-of-the-art in natural language processing, with the most well-known language models such as BERT[45] being based on transformer architecture.[46] While these new approaches are very promising, a critical knowledge gap exists namely, that limited experimental validation data was generated by synthesizing compounds and testing for activity for any of the aforementioned studies. Zhavoronkov et al.,[47] are among the earliest to have validated their generative approach by making or testing a few compounds[47] or finding structurally similar compounds from vendors.[48] In most cases, the molecules identified are generally structurally very similar to known actives. Generative models can explore the chemical space, propose molecules fitting design criteria and therefore validate this approach. However, default models may not lead to molecules in the desired chemical property space because either they stay close to the starting structure (if there was one) or they veer wildly off course and into non-synthesizable chemical space. Hence a single generative model may not cover all potential needs (hit discovery and lead optimization) for a company or group exploiting different targets and chemistries and this may require an array of different design approaches to be used.

1.2.1 Generative Applications

The Chemistry42 platform was launched in 2020 has been described in a recent application note (see also Chapter 2).[49] The generative design can be enabled for ligand-based drug design and structure-based drug design and it is suggested that 40+ models using different molecular representation are used to generate molecules which usually then converge over 3 days or more. It is mentioned that the performance of each generative model is monitored and recorded. Several case studies are presented including an earlier study from 2018 which described the generative tensorial reinforcement learning (GENTRL) model for DDR1 inhibitors. This model was trained on ZINC data and tuned on known DDR1 inhibitors and kinase inhibitors. The developed molecules were then filtered through structural filters before clustering, and pharmacophore models were used to select 40 molecules that were scored for synthesizability before 6 were synthesized. More than 50% of these had IC_{50} <1 μM and 2 had nM IC_{50}'s.[49] This study itself has come in for some criticism, suggesting the best hit was similar to known DDR1 inhibitors.[50]

Several AI approaches were applied by researchers at In Silico Medicine to identify a target for treating hepatocellular carcinoma and then generating molecules using a protein structure predicted with AlphaFold.[51] CDK20 was identified as it had a strong disease association and did not have an available crystal structure and few small molecule inhibitors. The AlphaFold predicted structure was used to identify potential binding sites and then a pocket-based generative approach was used to create 8,918 molecules with their commercially available Chemistry42 software and following docking and clustering seven compounds were selected for synthesis. From these, one compound (Figure 1.1) was identified

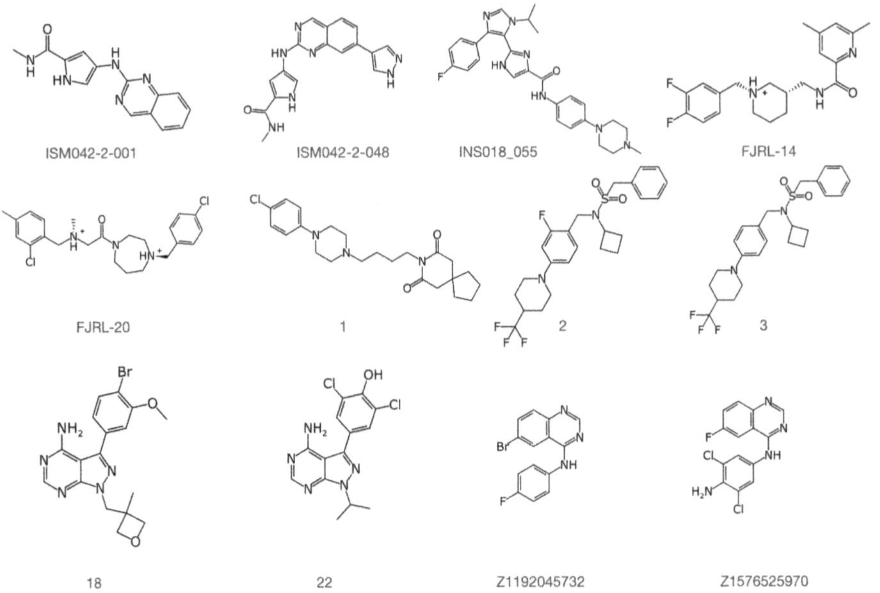

FIGURE 1.1 Molecules identified by generative approaches which were tested against various targets. ISM042-2-0015,[2] ISM042-2-0485,[2] INS018_0555,[3] FJRL-1455, FJRL-2055, 1, 2, 3,[57] 18, 22,[60] Z1192045732, Z1576525970.[67]

with a K_d of 9.2 μM (ISM042-2-001).[51] A second round of generative design resulted in 16 molecules of which 6 were tested with the best molecule (Figure 1.1) being ISM042-2-048 with K_d 566.7 nM and kinase IC_{50} 33.4 nM.[51] This molecule also had antiproliferative activity in Huh7 cells.

A similar computational workflow was applied to discover anti-fibrotic targets from lung fibrosis datasets and gene expression data (with high scores for several different measures).[52] These indicated TRAF-2 and NCK-interacting kinase (TNIK) as the number one anti-fibrotic target. Crystal structures of the TNIK kinase domain were then used with a structure-based approach using the Chemistry42 software with a two-point pharmacophore (hydrogen bond acceptor and hydrophobic feature), as well as physicochemical properties, medicinal chemistry filters and a synthetic accessibility score.[52] This resulted in molecules that were synthesized although it is not reported how many were made and tested. Ultimately, lead optimization to improve ADME properties led to INS018_055 (TNIK IC_{50} 7.8 nM). Kinase selectivity analysis suggested this molecule inhibited several other kinases as well. The molecule was also tested in cell models and shown to inhibit TGF-β as well as demonstrating efficacy in lung fibrosis, lung inflammation, kidney fibrosis and skin fibrosis models. The pharmacokinetics (PK) and tolerability in humans were then assessed and the compound is now in Phase II clinical trials.[52]

A 2023 minireview by In Silico Medicine authors of other generative chemistry in 2023 focused on 8 papers out of the over 50 that had been published in the preceding few years.[53] It was noted that most of the papers did not validate the models and were instead focused on model metrics. Also, it was suggested that molecules were generally similar to the training set. Several of the generative chemistry papers used as examples came in for heavy criticism, citing that the authors had described similar molecules previously, there was low novelty, or data is lacking to characterize compounds. In some cases, they also suggest that simpler cheminformatics tools or approaches could have delivered some of the molecules.[53] In most cases a full listing of molecules generated, and data are not provided which makes it even more difficult to assess how well a study performed as usually only a few structures are shown. This points to some of the difficulties of doing such work because how are you going to absolutely know for sure whether the structures generated are unique unless you check all patents, literature, and databases available? Those in small companies may not be able to access SciFinder because of the expense of this tool alone. If we are going to give author's the benefit of the doubt there is also the chance that while their paper is in review additional papers on similar molecules may be published and then of course it is too late. It was clear from this review that trivial differences between an existing molecule and a generative designed molecule will not be tolerated as novel enough, which is exactly the criticism used by others.[50]

A modified version of the GENTRL architecture (variational autoencoder that uses a recurrent neural network and convolutional neural network decoder) was recently used to design k-opioid receptor (KOR) antagonists.[54] The group performing this pretrained their model with a subset of ZINC and a set of ~2,000 molecules from ChEMBL with KOR antagonist data. 1 million molecules were narrowed to 2,545 that fulfilled various criteria then docked using Glide XP. Five molecules were identified for synthesis, and subsequent testing *in vitro* indicated two (Figure 1.1) had K_i of 6.46 μM (FJRL-14) and 7.59 μM (FJRL-20).[54] Based on their similarity to molecules in ChEMBL, it was suggested that these molecules were 'novel'.

Different examples of generative approaches have been applied in various scenarios. For example, one is trained on the active molecules in ChEMBL ($EC_{50} < 1$ μM) and uses a language model which implements an RNN model with LSTM to produce SMILES structures.[55] Data augmentation is proper when there is limited data, and this entails creating multiple examples of the same molecule. Sampling temperature was also varied which governs the randomness of the token and hence increases molecule diversity. By controlling the augmentation and temperature, the optimal settings for generative design with the language model were reached. The enrichment of molecules or transfer learning was achieved using molecules from ChEMBL and also libraries of natural products.[55] The combination of these efforts demonstrated that new molecules could be created however none of those described were synthesized or tested.

As SMILES can be generated in any direction, bidirectional RNNs have also been demonstrated as SMILES generators using several different algorithms and evaluated using uniqueness, validity and novelty, scaffold diversity, and biological and chemical relevance.[56] BIMODAL was found to perform the best using these various metrics and this method consisted of a 7 layer network, suggesting that bidirectional RNNs may be of utility for *de novo* design.[56]

The beam search algorithm can be used as an alternative approach to temperature sampling, allowing for generative design and prioritization.[57] This was demonstrated with prospective validation to produce retinoic acid-related orphan receptor (ROR) ligands. The ChEMBL pretrained model was fine-tuned with 255 RORγ ligands and then a further tuning with four natural product RORγ ligands. Synthetic accessibility was determined using IBM RXN. The beam search approach was used to explore the chemical space outside of the molecules in the fine-tuning set as molecules were found to be diverse. From the five best designs, three molecules were synthesized, and all had μM to sub μM IC_{50} against RORγ[58] (1 = 4.6 μM, 2 = 0.37 μM, 3 = 0.68 μM) (Figure 1.1) with Tanimoto similarity ranging from 0.28 to 0.71. Limitations of the beam search are the decreased number of designs sampled versus temperature sampling.

An approach to improve the language models has used the perplexity score to assess the goodness of the molecules designed.[58] This essentially works like a similarity metric to the training set, and measures how well it captured the underlying training set data and therefore can be used to confirm it matches the objectives. This has been demonstrated with an RNN with LSTM pretrained with ChEMBL and ten random targets with (pCHEMBL data larger than 6 – less than 1 μM) were then used to fine tune the models. Besides perplexity, measures of chemical similarity using Morgan and topological fingerprints were used, and these suggest that perplexity captures substructure and pharmacophore features as well as other information. In this study, molecular sampling (multinomial versus beam) and pretraining were also assessed.[58] Perplexity was shown to provide a measure of quality assessment for molecules produced by this generative approach.[58] As no molecules were synthesized or tested, this remains an open question.

There have been efforts to integrate automated synthesis and molecular design, including one that designed liver X receptor agonists.[59] An LSTM was pre-trained on 656,070 commercially available molecules from four vendors and fine-tuned on 40 LXRα agonists, which acted as the molecule generator, while a virtual reaction filter enabled the 17 reactions that were possible with the desktop microfluidics system used and HPLC-MS used to monitor the reactions. Twenty-five of 41 molecules could be synthesized, and 2 others could be purchased.[59] Seventeen of the compounds showed greater or equal to threefold LXR activation and potencies of the compounds were generated. Compound 17 had the highest selectivity of LXRβ and an EC_{50} of 0.21 μM. These results suggested the potential promise of the approach for fast design-make-test cycles requiring minimal human interference (data curation for pretraining and fine-tuning) such that the approach could be modified for other applications. There is still plenty of scope for improving the approach to increase diversity of molecules and explore more chemical space.[59]

A generative approach using a chemical language model (CLM) was used to develop ligands for the phosphoinositide 3-kinase (PI3Kγ).[60] This was trained on the US patent database, and then transfer learning was used by adding 46 PI3Kγ inhibitors from the Drug Target Commons database. Sixteen computer-generated molecules were purchased, and one of those had a sub μM K_d against PI3Kγ. Additional molecules that scored well were synthesized and tested, with two having higher affinity (compound 18, K_d = 52 nM and compound 22, K_d 13 nM) (Figure 1.1) for PI3Kγ.[60]

The many developments in chemical language models have also been reviewed (see also Chapter 3), highlighting some of the areas that still need development, including more collaborations in order to deploy and validate generative models.[61] Automated synthesis platforms would enable more validation with the drawback that they may be limited to certain chemistries. Leveraging more structure-based design functionality (electrostatics, shape, etc.) characteristics has been restricted so far by existing scoring functions and protein-ligand binding data. It is believed that approaches like few shot learning[62] when combined with language models could increase their utility. The chemical language of such large language models may also need to be modified or enhanced as we look at other molecules like peptides, proteins, and polymers.[61]

Large molecules like PROteolysis Targeting Chimeras (PROTACs) can be generated with graph-based generative models, and much of the prior work in this area has been reviewed.[63] The protac.db can be used to extract information to build a model to predict protein degradation activity. GraphINVENT was used to build a generative model for all three parts of a PROTAC, using 4,120 molecules from protac.db then fine-tuned with the protein degradation model. This approach was applied to IRAK3 degradation and 82% of the final sampled models were predicted as active. However, no experimental validation was performed to confirm these predictions.[63]

The development of new graph generative models includes MolGrow, which represents a hierarchical normalizing flow model for generating graphs that increased graph size during sampling after starting from a node.[64] A fragment-orientated atom ordering method is used and the model has been applied for distribution learning and property optimization and was benchmarked on the MOSES dataset. On distribution learning, MolGrow outperformed all other graph-based approaches on all metrics, whereas this was outperformed by SMILES-based methods.[64] Again, this approach was not validated by the synthesis and testing of compounds.

A DNN was used with a graph-based architecture called hydrogen count labeled graph-based defactorization (HyFactor) that was developed using an approach similar to the InChI notation to reduce GPU memory and the time for model training.[65] HyFactor uses implicit hydrogen atom counts instead of bond counts, which avoids molecule standardization issues. The efficiency of the architecture was compared to GAE using benchmarking with ZINC250K, ChEMBL, and MOSES. HyFactor had high reconstruction rates for ZINC and ChEMBL, although as the size increased the error also increased which may be reduced with data augmentation. Uniqueness and novelty of structures were found to increase with noise.[65]

Another graph-based approach is MoLeR, which supports using a molecular scaffold (fragments) as a seed for generative design and compares well to other methods (CGVAE, JT-VAE, and HierVAE) on molecular optimization but outperforms scaffold-based tasks.[66] Training data from GuacaMol was used to train MoLeR, and molecular swarm optimization was used for latent space optimization. MoLeR was faster than the baseline methods at molecule generation. In an unconstrained generation, MoLeR outperformed the baseline methods using Frechet ChemNet Distance. Scaffold-constrained generation, unconstrained optimization and scaffold-constrained optimization were also undertaken where good performance was observed.[66]

Several groups have used deep-generative neural networks with reinforcement learning. For example, a deep-recurrent neural network generative model was pretrained with

ChEMBL to produce valid SMILES[67], and reinforcement learning was used via the policy gradient algorithm. Several steps were taken (transfer learning, experience replay, and real-time reward shaping) to balance the exploration and exploitation modes of reinforcement learning. Data from ChEMBL for EGFR inhibitors were used to build a random forest machine-learning model. In order to validate their approach, they matched 17 compounds which were analogs of quinazoline with those in Enamine REAL and subsequently tested them *in vitro*. Two of these (Figure 1.1) had $IC_{50} < 100\,nM$, similar to the control used. It should be noted that these molecules have almost identical analogs in the training set. It was also suggested that the hit rate was comparable to virtual screening, yet it did not require a medicinal chemist.[67] The latter observation may indicate that the generative approach is suitable for selecting compounds with already known structures, but if you need novelty, perhaps the medicinal chemist would also be useful!

One toolkit for deep learning called OpenChem offers an array of tools using PyTorch and was illustrated with a generative RNN model for producing graphs and maximizing the melting temperature.[68] The model was pretrained on ChEMBL to learn the graphs and then a model used to predict melting temperature. A graphCNN regression model had an RMS error of 39.5°C. No prospective prediction data was shown.[68]

We have recently described the commercially available MegaSyn, in which we demonstrated an LSTM-based model to generate ibogaine analogs.[69] This model is first trained on a subset of ChEMBL-28's ~2 million compounds.[70] When trained, the model builds drug-like molecules and can be queried to generate compounds that fall within ChEMBL's chemical-space. Next, we applied transfer-learning[71] by training for an epoch on a natural product library.[72] The LSTM model was refined using a hill-climb maximum-likelihood estimator algorithm.[73] The algorithm starts by generating 10,000 compounds from the model. The compounds generated are then scored according to an objective reward function. The top 10% of ranked compounds are reserved and fed back into the model for training. In this way, the model starts by generating drug-like compounds and is re-trained on the top-scoring compounds until it finds a local minima of chemical space with the desired chemical properties. We trained our model using the hill climb algorithm for 15 epochs. For our scoring reward function, we then used Tanimoto similarity to the CANVASS library[72] (>0.2), an activity model against 5-HT_{2A} (agonist, predicted active), and off-target models for hERG, 5-HT_{1A}, 5-HT_{1F}, 5-HT_{2C} (predicted inactive). We also optimized for Tanimoto similarity > 0.6 when compared to Ibogaine and a lower cLogP than Ibogaine. 100,000 virtual molecules were generated from the final model then we assessed the top 50. Most had lower cLogP compared with ibogaine. All top generated molecules also possessed improved MPO scores[74,75] versus ibogaine. Our generative model also produced the known psychoplastogen, Tabernanthalog from the ibogaine structure[76] as well as many other analogs, suggesting it is capable of discovering new molecules with desirable properties that have been synthesized previously.

1.2.2 Synthesizability and Retrosynthetic Analysis

One of the big challenges of generative approaches is the synthesizability of the proposed molecules (see also Chapter 4), which is not an issue when you just use machine learning for virtual scoring of vendor available molecules. Efforts to determine the synthesizability assess synthetic pathways or structural complexity, the latter being a metric that can be readily implemented. For synthetic pathway assessment, there is now an array of approaches described that includes computer-assisted synthesis,[77–79] retrosynthesis[80–85], and synthetic viability tools (e.g. AutoGrow 3,[86] chemical stability[87] and others[88] in order to eliminate invalid options). For example, several efforts have been to train a neural network with millions of reactions in order to learn synthetic complexity, leading to scores like SCScore.[89] A recent study assessed synthesizability using an open-source retrosynthesis approach called ASKCOS.[90] Different generative algorithms were compared and benchmarked with different datasets like MOSES, ChEMBL, ZINC. The agreement between ASKCOS and synthesizability methods had higher AUC for SA_Score > SMILES length > SCScore. It was found that biasing a model by training on more synthesizable data performs well with distribution learning but not goal-directed learning. Goal-directed learning was not as sensitive to the starting compounds, and when biased by SA_Score, the fraction of synthesizable compounds in the top 100 candidates dramatically increased. It is important to note that there was no experimental validation of this work, and it was completely computational.[90]

Synthesis planning for multiple targets is complex. This can be solved by treating the pathway selection as a network flow problem and designing a decomposition strategy that accelerates numerical convergence while improving the solutions.[91] ASKCOS was used to perform retrosynthetic analysis to search for possible pathways. This creates a directed graph consisting of molecules and reactions. The ten most suitable reaction conditions for each reaction are produced, and the likelihood of success of the response is calculated by a reaction evaluation model developed using the USPTO database.[91] Mixed-integer linear programming has been used on the complete chemical reaction network, which avoids any information loss and increases flexibility for exploring reaction conditions, the downside, however, is the increased combinatorial complexity. This approach was demonstrated on several molecule libraries ranging from 2 to 48 targets and from 500 to 7,000 reactions. A weighted combination of three objectives was used, including a number of unique starting materials, the number of catalysts, solvents, and reagents (c/s/r), as well as the probability of the synthesis plan failing.[91] The solving of the optimization problem resulted in the sharing of chemicals between the syntheses of different targets reducing the number of starting materials and c/s/r. There are some limitations of the approach, including neglecting chiral information, and minimization of starting materials may lead to lower scoring reactions being included.[91]

Pharmaceutical companies have also made chemical reaction data public, for example chemical reactions (a set of 1,929,251 reactions) have been extracted from patents by a group at Eli Lilly[92], and a set of reactions (~45 common reactions) has been detailed by a group at AstraZeneca.[93] These can be used to form the basis of retrosynthesis methods.[69]

Combining enzymatic and non-enzymatic reactions may enable a more efficient synthesis for a molecule.[94] In order to do this computationally enzymatic reaction templates were extracted from a reaction database (BKMS, containing 37,000 enzyme-catalyzed reactions of which 4,196 were unique and not in the synthetic dataset) then used to train a neural network before combining with a synthetic synthesis planner like ASKCOS. A multi-step search algorithm was used to prioritize retrosynthetic steps while balancing synthetic and enzymatic steps to create a hybrid search. It was found that this could lead to shorter pathways as multiple synthetic steps were removed by enzymatic steps. Several case studies (dronabinol and (R,R)-formoterol) were provided using the hybrid approach suggesting enzymatic transformations that were innovative, indicating the potential to accelerate identification for new synthetic routes.[94]

As with the proliferation of generative algorithms, it is also difficult to evaluate chemical synthesis planning algorithms as they become more widely available. One recent comparison suggested that differences were small. Specifically, Monte Carlo Tree Search (MCTS) methods and the Retro algorithm were compared on four sets of test molecules and metrics such as a number of distinct solutions found and time at which a solution is found. As there is likely little difference between these methods, it suggests the need to develop new ones.[95]

RetroGNN is a new method to estimate synthesizability which searches for routes for a large number of random molecules in synthesis planning software; this is then used to train a graph neural network, which is then used to predict for a target molecule, the outcome of the synthesis planner.[96] This method was benchmarked and suggested as useful for generative drug discovery as it could find molecules that possessed the desired activity faster and were predicted to be easier to synthesize. Specifically, RetroGNN was trained on 50,000 M1 scores from the molecule. One retrosynthesis planning software was able to predict this score, 10^5 times faster. Examples of multiobjective optimization tasks were used to search for drug-like molecules, using three HIV targets. An antibiotic design example using RetroGNN produced synthesizable molecules compared to the SAScore, indicating that it could not only be used for *de novo* design but also as a guide for synthesis.[96]

Reinforcement learning has been used to improve single-step reaction predictors to create planning with dual value networks (PDVN), a policy learning framework as an online training algorithm.[97] This was benchmarked with the USPTO dataset and was shown to improve the success rate of Retro and RetroGraph and found shorter synthesis routes. ChEMBL and GDB17 were also used to create more challenging datasets and these yielded improvements in the number of solved targets over algorithms without the PDVN, were also used.[97]

Software to predict chemistry synthesis can be split into several areas including reaction deployment, development, and discovery, and these areas have benefited from machine learning methods.[98] Reaction deployment uses algorithms or statistical approaches for retrosynthetic planning and outcome prediction and is well explored and has been adopted by the industry. These could include one-step retrosynthetic prediction or multistep retrosynthesis. Reaction development uses predictive models to identify new synthetic processes, including types of reactions and conditions. Reaction discovery can be used to elucidate unknown mechanisms and develop new method. These areas are less well developed. Challenges with these approaches are that little is understood about the extrapolation of these methods and they are generally black boxes which complicate interpretability.[98] In summary, there is still plenty of scope for further development in this area.

1.2.3 Benchmarking

Several benchmark dataset resources, including MOSES[99] and GuacaMol[100], have been introduced in the literature in recent years. For example, MOSES provided a standardized dataset (based on ZINC clean leads) with evaluation metrics (fraction of valid and unique, novelty, filters, fragment similarity, scaffold similarity, similarity to nearest neighbor, internal diversity, Frechet ChemNet distance and properties distribution) as well as models (Character-level recurrent neural network (CharRNN), variational autoencoder (VAE) and adversarial autoencoder, Junction Tree VAE, Latent vector-based generative adversarial network, and more as baselines). The ChaRNN performed the best based on the metrics.[99] As the use of generative approaches continues to expand and the complexity increases, one would also imagine that additional benchmark sets will be needed and created.

1.3 THE FUTURE OF GENERATIVE APPROACHES

In order to demonstrate a self-driving laboratory (see also Chapter 10) machine-learning generative algorithms, machine-learning property prediction, computer-aided synthesis planning, automated chemical synthesis, as well as purification and characterization robotics have been integrated to demonstrate autonomous design-make-test-analyze cycles to exploit and explore chemical space in order to optimize dye-like molecules.[101] While this was not a drug discovery example, it very nicely illustrated how it could propose, synthesize, and characterize 303 previously unreported dye-like molecules and, at the same time showed that it could explore structure-property space. Common to drug discovery and materials science de novo design projects, while the property prediction model training sets were sizeable for absorption, lipophilicity, and photostability, they did not, however, extrapolate well for previously unexplored scaffolds. As described elsewhere, the frequently used synthesizability metrics did not show an increase in the quality of the reaction planning and were subsequently not explored. Human input was still required for error recovery and materials restocking.[101]

Photocatalysis is used in some synthetic methods for pharmaceutical and other chemicals and uses light to drive reactivity, but it needs to be optimized, replicated, and scaled.[102] An example of a self-driving laboratory using automated flow chemistry is the development of RoboChem, which is a platform for self-optimization, intensification, and scale-up of photocatalysis in flow.[102] On the software side, this approach uses Bayesian optimization to explore parameter space. Such an approach increases safety and releases scientists from reaction optimization and intensification tasks. One could imagine how generative approaches could be used earlier in the process to design molecules for synthesis with RoboChem.[102]

As outlined at the outset, perhaps the biggest challenge generative approaches face is convincing scientists that they offer credible ideas of molecules that are synthesizable. The slow accumulation of examples of prospectively predicted, designed, synthesized, and ultimately tested molecules will build into a credible validation of this approach. The few examples of molecules shown here (Figure 1.1) is a starting point, and there needs to be a balanced examination of the novelty of the molecules produced in the future in order to set realistic expectations of what the technology can do in the hands of both experts and non-experts alike. At that point, we may be able to escape both serendipity and Edisonian approaches and embrace the generative age of drug discovery.

FUNDING

We kindly acknowledge NIH funding from R44GM122196-02A1 from NIGMS and 1R44ES031038-01 from NIEHS for our machine learning software development and applications. "Research reported in this publication was supported by the National Institute of Environmental Health Sciences of the National Institutes of Health under Award Number R44ES031038. We also acknowledge 1R43DA055419-01 from NIDA. The content is solely the responsibility of the authors and does not necessarily represent the official views of the National Institutes of Health."

REFERENCES

1. Ban, T. A. The role of serendipity in drug discovery. *Dialogues Clin Neurosci* **2006**, *8* (3), 335–344. DOI:10.31887/DCNS.2006.8.3/tban.
2. Alves, P. L.; Abdalla, F. M. F.; Alponti, R. F.; Silveira, P. F. Anti-obesogenic and hypolipidemic effects of a glucagon-like peptide-1 receptor agonist derived from the saliva of the Gila monster. *Toxicon* **2017**, *135*, 1–11. DOI:10.1016/j.toxicon.2017.06.001.
3. Paul, S. M.; Mytelka, D. S.; Dunwiddie, C. T.; Persinger, C. C.; Munos, B. H.; Lindborg, S. R.; Schacht, A. L. How to improve R&D productivity: The pharmaceutical industry's grand challenge. *Nat Rev Drug Discov* **2010**, *9* (3), 203–214.
4. Wouters, O. J.; McKee, M.; Luyten, J. Estimated research and development investment needed to bring a new medicine to market, 2009–2018. *JAMA* **2020**, *323* (9), 844–853. DOI:10.1001/jama.2020.1166.
5. Henderson, R. H.; French, D.; Stewart, E.; Smart, D.; Idica, A.; Redmond, S.; Eckstein, M.; Clark, J.; Sullivan, R.; Keeling, P.; Lawler, M. Delivering the precision oncology paradigm: Reduced R&D costs and greater return on investment through a companion diagnostic informed precision oncology medicines approach. *J Pharm Policy Pract* **2023**, *16* (1), 84. DOI:10.1186/s40545-023-00590-9.
6. Kauvar, L. M.; Laborde, E. The diversity challenge in combinatorial chemistry. *Curr Opin Drug Disc Dev* **1998**, *1*, 66–70.
7. Sittampalam, G. S.; Iversen, P. W.; Boadt, J. A.; Kahl, S. D.; Bright, S.; Zock, J. M.; Janzen, W. P.; Lister, M. D. Design of signal windows in high throughput screening assays for drug discovery. *J Biomolecular Screening* **1997**, *2*, 159–169.
8. Banks, M.; Binnie, A.; Fogarty, S. High throughput screening using fully integrated robotic screening. *J Biomolecular Screening* **1997**, *2*, 133–135.
9. Zhang, L.; Chen, C.; Fu, J.; Lilley, B.; Berlinicke, C.; Hansen, B.; Ding, D.; Wang, G.; Wang, T.; Shou, D.; et al. Large-scale phenotypic drug screen identifies neuroprotectants in zebrafish and mouse models of retinitis pigmentosa. *Elife* **2021**, *10*, e57245. DOI:10.7554/eLife.57245.
10. Takakusagi, Y.; Takakusagi, K.; Sakaguchi, K.; Sugawara, F. Phage display technology for target determination of small-molecule therapeutics: An update. *Expert Opin Drug Discov* **2020**, *15* (10), 1199–1211. DOI:10.1080/17460441.2020.1790523.
11. Erlanson, D. A.; McDowell, R. S.; O'Brien, T. Fragment-based drug discovery. *J Med Chem* **2004**, *47* (14), 3463–3482. DOI:10.1021/jm040031v.

12. Velmurugan, D.; Pachaiappan, R.; Ramakrishnan, C. Recent trends in drug design and discovery. *Curr Top Med Chem* **2020**, *20* (19), 1761–1770. DOI:10.2174/1568026620666200622150003.
13. Zhu, L.; Chen, X.; Abola, E. E.; Jing, L.; Liu, W. Serial crystallography for structure-based drug discovery. *Trends Pharmacol Sci* **2020**, *41* (11), 830–839. DOI:10.1016/j.tips.2020.08.009.
14. Subramaniam, S.; Earl, L. A.; Falconieri, V.; Milne, J. L.; Egelman, E. H. Resolution advances in cryo-EM enable application to drug discovery. *Curr Opin Struct Biol* **2016**, *41*, 194–202. DOI:10.1016/j.sbi.2016.07.009.
15. Schneider, G. Virtual screening: An endless staircase? *Nat Rev Drug Discov* **2010**, *9* (4), 273–276.
16. Walters, W. P.; Stahl, M. T.; Murcko, M. A. Virtual screening-an overview. *Drug Discov Today* **1998**, *3*, 160–178.
17. Wang, Y.; Gao, Y.; Pan, Y.; Zhou, D.; Liu, Y.; Yin, Y.; Yang, J.; Wang, Y.; Song, Y. Emerging trends in organ-on-a-chip systems for drug screening. *Acta Pharm Sin B* **2023**, *13* (6), 2483–2509. DOI:10.1016/j.apsb.2023.02.006.
18. Leung, E. L.; Cao, Z. W.; Jiang, Z. H.; Zhou, H.; Liu, L. Network-based drug discovery by integrating systems biology and computational technologies. *Brief Bioinform* **2013**, *14* (4), 491–505. DOI:10.1093/bib/bbs043.
19. Dorel, M.; Barillot, E.; Zinovyev, A.; Kuperstein, I. Network-based approaches for drug response prediction and targeted therapy development in cancer. *Biochem Biophys Res Commun* **2015**, *464*, 386–391. DOI:10.1016/j.bbrc.2015.06.094.
20. Lewis, R.; Guha, R.; Korcsmaros, T.; Bender, A. Synergy maps: Exploring compound combinations using network-based visualization. *J Cheminform* **2015**, *7*, 36. DOI:10.1186/s13321-015-0090-6.
21. Zhang, S. Computer-aided drug discovery and development. *Methods Mol Biol* **2011**, *716*, 23–38. DOI:10.1007/978-1-61779-012-6_2.
22. Lessing, A.; Petrov, D.; Scheuermann, J. Advancing small-molecule drug discovery by encoded dual-display technologies. *Trends Pharmacol Sci* **2023**, *44* (11), 817–831. DOI:10.1016/j.tips.2023.08.006.
23. von Eichborn, J.; Murgueitio, M. S.; Dunkel, M.; Koerner, S.; Bourne, P. E.; Preissner, R. PROMISCUOUS: A database for network-based drug repositioning. *Nucleic Acids Res* **2010**, *39*, D1060–D1066.
24. Ekins, S. The next era: Deep learning in pharmaceutical research. *Pharm Res* **2016**, *33*, 2594–2603.
25. Korotcov, A.; Tkachenko, V.; Russo, D. P.; Ekins, S. Comparison of deep learning with multiple machine learning methods and metrics using diverse drug discovery datasets. *Mol Pharm* **2018**, *14*, 4462–4475.
26. Kadurin, A.; Nikolenko, S.; Khrabrov, K.; Aliper, A.; Zhavoronkov, A. druGAN: An advanced generative adversarial autoencoder model for de novo generation of new molecules with desired molecular properties in silico. *Mol Pharm* **2017**, *14* (9), 3098–3104. DOI:10.1021/acs.molpharmaceut.7b00346.
27. Gupta, A.; Muller, A. T.; Huisman, B. J. H.; Fuchs, J. A.; Schneider, P.; Schneider, G. Generative recurrent networks for de novo drug design. *Mol Inform* **2018**, *37* (1–2), 1700111. DOI:10.1002/minf.201700111.
28. Raisch, S.; Fomina, K. Combining human and artificial intelligence: Hybrid problem-solving in organizations. *Acad Manage Rev* **2023**. https://journals.aom.org/doi/10.5465/amr.2021.0421
29. Anstine, D. M.; Isayev, O. Generative models as an emerging paradigm in the chemical sciences. *J Am Chem Soc* **2023**, *145* (16), 8736–8750. DOI:10.1021/jacs.2c13467.
30. Olivecrona, M.; Blaschke, T.; Engkvist, O.; Chen, H. Molecular de-novo design through deep reinforcement learning. *J Cheminf* **2017**, *9* (1), 48. DOI:10.1186/s13321-017-0235-x.

31. Segler, M. H. S.; Kogej, T.; Tyrchan, C.; Waller, M. P. Generating focused molecule libraries for drug discovery with recurrent neural networks. *ACS Cent Sci* **2018**, *4* (1), 120–131. DOI:10.1021/acscentsci.7b00512.
32. Gomez-Bombarelli, R.; Wei, J. N.; Duvenaud, D.; Hernandez-Lobato, J. M.; Sanchez-Lengeling, B.; Sheberla, D.; Aguilera-Iparraguirre, J.; Hirzel, T. D.; Adams, R. P.; Aspuru-Guzik, A. Automatic chemical design using a data-driven continuous representation of molecules. *ACS Cent Sci* **2018**, *4* (2), 268–276. DOI:10.1021/acscentsci.7b00572.
33. Kang, S. G.; Morrone, J. A.; Weber, J. K.; Cornell, W. D. Analysis of training and seed bias in small molecules generated with a conditional graph-based variational autoencoder horizontal line insights for practical AI-driven molecule generation. *J Chem Inf Model* **2022**, *62* (4), 801–816. DOI:10.1021/acs.jcim.1c01545.
34. Prykhodko, O.; Johansson, S. V.; Kotsias, P. C.; Arus-Pous, J.; Bjerrum, E. J.; Engkvist, O.; Chen, H. A de novo molecular generation method using latent vector based generative adversarial network. *J Cheminform* **2019**, *11* (1), 74. DOI:10.1186/s13321-019-0397–9.
35. Hochreiter, S.; Schmidhuber, J. Long short-term memory. *Neural Comput* **1997**, *9*, 1735–1780.
36. Blaschke, T.; Olivecrona, M.; Engkvist, O.; Bajorath, J.; Chen, H. Application of generative autoencoder in de novo molecular design. *Mol Inform* **2018**, *37* (1–2), 1700123. DOI:10.1002/minf.201700123.
37. Sanchez-Lengeling, B.; Outeiral, C.; Guimaraes, G. L.; Aspuru-Guzik, A. Optimizing distributions over molecular space. An Objective-Reinforced Generative Adversarial Network for Inverse-design Chemistry (ORGANIC). 2017. https://chemrxiv.org/engage/chemrxiv/article-details/60c73d91702a9beea7189bc2.
38. Winter, R.; Montanari, F.; Steffen, A.; Briem, H.; Noé, F.; Clevert, D.-A. Efficient multi-objective molecular optimization in a continuous latent space. *Chem Sci* **2019**, *10* (34), 8016–8024. DOI:10.1039/C9SC01928F.
39. Krenn, M.; Häse, F.; Nigam, A.; Friederich, P.; Aspuru-Guzik, A. Self-referencing embedded strings (SELFIES): A 100% robust molecular string representation. *Mach Learn: Sci Technol* **2020**, *1* (4), 045024. DOI:10.1088/2632-2153/aba947.
40. Jin, W.; Barzilay, R.; Jaakola, T. Junction tree variational autoencoder for molecular graph generation. 2019. https://arxiv.org/pdf/1802.04364.pdf.
41. Maziarka, L.; Pocha, A.; Kaczmarczyk, J.; Rataj, K.; Danel, T.; Warchol, M. Mol-CycleGAN: A generative model for molecular optimization. *J Cheminform* **2020**, *12*, 2.
42. Gupta, A.; Muller, A. T.; Huisman, B. J. H.; Fuchs, J. A.; Schneider, P.; Schneider, G. Erratum: Generative recurrent networks for de novo drug design. *Mol Inform* **2018**, *37* (1–2), 1880141. DOI:10.1002/minf.201880141.
43. Bjerrum, E. J.; Threlfall, R. Molecular generation with recurrent neural networks (RNNs). *arXiv* **2017**, 1705.04612.
44. Domenico, A.; Nicola, G.; Daniela, T.; Fulvio, C.; Nicola, A.; Orazio, N. De novo drug design of targeted chemical libraries based on artificial intelligence and pair-based multiobjective optimization. *J Chem Inf Model* **2020**, *60* (10), 4582–4593. DOI:10.1021/acs.jcim.0c00517.
45. Devlin, J.; Chang, M.-W.; Lee, K.; Toutanova, K. BERT: Pre-training of deep bidirectional transformers for language understanding. *arXiv* **2018**, 1810.04805.
46. Vaswani, A.; Shazeer, N.; Parmar, N.; Uszkoreit, J.; Jones, L.; HGomez, A. N.; Kaiser, L.; Plusukhin, I. Attention is all you need. *arXiv* **2017**, 1706.03762.
47. Zhavoronkov, A.; Ivanenkov, Y. A.; Aliper, A.; Veselov, M. S.; Aladinskiy, V. A.; Aladinskaya, A. V.; Terentiev, V. A.; Polykovskiy, D. A.; Kuznetsov, M. D.; Asadulaev, A.; et al. Deep learning enables rapid identification of potent DDR1 kinase inhibitors. *Nat Biotechnol* **2019**, *37* (9), 1038–1040. DOI:10.1038/s41587-019-0224-x.

48. Putin, E.; Asadulaev, A.; Vanhaelen, Q.; Ivanenkov, Y.; Aladinskaya, A. V.; Aliper, A.; Zhavoronkov, A. Adversarial threshold neural computer for molecular de novo design. *Mol Pharm* 2018, *15* (10), 4386–4397. DOI:10.1021/acs.molpharmaceut.7b01137.
49. Ivanenkov, Y. A.; Polykovskiy, D.; Bezrukov, D.; Zagribelnyy, B.; Aladinskiy, V.; Kamya, P.; Aliper, A.; Ren, F.; Zhavoronkov, A. Chemistry42: An AI-driven platform for molecular design and optimization. *J Chem Inf Model* **2023**, *63* (3), 695–701. DOI:10.1021/acs.jcim.2c01191.
50. Walters, W. P.; Murcko, M. Assessing the impact of generative AI on medicinal chemistry. *Nat Biotechnol* **2020**, *38* (2), 143–145. DOI:10.1038/s41587-020-0418-2.
51. Ren, F.; Ding, X.; Zheng, M.; Korzinkin, M.; Cai, X.; Zhu, W.; Mantsyzov, A.; Aliper, A.; Aladinskiy, V.; Cao, Z.; et al. AlphaFold accelerates artificial intelligence powered drug discovery: Efficient discovery of a novel CDK20 small molecule inhibitor. *Chem Sci* **2023**, *14* (6), 1443–1452. DOI:10.1039/d2sc05709c.
52. Ren, F.; Aliper, A.; Chen, J.; Zhao, H.; Rao, S.; Kuppe, C.; Ozerov, I. V.; Zhang, M.; Witte, K.; Kruse, C.; et al. A small-molecule TNIK inhibitor targets fibrosis in preclinical and clinical models. *Nat Biotechnol* **2024**. https://pubmed.ncbi.nlm.nih.gov/38459338/
53. Ivanenkov, Y.; Zagribelnyy, B.; Malyshev, A.; Evteev, S.; Terentiev, V.; Kamya, P.; Bezrukov, D.; Aliper, A.; Ren, F.; Zhavoronkov, A. The Hitchhiker's guide to deep learning driven generative chemistry. *ACS Med Chem Lett* **2023**, *14* (7), 901–915. DOI:10.1021/acsmedchemlett.3c00041.
54. Salas-Estrada, L.; Provasi, D.; Qiu, X.; Kaniskan, H. U.; Huang, X. P.; DiBerto, J. F.; Lamim Ribeiro, J. M.; Jin, J.; Roth, B. L.; Filizola, M. De novo design of kappa-opioid receptor antagonists using a generative deep-learning framework. *J Chem Inf Model* **2023**, *63* (16), 5056–5065. DOI:10.1021/acs.jcim.3c00651.
55. Moret, M.; Friedrich, L.; Grisoni, F.; Merk, D.; Schneider, G. Generative molecular design in low data regimes. *Nat Mach Intell* **2020**, *2* (3), 171–180. DOI:10.1038/s42256-020-0160-y.
56. Grisoni, F.; Moret, M.; Lingwood, R.; Schneider, G. Bidirectional molecule generation with recurrent neural networks. *J Chem Inf Model* **2020**, *60* (3), 1175–1183. DOI:10.1021/acs.jcim.9b00943.
57. Moret, M.; Helmstadter, M.; Grisoni, F.; Schneider, G.; Merk, D. Beam search for automated design and scoring of novel ROR ligands with machine intelligence. *Angew Chem Int Ed Engl* **2021**, *60* (35), 19477–19482. DOI:10.1002/anie.202104405.
58. Moret, M.; Grisoni, F.; Katzberger, P.; Schneider, G. Perplexity-based molecule ranking and bias estimation of chemical language models. *J Chem Inf Model* **2022**, *62* (5), 1199–1206. DOI:10.1021/acs.jcim.2c00079.
59. Grisoni, F.; Huisman, B. J. H.; Button, A. L.; Moret, M.; Atz, K.; Merk, D.; Schneider, G. Combining generative artificial intelligence and on-chip synthesis for de novo drug design. *Sci Adv* **2021**, *7* (24), eabg3338. DOI:10.1126/sciadv.abg3338.
60. Moret, M.; Pachon Angona, I.; Cotos, L.; Yan, S.; Atz, K.; Brunner, C.; Baumgartner, M.; Grisoni, F.; Schneider, G. Leveraging molecular structure and bioactivity with chemical language models for de novo drug design. *Nat Commun* **2023**, *14* (1), 114. DOI:10.1038/s41467-022-35692-6.
61. Grisoni, F. Chemical language models for de novo drug design: Challenges and opportunities. *Curr Opin Struct Biol* **2023**, *79*, 102527. DOI:10.1016/j.sbi.2023.102527.
62. Stanley, M.; Bronskill, J. F.; Maziarz, K.; Misztela, H.; Lanini, J.; Segler, M.; Schneider, N.; Brockschmidt, M. FS-Mol: A few-shot learning dataset of molecules. In *NeurIPS 2021*, 2021. https://openreview.net/forum?id=701FtuyLlAd
63. Nori, D.; Coley, C. W.; Mercado, R. De novo PROTAC design using graph-based deep generative models. *arXiv* **2022**, 2211.02660.

64. Kuznetsov, M.; Polykovskiy, D. MolGrow: A graph normalizing flow for hierarchical molecular generation. *arXiv* **2021**, 2106.05856.
65. Akhmetshin, T.; Lin, A.; Mazitov, D.; Zabolotna, Y.; Ziaikin, E.; Madzhidov, T.; Varnek, A. HyFactor: A novel open-source, graph-based architecture for chemical structure generation. *J Chem Inf Model* **2022**, *62* (15), 3524–3534. DOI:10.1021/acs.jcim.2c00744.
66. Maziarz, K.; Jackson-Flux, H.; Cameron, P.; Sirockin, F.; Schneider, N.; Stiefl, N.; Segler, M.; Brockschmidt, M. Learning to extend molecular scaffolds with structural motifs. *arXiv* **2021**, 2103.03864.
67. Korshunova, M.; Huang, N.; Capuzzi, S.; Radchenko, D. S.; Savych, O.; Moroz, Y. S.; Wells, C. I.; Willson, T. M.; Tropsha, A.; Isayev, O. Generative and reinforcement learning approaches for the automated de novo design of bioactive compounds. *Commun Chem* **2022**, *5* (1), 129. DOI:10.1038/s42004-022-00733-0.
68. Korshunova, M.; Ginsburg, B.; Tropsha, A.; Isayev, O. OpenChem: A deep learning toolkit for computational chemistry and drug design. *J Chem Inf Model* **2021**, *61* (1), 7–13. DOI:10.1021/acs.jcim.0c00971.
69. Urbina, F.; Lowden, C. T.; Culberson, J. C.; Ekins, S. MegaSyn: Integrating generative molecular design, automated analog designer, and synthetic viability prediction. *ACS Omega* **2022**, *7* (22), 18699–18713. DOI:10.1021/acsomega.2c01404.
70. Gaulton, A.; Hersey, A.; Nowotka, M.; Bento, A. P.; Chambers, J.; Mendez, D.; Mutowo, P.; Atkinson, F.; Bellis, L. J.; Cibrian-Uhalte, E.; et al. The ChEMBL database in 2017. *Nucleic Acids Res* **2017**, *45* (D1), D945–D954. DOI:10.1093/nar/gkw1074.
71. Goh, G. B.; Siegel, C.; Vishnu, A.; Hodas, N. O. Using rule-based labels for weak supervised learning: A ChemNet for transferable chemical property prediction. *arXiv* **2017**, 1712.02734.
72. Kearney, S. E.; Zahoránszky-Kőhalmi, G.; Brimacombe, K. R.; Henderson, M. J.; Lynch, C.; Zhao, T.; Wan, K. K.; Itkin, Z.; Dillon, C.; Shen, M.; et al. Canvass: A crowd-sourced, natural-product screening library for exploring biological space. *ACS Cent Sci* **2018**, *4* (12), 1727–1741. DOI:10.1021/acscentsci.8b00747.
73. Neil, D.; Segler, M. H. S.; Guasch, L.; Ahmed, M.; Plumbley, D.; Sellwood, M.; Brown, N. Exploring deep recurrent models with reinforcement learning for molecule design. In *ICLR 2018 Conference*, Vancouver, 2018.
74. Urbina, F.; Zorn, K. M.; Brunner, D.; Ekins, S. Comparing the Pfizer central nervous system multiparameter optimization calculator and a BBB machine learning model. *ACS Chem Neurosci* **2021**, *12* (12), 2247–2253. DOI:10.1021/acschemneuro.1c00265.
75. Wager, T. T., Hou, X., Verhoest, P. R., Villalobos, A. Moving beyond rules: The development of a central nervous system multiparameter optimization (CNS MPO) approach to enable alignment of druglike properties. *ACS Chem Neurosci* **2010**, *1* (6), 435–449. DOI:10.1021/cn100008c.
76. Cameron, L. P.; Tombari, R. J.; Lu, J.; Pell, A. J.; Hurley, Z. Q.; Ehinger, Y.; Vargas, M. V.; McCarroll, M. N.; Taylor, J. C.; Myers-Turnbull, D.; et al. A non-hallucinogenic psychedelic analogue with therapeutic potential. *Nature* **2021**, *589* (7842), 474–479. DOI:10.1038/s41586-020-3008-z.
77. Warr, W. A. A short review of chemical reaction database systems, computer-aided synthesis design, reaction prediction and synthetic feasibility. *Mol Inform* **2014**, *33* (6–7), 469–476. DOI:10.1002/minf.201400052.
78. Szymkuc, S.; Gajewska, E. P.; Klucznik, T.; Molga, K.; Dittwald, P.; Startek, M.; Bajczyk, M.; Grzybowski, B. A. Computer-assisted synthetic planning: The end of the beginning. *Angew Chem Int Ed Engl* **2016**, *55* (20), 5904–5937. DOI:10.1002/anie.201506101.
79. Badowski, T.; Molga, K.; Grzybowski, B. A. Selection of cost-effective yet chemically diverse pathways from the networks of computer-generated retrosynthetic plans. *Chem Sci* **2019**, *10* (17), 4640–4651. DOI:10.1039/c8sc05611k.

80. Segler, M. H. S.; Waller, M. P. Neural-symbolic machine learning for retrosynthesis and reaction prediction. *Chemistry* **2017**, *23* (25), 5966–5971. DOI:10.1002/chem.201605499.
81. Coley, C. W.; Barzilay, R.; Jaakkola, T. S.; Green, W. H.; Jensen, K. F. Prediction of organic reaction outcomes using machine learning. *ACS Cent Sci* **2017**, *3* (5), 434–443. DOI:10.1021/acscentsci.7b00064.
82. Shibukawa, R.; Ishida, S.; Yoshizoe, K.; Wasa, K.; Takasu, K.; Okuno, Y.; Terayama, K.; Tsuda, K. CompRet: A comprehensive recommendation framework for chemical synthesis planning with algorithmic enumeration. *J Cheminform* **2020**, *12* (1), 52. DOI:10.1186/s13321-020-00452-5.
83. Zheng, S.; Rao, J.; Zhang, Z.; Xu, J.; Yang, Y. Predicting retrosynthetic reactions using self-corrected transformer neural networks. *J Chem Inf Model* **2020**, *60* (1), 47–55. DOI:10.1021/acs.jcim.9b00949.
84. Lee, A. A.; Yang, Q.; Sresht, V.; Bolgar, P.; Hou, X.; Klug-McLeod, J. L.; Butler, C. R. Molecular transformer unifies reaction prediction and retrosynthesis across pharma chemical space. *Chem Commun (Camb)* **2019**, *55* (81), 12152–12155. DOI:10.1039/c9cc05122h.
85. Bai, R.; Zhang, C.; Wang, L.; Yao, C.; Ge, J.; Duan, H. Transfer learning: Making retrosynthetic predictions based on a small chemical reaction dataset scale to a new level. *Molecules* **2020**, *25* (10), 2357. DOI:10.3390/molecules25102357.
86. Durrant, J. D.; Lindert, S.; McCammon, J. A. AutoGrow 3.0: An improved algorithm for chemically tractable, semi-automated protein inhibitor design. *J Mol Graphics Model* **2013**, *44*, 104–112. DOI:10.1016/j.jmgm.2013.05.006.
87. Clark, A. M.; Dole, K.; Coulon-Spector, A.; McNutt, A.; Grass, G.; Freundlich, J. S.; Reynolds, R. C.; Ekins, S. Open source Bayesian models: 1. Application to ADME/Tox and drug discovery datasets. *J Chem Inf Model* **2015**, *55*, 1231–1245. DOI:10.1021/acs.jcim.5b00143.
88. Fukunishi, Y.; Kurosawa, T.; Mikami, Y.; Nakamura, H. Prediction of synthetic accessibility based on commercially available compound databases. *J Chem Inf Model* **2014**, *54* (12), 3259–3267. DOI:10.1021/ci500568d.
89. Coley, C. W.; Rogers, L.; Green, W. H.; Jensen, K. F. SCScore: Synthetic complexity learned from a reaction corpus. *J Chem Inform Model* **2018**, *58* (2), 252–261. DOI:10.1021/acs.jcim.7b00622.
90. Gao, W.; Coley, C. W. The synthesizability of molecules proposed by generative models. *J Chem Inf Model* **2020**, *60* (12), 5714–5723. DOI:10.1021/acs.jcim.0c00174.
91. Gao, H.; Pauphilet, J.; Struble, T. J.; Coley, C. W.; Jensen, K. F. Direct optimization across computer-generated reaction networks balances materials use and feasibility of synthesis plans for molecule libraries. *J Chem Inf Model* **2021**, *61* (1), 493–504. DOI:10.1021/acs.jcim.0c01032.
92. Watson, I. A.; Wang, J.; Nicolaou, C. A. A retrosynthetic analysis algorithm implementation. *J Cheminform* **2019**, *11* (1), 1. DOI:10.1186/s13321-018-0323–6.
93. Hartenfeller, M.; Eberle, M.; Meier, P.; Nieto-Oberhuber, C.; Altmann, K. H.; Schneider, G.; Jacoby, E.; Renner, S. A collection of robust organic synthesis reactions for in silico molecule design. *J Chem Inf Model* **2011**, *51* (12), 3093–3098. DOI:10.1021/ci200379p.
94. Levin, I.; Liu, M.; Voigt, C. A.; Coley, C. W. Merging enzymatic and synthetic chemistry with computational synthesis planning. *Nat Commun* **2022**, *13* (1), 7747. DOI:10.1038/s41467-022-35422-y.
95. Tripp, A.; Krzysztof, M.; Lewis, S.; Liu, G.; Segler, M. Re-evaluating chemical synthesis planning algorithms. 2022. https://openreview.net/pdf?id=8VLeT8DFeD.
96. Liu, C. H.; Korablyov, M.; Jastrzebski, S.; Wlodarczyk-Pruszynski, P.; Bengio, Y.; Segler, M. Retro GNN: Fast estimation of synthesizability for virtual screening and de novo design by learning from slow retrosynthesis software. *J Chem Inf Model* **2022**, *62* (10), 2293–2300. DOI:10.1021/acs.jcim.1c01476.

97. Liu, G.; Xue, D.; Xie, S.; Xia, Y.; Tripp, A.; Maziarz, K.; Segler, M.; Qin, T.; Zhang, Z.; Liu, T.-Y. Retrosynthetic planning with dual value networks. *arXiv* **2023**, 2301.13755.
98. Tu, Z.; Stuyver, T.; Coley, C. W. Predictive chemistry: Machine learning for reaction deployment, reaction development, and reaction discovery. *Chem Sci* **2023**, *14* (2), 226–244. DOI:10.1039/d2sc05089g.
99. Polykovskiy, D.; Zhebrak, A.; Sanchez-Lengeling, B.; Golovanov, S.; Tatanov, O.; Belyaev, S.; Kurbanov, R.; Artamonov, A.; Aladinskiy, V.; Veselov, M.; et al. Molecular sets (MOSES): A benchmarking platform for molecular generation models. *Front Pharmacol* **2020**, *11*, 565644. DOI:10.3389/fphar.2020.565644.
100. Brown, N.; Fiscato, M.; Segler, M. H. S.; Vaucher, A. C. GuacaMol: Benchmarking models for de novo molecular design. *J Chem Inf Model* **2019**, *59* (3), 1096–1108. DOI:10.1021/acs.jcim.8b00839.
101. Koscher, B. A.; Canty, R. B.; McDonald, M. A.; Greenman, K. P.; McGill, C. J.; Bilodeau, C. L.; Jin, W.; Wu, H.; Vermeire, F. H.; Jin, B.; et al. Autonomous, multiproperty-driven molecular discovery: From predictions to measurements and back. *Science* **2023**, *382* (6677), eadi1407. DOI:10.1126/science.adi1407.
102. Slattery, A.; Wen, Z.; Tenblad, P.; Sanjose-Orduna, J.; Pintossi, D.; den Hartog, T.; Noel, T. Automated self-optimization, intensification, and scale-up of photocatalysis in flow. *Science* **2024**, *383* (6681), eadj1817. DOI:10.1126/science.adj1817.

2 Generative Drug Discovery

Quentin Vanhaelen, Alex Aliper, and Alex Zhavoronkov

2.1 INTRODUCTION

The field of artificial intelligence (AI) and machine learning (ML) has witnessed many changes with respect to deep learning (DL) methods mostly enabled thanks to technological improvements and the increasing availability of very large training datasets. The recent successes of AI in different fields of medicine, life sciences and health care [1–3] have given promise that it can be deployed to support drug discovery and clinical pharmacology to solve a wide range of very challenging problems, including the discovery of new drugs for the treatment of human diseases. What makes drug discovery extremely complex is that it is a multi-dimensional, multi-search and optimization problem. For decades, scientists have worked on various approaches suitable for the reliable prediction of novel small-molecule drugs that potently bind to a disease-causing protein and alter its function.

Due to the almost unlimited number of molecular structures that can be generated *de novo* [4,5], standard computational drug design approaches tend to include limited numbers of fragments and/or employ sophisticated search strategies to sample hit compounds from a predefined area of the chemical space. Furthermore, standard *de novo* design methods often rely on explicit chemical knowledge accumulation in the form of synthesis rules or basic physical models. They are limited by our incomplete understanding of how molecules interact because scientists cannot tell conventional software how to find insights into data when they do not themselves know what elements of the data are most important and how they relate to one another. This explains in part why, despite the rapid advances in recent decades in high-throughput screening technologies, only a small fraction of the drug-like space has been investigated in the search for new drugs. The situation is also made difficult by the fact that our fundamental understanding of human disease, which can only be comprehended by combining the information from multiple data types, is still far from complete.

Researchers began using DL architectures to develop novel classes of algorithms for *de novo* drug design to explore the largely unexplored chemical space more efficiently while bypassing our incomplete understanding of many disease mechanisms. DL-based algorithms, often referred to as AI methods, have many variants, are flexible, and have the ability to treat information from the scientific literature and databases, as well as patient-level data. What makes DL so attractive is its ability to identify relevant patterns within complex, nonlinear data in an automatic fashion

DOI: 10.1201/9781003399346-3

with a reduced need for manual feature engineering. Being able to derive their insights into which data elements matter, DL-based methods can extract better predictions for a wider range of variables.

Nowadays, AI-enabled generative models for *de novo* molecular design are applied to directly generate molecular structures, readily synthesizable within a few reaction steps, with desired properties and/or activities (i.e. pharmacological activity) that are easily quantifiable, such as molecular weight, or more abstract, like toxicity and synthetic accessibility (SA). This design concept comprises molecule generation, molecule scoring, and molecule optimization. For drug discovery and medicinal chemistry specifically, this involves tasks in drug target and lead compound identification, drug design optimization against multiple property profiles of interest, and finally appropriate identifying synthetic routes. These new classes of *de novo* design algorithms constitute what is referred to as generative chemistry. There is a growing number of case studies in generative chemistry which resulted in generated compounds being synthesized and validated either *in vitro* and/or *in vivo*. These case studies provide an overview of the current capabilities of AI-enabled generative models. In addition to better success rates, the use of AI in drug discovery should lead to quicker and cheaper drug discovery and development, ultimately allowing novel drugs to reach the market faster [6]. A recently published perspective presented a systematic evaluation of studies that include synthesis and experimental in vitro validation in biochemical assays of the generated molecular structures in order to discuss the relevance of this type of approach from the viewpoint of medicinal chemistry [7].

This chapter is divided into the following parts: Section 2.2 reviews the 1D representations commonly used by many AI-enabled generative models. Section 2.3 reviews the most widely used algorithm architectures in the field of generative chemistry. It is widely acknowledged that good reward functions are critical for molecular generation and essential for molecular optimization. In Section 2.4, we discuss several proposed metrics for comparing generative models and the closely related topic of the proper definition of the applicability domain and selection of appropriate reward functions for molecular optimization. Section 2.5 reviews the progress in the development of benchmarking platforms for the training and validation of generative models. Section 2.6 discusses several optimization strategies used when training AI-enabled generative models. Section 2.7 discusses the Transformer architecture in more detail and reviews several recent AI-enabled models integrating this type of architecture to illustrate how Transformers can be combined with already-established architectures to improve model performance. Section 2.8 illustrates how the AI-enabled end-to-end pipelines for *de novo* drug design can be used to create novel molecular structures for novel targets. We end up with a short conclusion.

2.2 REPRESENTATION OF MOLECULAR STRUCTURES

The first step to use large datasets of molecular structures for the training and validation of AI-enabled generative models is to encode the molecular structures into a structured digital representation. Although the representation of small and relatively simple organic molecules does not pose significant issues with multiple methods being available for this task, the situation dramatically changes when considering molecular structures whose complex topology includes ring structures, non-standard valency/bonding, inorganic components, or symmetry. These complex topological features can cause problems such as molecular representations being noncanonical (i.e. multiple different representations for the same molecule) or being nonunique (i.e. multiple different molecules that are encoded into the same representation). Other issues encountered include assuming the wrong number of implicit hydrogen atoms or failing to capture tautomerism. Initially, one suggested using molecular fingerprints [8] to represent the molecular structures and the first published proof of concept of *de novo* drug design was based on this type of representation [9,10]. It became apparent that representing molecules using the molecular fingerprints suffered from two disadvantages. First, there is no one-to-one mapping from a molecule to the fingerprint, and second, the fingerprint representation contains less information about the topology of the molecular structures than other two-dimensional representations of the molecules, such as string representation. There are currently different classes of representations, and selecting the appropriate one usually depends on the context; see [11,12] for recent discussions on this matter. In most cases, the encoding is a two-step procedure. First, molecular structures are encoded as line notations, such as the Simplified Molecular-Input Line-Entry System (SMILES) [13,14], which is the most used approach to express molecular structures (see Figure 2.1). The encoding can also be carried out using Wiswesser Line Notation (WLN) [15], or SYBYL Line Notation (SLN) [16] formats. These line notations are transformed into digital representations such as numerical vectors or graphs. Techniques for expressing molecular structures in the form of strings have been widely applied for the construction of molecular information, especially within databases because string format is easier to handle than more elaborated format such as graph data. For instance, SMILES has an arrangement of characters according to grammar and context, like natural language, and that is why many techniques primarily developed in the field of Natural Language Processing (NLP) are applicable to inverse molecular design problems.

SMILES was the first encoding technique to be successfully used with a variational autoencoder (VAE) to create a continuous representation of molecules. This is important because a continuous representation allows for efficient navigation of the immense chemical space of possible molecules. SMILES notation provides a 1D representation of molecules as sequences of "tokens". The SMILES of a molecule is built through a depth-first traversal of the molecular structure, encoding atoms and how they connect. As the process of encoding a molecule into a string can start at different locations of the molecule, there exists a one-to-many relationship where a single molecule can be represented by several different SMILES. As such, canonicalization algorithms that generate what is known as canonical SMILES have been developed to ensure that a one-to-one relationship is possible. The SMILES syntax also presents an added difficulty because of rings and branches requiring symbols to occur in pairs which often leads to syntactically invalid SMILES strings. To transform the SMILES associated with molecular structures into an input suitable for generative models, a language is constructed by examining the characters the SMILES strings are composed of. Then, each character or token of the language is assigned to a unique number. Next, numerical vectors are encoded by matching

(a)

IUPAC name

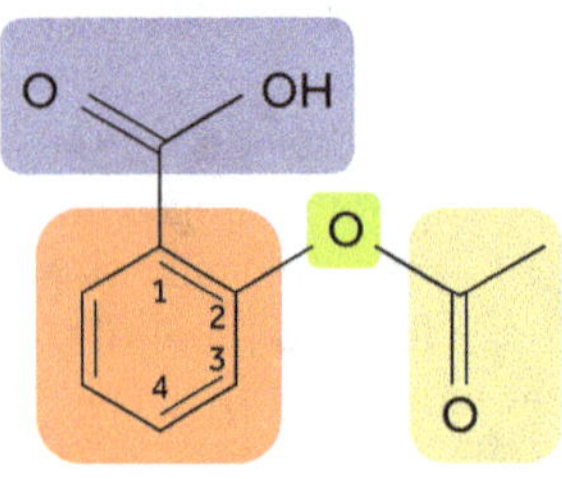

2-Acetyloxybenzoic acid

(b)

SMILES

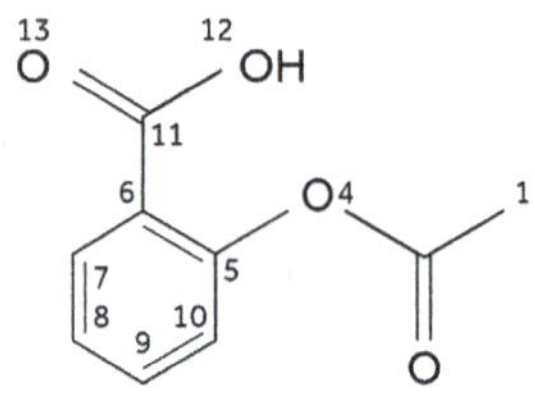

CC(=O)OC1=C(C=CC=C1)C(O)=O
1 2 3 4 5 6 7 8 9 10 1112 13

(c)

(1) Canonical order

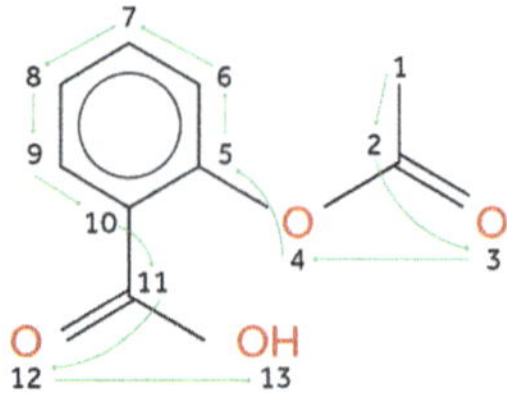

(2) Unrestricted random atom order

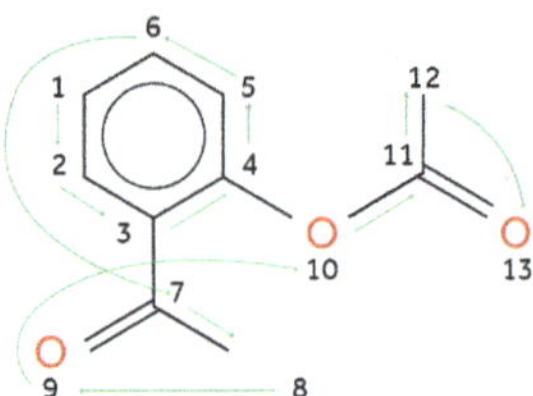

(3) Restricted random atom order

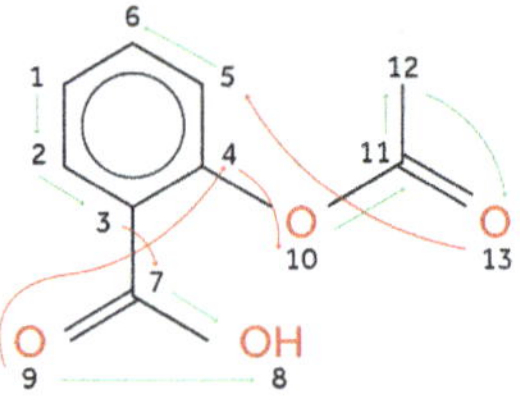

FIGURE 2.1 (a) Representation of molecular structures using IUPAC nomenclature. (b) Representation of molecular structures using the SMILES (c) the three different approaches used to encode molecular structures as SMILES string. (1) Canonical order (2) unrestricted random atom order (3) restricted random atom order.

the characters of the SMILES strings with the associated numbers of the language. These numerical vectors constitute the structured data used as inputs for training generative models. Interestingly, the one-to-many relationship between molecules and noncanonical SMILES, i.e. randomized SMILES (sometimes referred to as enumerated SMILES), can be leveraged to perform data augmentation when training AI-enabled generative models by allowing to expand a given data set with the various possible SMILES of the molecules it contains. In recent work, it was suggested that using randomized SMILES offered advantages when it comes to model optimization [17]. Besides, other SMILES representations have also been suggested to circumvent the limitations of the standard SMILES syntax. For instance, DeepSMILES [18] is an adaptation of the SMILES syntax focusing on two of the major causes of generating invalid SMILES, unmatched ring and parentheses closures.

The International Union of Pure and Applied Chemistry (IUPAC) introduced the International Chemical Identifier (InChI) system [19], which is a notation language that represents molecules as layered strings of characters and aims to be a unique encoding representation of a molecular structure. In the InChI format, molecules are encoded as predefined layers of information arranged in a predefined order. Although the InChI format is flexible in representing molecular structures, the attempts to develop AI-enabled generative models using molecules encoded in the InChI format were not successful. Studies showed that the InChI format led to poorer performance compared with similar models using SMILES, and experiments showed that models using InChI failed to correctly learn molecular structures [20]. Several reasons have been evoked, such as the added complexity of the InChI syntax, compared with SMILES [21]. Nonetheless, InChI provides an alternative unique identifier for molecular structures which can be exploited to derive a canonical SMILES.

Another representation of molecular structures that are often overlooked in the field of generative chemistry in favor of SMILES is the IUPAC naming system itself [22]. The IUPAC nomenclature constitutes a systematic terminology of naming organic molecules based on functional groups and moieties, which are commonly occurring clusters of connected atoms that have known chemical behaviors. IUPAC nomenclature uses words to represent functional groups, unlike most other string representations, which use letters/numbers. Although it is argued that IUPAC nomenclature can be very lengthy and does not specify the full structure of a compound, recent work has proposed that representations such as SMILES or molecular graphs are less suitable for molecular optimization because adding or removing arbitrary atoms has no intuitive meaning to chemists and is unlikely to allow for easy synthesis [23]. It was shown that IUPAC names can be used as a base representation for molecular modeling, as discussed in more detail below.

2.3 OVERVIEW OF GENERATIVE MODELS

Even when using AI-enabled generative models, *de novo* design of molecular structures is challenging because they must satisfy multiple constraints that are intuitive to domain experts but sometimes challenging to quantify. Moreover, generating molecules that are structurally close to a target class, but that are diverse, that is generating diverse molecules with desired properties are two diametrically opposed goals. For these reasons, *de novo* molecular design was, for many years, mainly a process of trial and error, with human expert knowledge and intuition about chemistry playing a major role. An important breakthrough came in 2014 with the creation of the generative adversarial network (GAN), a novel type of DL architecture which learns underlying data distribution in an unsupervised setting and demonstrated unprecedented capabilities to generate new objects with desired properties [24]. Insilico Medicine was among the first to publish a proof of concept in 2016 demonstrating how the capabilities of AI to identify nonlinear patterns within complex and often noisy biological datasets could be used to make reliable predictions of novel small-molecule drugs [9]. Various programs were initiated to leverage AI's unique capabilities to help accelerate drug discovery, and several milestones were quickly reached that showed the ability of AI to search regions of the chemical space that had remained unexplored so far using classical drug discovery approaches to produce novel small molecules with biological activity. The field of generative chemistry progressively took shape to foster the creation of new AI-enabled generative methods mainly for the goal-directed design of molecules [25]. In a more recent study, Insilico Medicine was able to significantly reduce the time needed to identify three preclinical candidates compared with the three to five years typically required [26]. This was made possible thanks to the support of compound synthesis services from contract research organizations (CROs) and expertise from academia and larger pharma partners. In a typical case of *de novo* molecular design, AI-enabled generative models must design molecules, create a ranked list by assessing their feasibility, perform conformational analysis, and identify the molecular structures featuring specific structural properties that are responsible for the affinity toward the target of interest. Various types of AI-enabled generative models are now available for directing and controlling the generation of molecules towards compounds with pre-defined chemical properties and desired activities, meeting multiple desired target conditions. The commonly used architectures can be roughly classified into three categories (see Figure 2.2) based on recurrent neural networks (RNNs) [27,28], autoencoders (AEs), with, for instance, variational autoencoders (VAEs) [29,30], and generative models based on generative adversarial networks (GANs) which learn underlying data distribution in an unsupervised setting [31]. Excellent reviews providing comprehensive analysis of the mathematical fundamentals behind these methods are published elsewhere [32] and detailed lists of representative AI-enabled generative models are available in [11,33,34]. Over time, generative models have been further improved and combined for better efficiency. For instance, with the introduction of memory augmented memory augmented RNN or with reinforcement learning (RL) and transfer learning (TL), that allow to alter the probability of generating molecules with specific properties either after or during training, see Figure 2.3. Using those novel learning techniques, one has published models with TL being used to fine-tune RNNs to design drugs for specific targets and to generate molecules that are structurally similar to drugs with known activities against particular targets.

The original GAN architecture suffered from two issues when used for *de novo* molecular design. First, a GAN generates real-valued continuous data, but it is not appropriate for indirect sequence generation of discrete tokens such as SMILES strings. Second, a GAN can only give the score/loss of an entire string. Balancing the current score of a partially generated subsequence with the future score of the complete sequence is a non-trivial task. GAN-based models employing RNNs, especially long-short-term memory (LSTM), a widely studied, popular architecture, as generators were proposed to address these problems. For instance, SeqGAN [35], which also uses RL to facilitate the generation of discrete data, and ORGAN [36] which is a SeqGAN-based model that accounts for chemical properties such as the solubility and drug-likeness of generated molecules. However, GAN-based models that use an RNN as a generator for the design of molecular structures with SMILES representations have limited capabilities to extract latent features from a long sequence with rich semantic information such as SMILES strings. The limited capability of these models to capture long-range dependency is problematic because the molecular structures expressed in the SMILES format often have relatively long sequences.

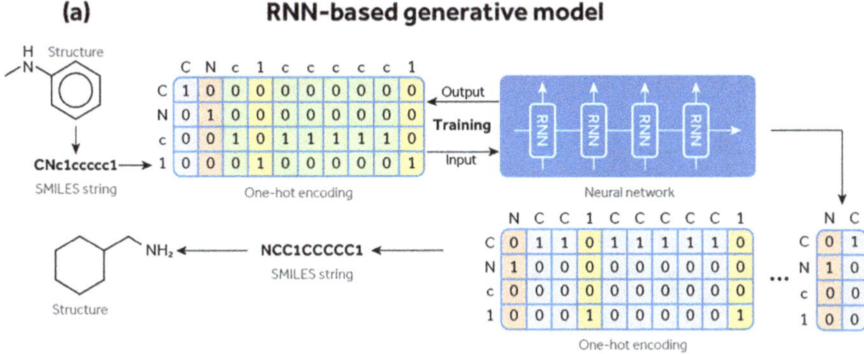

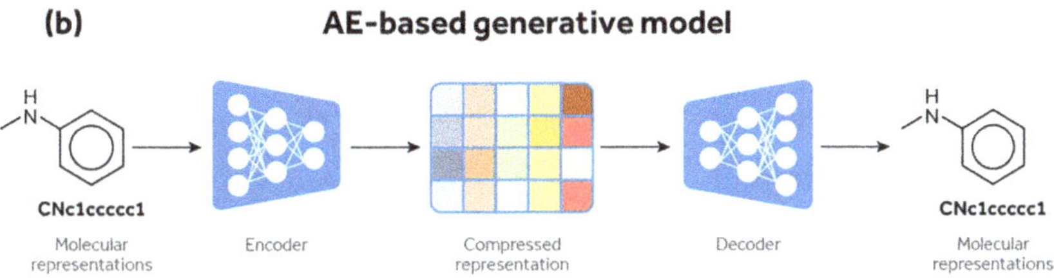

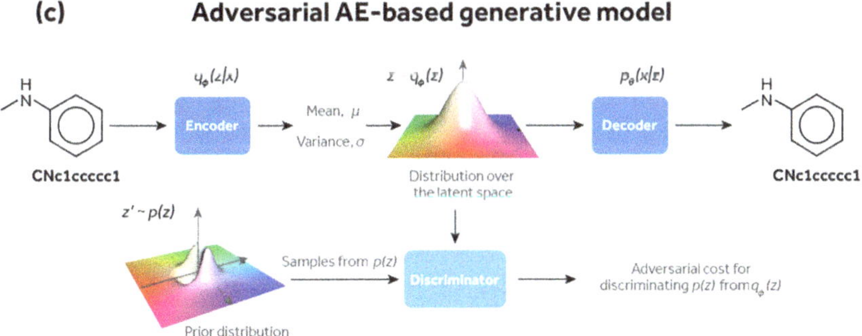

FIGURE 2.2 There are currently three major classes of AI-enabled generative models using SMILES representation of molecules as inputs. (a) RNN-based generative model (b) AE-based generative model, and (c) adversarial-based generative model. Each of these architectures has advantages and can also be complemented with additional modules, such as TL and RL modules, to improve the efficacy of the generative process depending on the characteristics of the task.

Consequently, it is more difficult for GAN based on RNNs to design a molecular structure with complex rings [37] because highly cyclic molecules have long sequence representations and a stricter syntax than acyclic molecules. It means that even slight modifications in the SMILES syntax can lead to the generation of invalid structures or structures with chemical properties that differ from those expected. Another issue is that RNNs cannot work on GPU implementations because the current iteration must be computed after the previous time step, which is not conducive

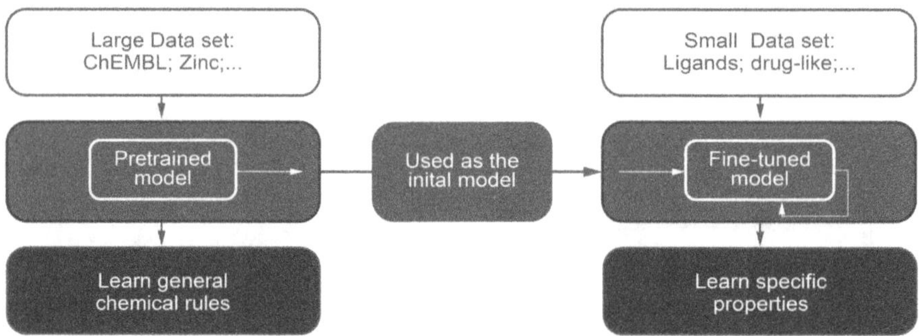

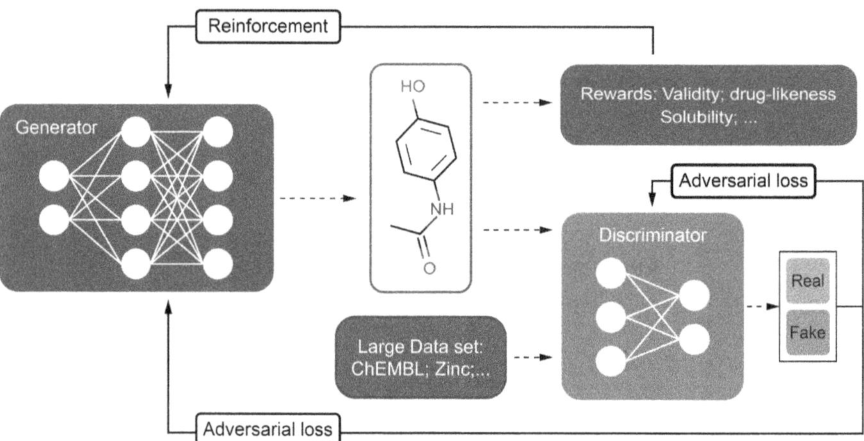

FIGURE 2.3 (Top) Transfer learning. A generative model is first trained on large datasets to learn the general chemical rules that apply to large classes of molecules. This model is then fine-tuned on datasets corresponding to pre-selected types of structures appropriate for targets of interest to become able to generate structures closer to drugs with known activities against these predefined targets (Bottom) Reinforcement learning. Example of integration of RL within a GAN architecture. Molecular structures created by the generator module are evaluated using metrics for drug-likeness, solubility, and other relevant properties. The generator is being rewarded as the properties of the molecules improve and it keeps exploring the most suitable area of the chemical space.

to exploring the near-infinite chemical spaces of big data. Recently, a novel type of architecture, referred to as Transformer, was suggested to circumvent the limitations posed by RNNs. Transformer was initially aimed at natural language processing (NLP) problems, where the network input is a series of high-dimensional embeddings representing words or word fragments. A transformer [38] is a self-attention-based neural network architecture that can capture semantic features in sentences using a self-attention mechanism alone without the need of an RNN. Transformers can solve the limitations of traditional RNNs in iterative calculations and use the self-attention mechanism to capture useful syntax information. Architectures combining transformers with either GAN or encoder-decoder architectures can be utilized for AI-enabled generation of molecular structures whenever the generation task is formalized as a kind of natural language processing that treats SMILES strings as sentences. One has integrated transformers with different types of architecture, such as GAN and AE, and these models have demonstrated the effectiveness of this approach although they also face their own challenges when applied for *de novo* drug design.

2.4 DEVELOPMENT OF APPLICABILITY DOMAINS FOR AI-ENABLED GENERATIVE MODELS

Generative models used for goal-directed design of molecules with a desired profile are known for sometimes generating unrealistic, not synthesizable, or unstable structures. For instance, the pioneering molecular autoencoder work resulted in molecules which were difficult to synthesize or contained highly labile (reactive or unstable) groups which would rapidly break apart in the body and thus were not viable drugs. An important direction of research is concerned with the development of systematic and robust methods to assess the performance of the AI-enabled models and for rigorously evaluating and comparing generated molecular structures, which, considering the rapid growth of this field, is essential to help guide future work. Methods to constrain AI-enabled models to generate structures in reasonable portions of the chemical space are thus required. Issues commonly encountered in earlier work on *de novo* design of molecular structures can be mitigated when using appropriate reward functions that lead to generated molecules which meet the minimum following requirement: Diversity: the set of molecules generated is diverse enough to be interesting. Novelty: i.e. the probability of generating a new molecule that does not exist in the training data, so the model does not simply reproduce molecules in the training set. Stability: the molecules are stable in the target environment and not highly reactive. Synthesizability: the molecules can be synthesized. Non-triviality: the molecules are not degenerate or trivial solutions to maximizing the reward function. Good properties: the molecules have the properties desired for the application at hand.

Establishing standardized metrics requires the definition of applicability domains (AD) for generative models in a similar fashion to the ones already applied for predictive models. In [33] the authors were concerned with the search for an AD definition suited to generative models that could take into account the drug-likeness of a molecule. They explored ADs suited for designing drug-like molecules using goal-oriented generation algorithms in the context of lead optimization. They used a SMILES-based LSTM, an architecture adapted for the development of a generative AD. They trained this model on three lead-optimization datasets to study ADs. The appreciation of whether a molecule is structurally like the training set is dependent both on the molecular descriptors and on the measure of similarity used. Various types of molecular descriptors were considered, including Extended-Connectivity Fingerprints (ECFP) [39], Atom-Pair (AP) fingerprints [40], the Quantitative Estimate of Drug-Likeness score (QED) [41], which is a reference for gauging the drug-likeness of a molecular structure and molecular descriptors based on a combination of physio-chemical descriptors. Two similarity measures were considered.

The first one, a range-based method, is the bounding box approach [42] and the second one is the Tanimoto distance, a similarity measure widely used in cheminformatics [43]. Several ADs were defined, each made of a similarity measure and a set of descriptors or a combination of a pair of descriptors and similarity measures. SMILES validity was used as a baseline AD. The evaluation of the generated molecules was based on three properties. First, the diversity of generated compounds was evaluated by combining the measure of the internal diversity based on the Tanimoto dissimilarity coefficient together with the entropy of the repartition of generated molecules within the clusters. This provides a good insight into the molecular diversity of the generated sets. Second, for each AD, one assessed the ability of the generative algorithm to retrieve actives from the test set. Indeed, testing whether the generative algorithm can retrieve unseen known actives constitutes the best proxy to evaluate its ability to generate novel bioactive molecules, which is the objective of goal-directed generation in the context of lead optimization. Third, QED and the SA score (SAS) were used to measure the quality of the generated compounds in a medicinal chemistry context. The results emphasize the importance of using an adequate AD when using generative algorithms for molecular design. The main observations and take-away messages of this study can be summarized as follows. Generally, combining several descriptors and similarity measures allows us to define ADs that perform well in different training settings. Nevertheless, classic ADs used in QSAR modeling (e.g. Tanimoto similarity on ECFP4 fingerprints) are insufficient to discriminate molecular structures designed using generative models. Furthermore, measures of drug-likeness such as QED can be optimized in unintended ways and taken alone; they are not valid AD for generative models. Different good AD definitions can lead to the exploration of different regions of the chemical space. In terms of diversity, suitable ADs generate sets of molecules that fit well within the original dataset used, while ADs that are not stringent enough generate sets of molecules that overfit specific regions of chemical space. Good AD definitions lead to higher diversity in addition to higher quality of the generated structures. Good ADs explore the vicinity of the original training set, with close neighbors of generated molecules showing an enrichment towards the actives of the dataset. Counter-intuitively, good ADs are associated with lower rewards. These results suggest that an AD definition that is insufficient to constrain generative models leads to the over-exploitation of narrow regions of the chemical space, often with the addition of non-drug-like patterns to a high-scoring molecular structure. The constraints associated with good ADs prevent generative algorithms from over-exploiting a specific region of the chemical space, leading to a wider distribution of rewards. Finally, the results highlighted the importance of choosing a carefully curated training dataset. The training set needs to have only molecules that are considered as reasonable molecules. If this is not the case, for instance, if the training set includes results from a high-throughput screening campaign, all of which would not be deemed reasonable starting points for a lead-optimization program, the applicability domains defined with respect to the training set might be insufficient to generate only reasonable molecules. The appropriate definition of an AD also depends on the context of the program being carried out. In this study, ADs were defined in a lead-optimization context, where the chemical space explored is focused on a narrow set of chemical series, and novelty is not a critical feature, but when using generative models in distribution learning programs, where the goal is to generate libraries of compounds for downstream task, other AD definitions could be more suitable as distribution learning aims at exploring a diverse chemical space.

2.5 BENCHMARKING PLATFORMS

The development of benchmarking platforms to evaluate AI-enabled generative model performance using standardized criteria started with AI/ML being used for predicting molecular properties has been the subject of a lot of efforts. A first example of this kind was the platform MoleculeNet that provides a benchmark to compare the utility of different regression modeling techniques across a wide range of property prediction problems. The same needs that quickly appeared in the more recent field of AI-enabled generative chemistry were also addressed with many initiatives, for example the Python software package called GuacaMol [44] which contains a large set of optimization benchmarking methods for drug discovery and benchmarking models for *de novo* molecular design for goal-oriented generation tasks. Another benchmarking platform in the form of a Python package called DiversityNet benchmark was released by Benhenda et al. [45]. DiversityNet implements several generative models of the three main classes (VAEs, RNNs, and several flavors of GANs), and provides a set of metrics that primarily evaluate the diversity and the quality of the generated molecules through multi-objective tasks. The DiversityNet platform aims at standardizing the validation of the generated molecular structures and to that end, it facilitates the sharing of fine-tuned open-source implementations of AI enabled generative models. A particularly successful benchmarking platform is Molecular Sets (MOSES) [46], which provides users with tools to evaluate the learning performance of a large panel of generative models. To assess whether the AI-enabled generative models can generate new molecules, it uses criteria such as validity, uniqueness, internal diversity, filters, and novelty rates, along with the internal diversity and the fraction of generated molecular structures that successfully pass structural filters for molecular quality. MOSES includes baseline models and standardized data set with a recommended train, test, and scaffold test split. The platform provides metrics to evaluate how well the model learned features of the training datasets. Metrics such as the Fréchet ChemNet Distance [47], the distance between the distribution of various physicochemical properties, Fragment similarity (Frag), Scaffold similarity (Scaf), and the nearest neighbor Tanimoto similarity (SNN) [48] help to capture more abstract chemical and biological similarities, while the cosine similarity of Bemis–Murcko scaffolds [49] and the cosine similarity of BRICS fragments help compare molecules at a substructure level.

2.6 OPTIMIZATION STRATEGIES IN GENERATIVE CHEMISTRY

In [17], the authors showed how to optimize model performance by choosing randomized SMILES rather than the canonical SMILES as a molecule representation. They performed a benchmark on RNN-based models trained with different SMILES variants (canonical SMILES, randomized SMILES, and DeepSMILES), using subsets of different sizes of the GDB-13 database [50] to explore the data amplification capabilities of randomized SMILES. In this study, the performance of the two most used recurrent cell architectures (LSTM and gated recurrent unit (GRU)) was compared. To assess the properties of the output domain, metrics were developed that define how well a model has generalized the training set. In this study, the generated chemical space is evaluated with respect to its uniformity (equal probability of sampling), completeness (sampling all molecules from GDB-13), and closedness (only molecules from GDB-13 are sampled). Furthermore, the physicochemical properties of the molecules sampled from the different SMILES variants were evaluated using the benchmarking platform MOSES. Properties evaluated include the molecular weight, the octanol-water partition coefficient (logP), SAS, QED, Natural-Product likeness score (NP), and Internal Diversity. In this study, the GRU cells have not shown any improvement whatsoever compared to the LSTM cells and even though the training time per epoch of the GRU cells is lower, LSTM models are able to converge in fewer epochs. GRU cells are widely used and provide a noticeable speed improvement, but studies concluded that in some circumstances, they perform worse. GRU cells were thus dropped because of their consistently lower performance with all configurations and types of SMILES used. The best canonical SMILES model was only able to enumerate 72.8% of GDB-13 compared to the 83.0% of the restricted randomized SMILES. Furthermore, the models trained with restricted randomized variants had a more complete and more closed domain than those trained with the unrestricted variant. Moreover, randomized SMILES without data augmentation performed better than the models trained with canonical SMILES but worse than models using randomized SMILES with data augmentation. This indicates that not using the canonical representation constraint makes better models but also that data augmentation has a positive impact on the training process. Overall, the models using LSTM cells trained with 1 million restricted randomized SMILES are the best performers in the sense that they can generalize to larger chemical spaces and can more accurately represent the target chemical space. An explanation suggested by the authors is that a SMILES molecular generative model learns by finding patterns in the SMILES strings from the training set with the goal of generalizing a model that can obtain all the SMILES in the training set with the highest possible probability. The procedure is the same with any SMILES variant but when the canonical representation is used, the model learns to generate one linear representation of each molecule obtained through a canonicalization algorithm. This means that the model must learn not only to generate valid SMILES strings but also to generate those in the canonical form.

Besides the choice of the molecule representation, AI-enabled generative model performance can be improved by combining various optimization methods while considering that these optimization methods might be ineffective or even worsen the performance if they are not correctly configured. It is thus important to carefully evaluate how to combine optimization methods to design better AI-enabled generative models. In [51], the authors tested combinations of three techniques to propose a procedure for the design of Convolutional Neural Network (CNN) models on different properties of molecules. First, the dynamic batch size (DB) strategy for different enumeration ratios of the SMILES. Indeed, augmented data by the restricted enumeration of SMILES representation of each compound gives the characteristic of redundancy, which helps to maintain the generalization performance as the small batch size while enjoying the benefit of a large batch size. Second, Bayesian optimization (BO) for hyperparameter optimization. When performing hyperparameter optimization, one must deal with multiple combinations of hyperparameter values that are often complex and high dimensional, with interactions that are difficult to understand. Automated optimization methods include grid search and random selection. However, Bayesian optimization has emerged as a reliable alternative. Third, TL is used to pass the knowledge from a related task that has been learned. For the same reasons, encoding relevant domain-specific information into the model can be used to bootstrap the training of a deep neural network and increase the overall model accuracy. Here, the authors propose feature learning using chemical features obtained by a feedforward neural network, which are concatenated with the learned molecular feature vector. The authors tested the combinations of DB, BO, hybrid representation with Molecular ACCess System (MACCS) fingerprint [52], and hybrid representation with 200 RDKit features. An advantage of the dynamic batch size strategy is reducing the training time, and this optimization technique was implemented first and other optimization techniques were built on top of it. The optimized version of the CNN was compared with the performance of Graph Convolutional Network (GCN) and Random Forest (RF) models. The results showed that the best model with hybrid representation demonstrated better performance when using BO combined with DB tuning. However, the authors also uncovered several restrictions and conditions to ensure that the optimized methods could provide the expected benefit. They concluded that increasing the batch size can benefit the model training in the enumeration dataset, but the batch should be carefully increased instead of being simply proportional to the enumeration ratio. The results obtained when trying to generalize the optimized hyperparameters of the model on the original dataset to the model on the enumerated dataset showed that the optimized hyperparameters are specific to the dataset configuration and the optimized hyperparameters must be found on the same configurations, including the enumeration ratio of the dataset. The effect, also dataset dependent, of the hybrid representation of the molecular features on the enumerated dataset is that it leverages both the advantages of automatic feature extraction and classical molecular representation, which is known to improve the performance of the model. There are two main limitations when utilizing only raw representations to develop models. One limitation is that the models are unable to learn to identify and extract all the features of a molecule due to little training data, and they are susceptible to overfitting artifacts in the data. This limitation can be addressed by SMILES notation enumeration. The second limitation is that the encoding processes can capture only local information and result in a molecular representation that is fundamentally local rather than global in nature. This makes it difficult to predict properties that depend more on the global features, and Transformers should be considered to handle this issue. The best results were obtained when the optimization techniques were integrated with enumeration, the most beneficial optimization techniques, in light of DB, considering that although the redundancy of the enumerated dataset can be employed to enlarge the batch size, excessively enlarging the batch size leads to poorer performance.

Generative model optimization, training procedure, as well as the properties of the generated molecules, depends on multiple intertwined factors, and this advocates for the development of formatted guidelines for the proper assembly of datasets and standardized procedures for hyperparameter tuning to evaluate generative model performance, which is context-dependent. We summarized in Figure 2.4 different interconnected points which must be considered to properly configure generative models and ensure the successful generation of novel molecular structure. First, the aim and scope of the experiment must be clearly defined because the definition of appropriate ADs depends on whether one is working in a lead-optimization context or distribution learning programs. For example, in [53], the authors released a web interface providing users with the ability to generate molecules using a restricted number of AI-enabled generative models designed specifically to handle lead optimization tasks. Second, one should carefully evaluate what is the most adapted generative model because there are classes of AI-enabled generative models that are more suitable for the generation of the bulk of molecules, while others are more convenient for the targeted generation of specific molecules. Conditional Variational Autoencoder can be regarded as a specialized algorithm for the generation of molecules displaying specific properties, while CDN is designed to generate similar yet diverse molecules

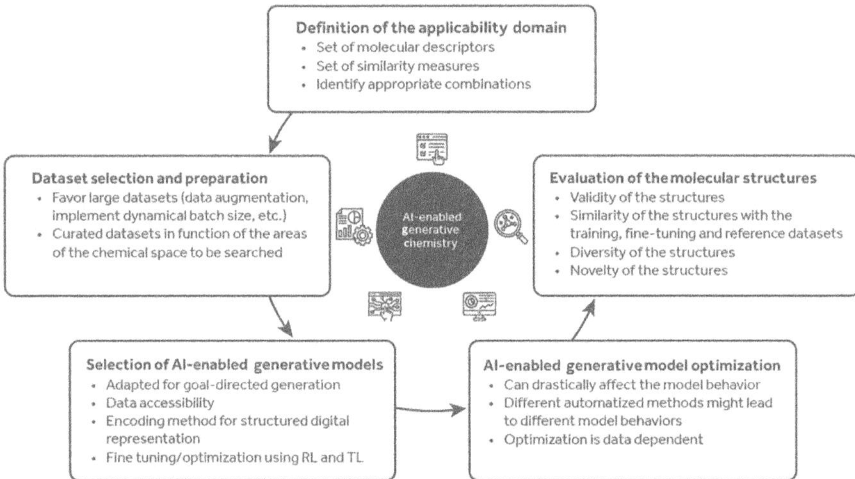

FIGURE 2.4 Previous experience in the field of AI-based generative chemistry shows that the design of a successful AI-enabled generative experiment and the proper evaluation of the generated molecular structures require to follow a multiple-step process that should include (1) The definition of an AD appropriate to the type of task. (2) The preparation of large datasets which should be properly curated and filled with molecules corresponding, in terms of properties, to the areas of the chemical space to be searched. (3) The selection of a suitable AI-based architecture for the generative model. Previous studies showed that models adapted for distribution learning are not necessarily suitable for goal-oriented generation. The architecture should be thought of as functions of the encoding method used to represent the molecular structures as input and output. Other modules, such as TL or RL for optimization contribute to improving the quality of the generated molecules and should be considered. (4) Multiple strategies have been suggested to optimize the generative model, but they should be chosen and combined carefully because they can potentially strongly affect the model behavior. One should keep in mind that most of these optimization procedures are data-dependent. (5) There are many aspects to be covered when evaluating the generated molecules, some of them might seem to be contradictory in nature. Appropriate metrics should be used and combined to provide an optimal evaluation of the output, according to the goal of the experiment.

when compared to a particular prototype. Third, one should choose the right training datasets for training and validation. The training set should be carefully curated and contain only molecules that are considered reasonable molecules. The size and composition of the training set are also important to ensure a proper calibration of the generative models and allow the use of optimization techniques such as DB size tuning. An AD defined using inappropriate training sets might lead to poor evaluation of the generated molecules and the properties of the molecules can vary dramatically depending on the combination of algorithms and training sets used. Finally, the fine-tuning of the generative model, either through automatized training, optimization methods such as BO, or manual setting of hyperparameters, should be done with caution. This is true even for classical ML algorithms in the context of relatively simple classification tasks. Indeed, in this regard, it was shown that hyperparameter tuning cannot only strongly affect quantitatively the classification but also its outcome [54].

2.7 DEEP LEARNING MODELS USING TRANSFORMERS FOR GENERATIVE CHEMISTRY

De novo molecular design using ML can be of limited use when the knowledge of experts about structure-activity relationships and external factors like patentability are important to consider in the design process. These constraints are often expressed by providing known portions of the molecular structure. For example, one could be interested in a particular scaffold because it has favorable intellectual property attributes, or certain parts of a drug may be needed for the desired biological activity, while other parts can be modified to increase bioavailability. To address these types of situations, one designed a generative model, referred to as Controllable Characteristic-Conditioned Chemical Changer with T5 (C5T5) [23], able to make localized modifications to a molecular structure that change its physical properties in a desired way. Together with this peculiar model, the authors proposed a novel self-supervised pre-training method for generative modeling of organic molecules that allows domain experts to better control the molecular optimization process while also providing more understandable predictions than prior methods. Interestingly, this method operates on IUPAC names [55–57] rather than SMILES. By using a more interpretable molecular representation, the method aims at addressing the fact that molecular optimization is a difficult problem because it requires modifying, with localized edits and without making it too difficult to synthesize, a molecule that already satisfies several requirements that need to be preserved. The use of IUPAC names allows interpretable targeted modifications to molecules that lead to desired changes across several physical properties. This allows C5T5 to use the IUPAC name base representation to support targeted modifications to existing molecules by enabling transformers to make zero-shot select-and- replace edits, altering organic substances towards desired property values. The training method is inspired by TL techniques [58]. The T5 model is trained in a self-supervised fashion on a large dataset of molecules and estimates of their molecular property values whereas novel molecules are generated from the output of the decoder module of the T5 model. The effectiveness of the C5T5 framework was demonstrated on different molecular optimization tasks for which C5T5 was trained to make localized modifications that affect four properties used to estimate bioavailability of a candidate drug, namely, the distribution coefficients (logD), logP, PSA, and refractivity [59]. This study showed that the localized changes proposed by the C5T5 model can control the property value as desired. Positive results were also obtained when multiple areas of the molecules had to be modified together to achieve the desired property changes.

As discussed in the introduction, AI-enabled generative models based on RNN exhibit limitations in capturing long-range dependency, resulting in a high invalid percentage in generated molecules. In [60], the authors aimed at generating novel potent BRAF inhibitors. To that end, they implemented a novel ligand-based *de novo* molecular design approach integrating Transformers to increase the capacity of handling large sequence data. A Transformer-encoder-based generator was trained to learn the grammatical rules of known drug molecules and TL was used to fine tune the generative model by introducing the prior knowledge of drugs with known activities against targets into the generative model to construct new molecules similar to the known ligands. An RL module was used to optimize the parameters of the generator to create small molecules with desirable activity and with drug-like properties that are expected to bind well with the target. A dataset of approximately 1.6 million small molecules represented in canonical SMILES with a length of 100 or less was created for training. Three generative models were tested: Transformer-based, GRU-based, and bidirectional GRU-based models. The authors trained a stack-augmented GRU model on the same dataset and tested the effect of different layers of GRU on generating valid molecular percentages. Unlike Transformer structures, the expressive power of the GRU cannot be increased by deepening the network. Therefore, only one layer of GRU was used for molecular generation in our experiment. It was found in the experiment that the bidirectional GRU did not improve the performance of the generative model.

The study showed that the generative model based on the Transformer was superior to the generative model using GRU in terms of the stability of the training process and has higher accuracy of generating valid molecules on the validation set. The Transformer was also superior in terms of the performance of RL. The generative model based on the Transformer has improved the percentage of generating chemically valid molecules (from 95.6% to 98.2%), the structural diversity and SAS of the generated molecules. The Transformer model also outperformed the GRU-based RNN in capturing the long-range dependency of small molecules. In addition, the samples generated by the generative model almost covered the entire chemical space occupied by BRAF inhibitors, which proves that the Transformer-based *de novo* drug design method is successful under "low data" conditions and the Transformer-based generative model has the potential to generate BRAF inhibitors with novel structures and higher activity. Finally, molecular docking and binding mode analysis proved that our model could generate quality candidate compounds for BRAF.

2.8 USING THE AI-ENABLED PLATFORM FOR *DE NOVO* DRUG DESIGN CHEMISTRY42 TO GENERATE NOVEL TARGETS AGAINST CDK20

The interplay between the study of the biological mechanisms of a disease, the identification of appropriate targets, and the design of suitable drug-like compounds is one of the major drivers behind the assembly of fully integrated AI-driven end-to-end drug discovery pipelines undertaken by AI-native drug discovery companies because this type of infrastructure would make much easier not only to optimize and accelerate the design and validation of novel small drug molecules but also to identify and validate novel promising targets in various therapeutic areas. A recent case study illustrating how platforms leveraging AI/ML capabilities for drug *de novo* design can be effectively used toward this endeavor was recently published [61]. The purpose of the study was to design potent molecular structures against Cyclin-dependent kinase 20 (CDK20) using Chemistry42, a well-established integrated platform combining state-of-the-art AI/ML technologies with computational and medicinal chemistry methodologies for the *de novo design* of small molecules (https://www.chemistry42.com/) [62]. The Chemistry42 platform integrates SBDD and LBDD methods and allows the configuration of generative experiments with many structural properties and predefined reward functions and optimization functionalities to be calibrated by the users. The platform includes state-of-the-art generative models of all categories mentioned above [10,63–65]. CDK20 was recently identified using the online platform for target identification PandaOmics (https://www.pandaomics.com/) [66–70] as a promising novel therapeutic target against hepatocellular carcinoma (HCC), a disease associated with liver cancers which still lack effective treatments. It is worth noting that there is a limited number of CDK20 inhibitors. This is partially due to the limited availability of experimental structure information about this target and the lack of 3D structure information. Using the protein structure predicted by AlphaFold as an input, the SBDD method implemented within the Chemistry42 platform was used for the design and optimization of novel molecules with predefined drug-like properties against the target CDK20. A total of 8,918 molecules were generated, and after several filtering steps, including molecular docking and clustering, seven molecular structures were selected for synthesis and underwent biological testing. One compound was found to elicit a Kd value of 9.2 ± 0.5 mM ($n = 3$) in CDK20 kinase binding assay. An overview of the end-to-end integrated pipeline, including the *de novo* drug design, molecule synthesis, and experimental validation is given in Figure 2.5.

2.9 CONCLUSION

Leveraging on the progress made in AI-enabled generative chemistry and in the maturation of a dynamical ecosystem made of large-scale databases and standardized benchmarking procedures, AI-native companies began developing technologies to foster massive disruptions in small molecule drug discovery, and private and public market investors have invested to support these new actors [71]. In addition to these breakthroughs in AI/ML, the field of drug discovery and development begins to witness a second wave of innovations with the quickly emerging field of quantum computing, which has already shown promise in various applications including quantum chemistry and AI/ML. While quantum generative adversarial network (QuGAN) provided the first theoretical framework of quantum adversarial learning [72], one also started to actively explore the possibilities offered by hybrid quantum-classical GAN for *de novo* drug design [73].

AI-enabled generative chemistry has contributed to enhancing the diversity of molecular structures targeting well-known or even novel biological mechanisms associated with various diseases, and one witness a steady improvement in early discovery efficiency and productivity with examples of novel structures, identified by exploring previously uncharted areas of the chemical space, undergoing preclinical

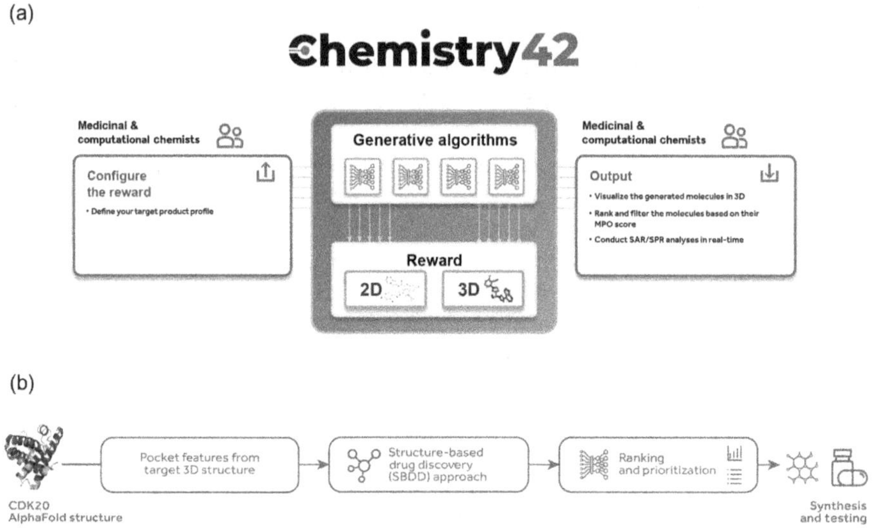

FIGURE 2.5 (a) Chemistry42 is a platform specifically designed to accelerate the design and optimization of novel molecules with predefined drug-like properties. The Chemistry42 platform combines state-of-the-art artificial Intelligence techniques with computational and medicinal chemistry methodologies. The Chemistry42 platform is available through licensing or collaboration and is routinely used to efficiently generate novel molecular structures with optimized properties that can be validated through in vitro and in vivo studies. The Chemistry42 platform is one of the core components of the Pharma.ai drug discovery integrated platform developed by Insilico Medicine. (b) The pipeline to combine AlphaFold with Insilico Medicine end-to-end, and AI-powered drug discovery platforms PandaOmics and Chemistry42 in the drug discovery for hepatocellular carcinoma from target selection and hit generation to hit identification. A novel therapeutic target was identified that has AlphaFold-predicted but no experimentally determined structures.

studies, and progressing into clinical trials with shorter discovery and development timelines [74]. Among these AI-native companies, Insilico Medicine has recently announced that its compound INS018_055 has entered Phase II clinical trials. INS018_055 is a novel structure designed using an Insilico Medicine AI-enabled generative engine. The compound designed to help treat idiopathic pulmonary fibrosis (IPF) acts as an inhibitor of a novel target which was also identified using an AI-enabled target identification engine. Looking to take advantage of these AI-native drug discovery pipelines gaining maturity and momentum, major pharmaceutical companies launched discovery partnerships with AI-native drug discovery companies to pursue new development programs and develop essential healthcare tools [75].

REFERENCES

1. Ching T, Himmelstein DS, Beaulieu-Jones BK, Kalinin AA, Do BT, Way GP, et al. Opportunities and obstacles for deep learning in biology and medicine. *J R Soc Interface*. 2018;15: 20170387. doi:10.1098/rsif.2017.0387.
2. Davenport T, Kalakota R. The potential for artificial intelligence in healthcare. *Future Healthc J*. 2019;6: 94–98.

3. Esmaeilzadeh P. Use of AI-based tools for healthcare purposes: A survey study from consumers' perspectives. *BMC Med Inform Decis Mak.* 2020;20: 170.
4. Virshup AM, Contreras-García J, Wipf P, Yang W, Beratan DN. Stochastic voyages into uncharted chemical space produce a representative library of all possible drug-like compounds. *J Am Chem Soc.* 2013;135: 7296–7303. doi:10.1021/ja401184g.
5. Reymond J-L, Ruddigkeit L, Blum L, van Deursen R. The enumeration of chemical space. *Wiley Interdiscip Rev Comput Mol Sci.* 2012;2: 717–733.
6. Vamathevan J, Clark D, Czodrowski P, Dunham I, Ferran E, Lee G, et al. Applications of machine learning in drug discovery and development. *Nat Rev Drug Discov.* 2019;18: 463–477.
7. Ivanenkov Y, Zagribelnyy B, Malyshev A, Evteev S, Terentiev V, Kamya P, et al. The hitchhiker's guide to deep learning driven generative chemistry. *ACS Med Chem Lett.* 2023;14: 901–915. doi:10.1021/acsmedchemlett.3c00041.
8. Mouchlis VD, Afantitis A, Serra A, Fratello M, Papadiamantis AG, Aidinis V, et al. Advances in de novo drug design: From conventional to machine learning methods. *Int J Mol Sci.* 2021;22: 1676. doi:10.3390/ijms22041676.
9. Kadurin A, Aliper A, Kazennov A, Mamoshina P, Vanhaelen Q, Khrabrov K, et al. The cornucopia of meaningful leads: Applying deep adversarial autoencoders for new molecule development in oncology. *Oncotarget.* 2017;8: 10883–10890.
10. Kadurin A, Nikolenko S, Khrabrov K, Aliper A, Zhavoronkov A. dru GAN: An advanced generative adversarial autoencoder model for de novo generation of new molecules with desired molecular properties in silico. *Mol Pharm.* 2017;14: 3098–3104.
11. Sousa T, Correia J, Pereira V, Rocha M. Generative deep learning for targeted compound design. *J Chem Inf Model.* 2021;61: 5343–5361.
12. Wigh DS, Goodman JM, Lapkin AA. A review of molecular representation in the age of machine learning. *Wiley Interdiscip Rev Comput Mol Sci.* 2022;12: e1603. doi:10.1002/wcms.1603.
13. Weininger D. SMILES, a chemical language and information system. 1. Introduction to methodology and encoding rules. *J Chem Inf Model.* 1988;28: 31–36.
14. Weininger D, Weininger A, Weininger JL. SMILES. 2. Algorithm for generation of unique SMILES notation. *J Chem Inf Comput Sci.* 1989;29: 97–101.
15. Vollmer JJ. Wiswesser line notation: an introduction. *J Chem Educ.* 1983;60: 192.
16. Homer RW, Swanson J, Jilek RJ, Hurst T, Clark RD. SYBYL line notation (SLN): A single notation to represent chemical structures, queries, reactions, and virtual libraries. *J Chem Inf Model.* 2008;48: 2294–2307.
17. Arús-Pous J, Johansson SV, Prykhodko O, Bjerrum EJ, Tyrchan C, Reymond J-L, et al. Randomized SMILES strings improve the quality of molecular generative models. *J Cheminform.* 2019;11: 71.
18. O'Boyle N, Dalke A. DeepSMILES: An adaptation of SMILES for use in machine-learning of chemical structures. *ChemRxiv.* 2018. doi:10.26434/chemrxiv.7097960.v1.
19. Heller S, McNaught A, Stein S, Tchekhovskoi D, Pletnev I. InChI - the worldwide chemical structure identifier standard. *J Cheminform.* 2013;5: 7.
20. Winter R, Montanari F, Noé F, Clevert D-A. Learning continuous and data-driven molecular descriptors by translating equivalent chemical representations. *Chem Sci.* 2019;10: 1692–1701.
21. Gómez-Bombarelli R, Wei JN, Duvenaud D, Hernández-Lobato JM, Sánchez-Lengeling B, Sheberla D, et al. Automatic chemical design using a data-driven continuous representation of molecules. *ACS Cent Sci.* 2018;4: 268–276.
22. Favre HA, Powell WH. *Nomenclature of Organic Chemistry: IUPAC Recommendations and Preferred Names 2013.* Cambridge, England: Royal Society of Chemistry; 2011.
23. Rothchild D, Tamkin A, Yu J, Misra U, Gonzalez J. C5T5: Controllable generation of organic molecules with transformers. 2021. doi:10.48550/ARXIV.2108.10307.
24. Goodfellow IJ, Pouget-Abadie J, Mirza M, Xu B, Warde-Farley D, Ozair S, et al. Generative adversarial networks. 2014. doi:10.48550/ARXIV.1406.2661.

25. Vanhaelen Q, Lin Y-C, Zhavoronkov A. The advent of generative chemistry. *ACS Med Chem Lett.* 2020;11: 1496–1505.
26. Zhavoronkov A, Ivanenkov YA, Aliper A, Veselov MS, Aladinskiy VA, Aladinskaya AV, et al. Deep learning enables rapid identification of potent DDR1 kinase inhibitors. *Nat Biotechnol.* 2019;37: 1038–1040.
27. Gupta A, Müller AT, Huisman BJH, Fuchs JA, Schneider P, Schneider G. Generative recurrent networks for de novo drug design. *Mol Inform.* 2018;37: 1700111. doi:10.1002/minf.201700111
28. Suresh N, Chinnakonda Ashok Kumar N, Subramanian S, Srinivasa G. Memory augmented recurrent neural networks for de-novo drug design. *PLoS One.* 2022;17: e0269461.
29. Lim J, Ryu S, Kim JW, Kim WY. Molecular generative model based on conditional variational autoencoder for de novo molecular design. *J Cheminform.* 2018;10: 31.
30. Blaschke T, Olivecrona M, Engkvist O, Bajorath J, Chen H. Application of generative autoencoder in de novo molecular design. *Mol Inform.* 2018;37: 1700123. doi:10.1002/minf.201700123.
31. Tong X, Liu X, Tan X, Li X, Jiang J, Xiong Z, et al. Generative models for de novo drug design. *J Med Chem.* 2021;64: 14011–14027.
32. Elton DC, Boukouvalas Z, Fuge MD, Chung PW. Deep learning for molecular design—A review of the state of the art. *Mol Syst Des Eng.* 2019;4: 828–849. doi:10.1039/c9me00039a.
33. Langevin M, Grebner C, Guessregen S, Sauer S, Li Y, Matter H, et al. Impact of applicability domains to generative artificial intelligence. doi:10.26434/chemrxiv-2022-mdhwz.
34. Lopez R, Gayoso A, Yosef N. Enhancing scientific discoveries in molecular biology with deep generative models. *Mol Syst Biol.* 2020;16: e9198.
35. Yu L, Zhang W, Wang J, Yu Y. SeqGAN: Sequence generative adversarial nets with policy gradient. *Proceedings of the AAAI Conference on Artificial Intelligence*, 2017. doi:10.1609/aaai.v31i1.10804.
36. Sanchez-Lengeling B, Outeiral C, Guimaraes GL, Aspuru-Guzik A. Optimizing distributions over molecular space. An Objective-Reinforced Generative Adversarial Network for Inverse-design Chemistry (ORGANIC). doi:10.26434/chemrxiv.5309668.
37. Arús-Pous J, Blaschke T, Ulander S, Reymond J-L, Chen H, Engkvist O. Exploring the GDB-13 chemical space using deep generative models. *J Cheminform.* 2019;11: 20.
38. Rahimovich DR, Qaxramon O'g'li AS, Abdiqayum O'g'li SR. Application of transformer model architecture in the new drugs design. *2021 International Conference on Information Science and Communications Technologies (ICISCT)*, 2021. IEEE. doi:10.1109/icisct52966.2021.9670309.
39. Rogers D, Hahn M. Extended-connectivity fingerprints. *J Chem Inf Model.* 2010;50: 742–754.
40. Riniker S, Landrum GA. Similarity maps - A visualization strategy for molecular fingerprints and machine-learning methods. *J Cheminform.* 2013;5: 43.
41. Bickerton GR, Paolini GV, Besnard J, Muresan S, Hopkins AL. Quantifying the chemical beauty of drugs. *Nat Chem.* 2012;4: 90–98.
42. Bero SA, Muda AK, Choo YH, Muda NA, Pratama SF. Similarity measure for molecular structure: A brief review. *J Phys Conf Ser.* 2017;892: 012015.
43. Bajusz D, Rácz A, Héberger K. Why is Tanimoto index an appropriate choice for fingerprint-based similarity calculations? *J Cheminform.* 2015;7: 20.
44. Brown N, Fiscato M, Segler MHS, Vaucher AC. GuacaMol: Benchmarking models for de novo molecular design. *J Chem Inf Model.* 2019;59: 1096–1108.
45. Benhenda M, Bjerrum EJ, Yi H, Zaveri C. *DiversityNet: A Collaborative Benchmark for Generative AI Models in Chemistry.* Authorea. Authorea, Inc.; 2019. doi:10.22541/au.155751672.29626289.

46. Polykovskiy D, Zhebrak A, Sanchez-Lengeling B, Golovanov S, Tatanov O, Belyaev S, et al. Molecular sets (MOSES): A benchmarking platform for molecular generation models. *Front Pharmacol.* 2020;11: 565644.
47. Preuer K, Renz P, Unterthiner T, Hochreiter S, Klambauer G. Fréchet ChemNet distance: A metric for generative models for molecules in drug discovery. *J Chem Inf Model.* 2018;58: 1736–1741.
48. Anastasiu DC, Karypis G. Efficient identification of tanimoto nearest neighbors. *2016 IEEE International Conference on Data Science and Advanced Analytics (DSAA)*, 2016. IEEE. doi:10.1109/dsaa.2016.23.
49. Bemis GW, Murcko MA. The properties of known drugs. 1. Molecular frameworks. *J Med Chem.* 1996;39: 2887–2893.
50. Blum LC, Reymond J-L. 970 million druglike small molecules for virtual screening in the chemical universe database GDB-13. *J Am Chem Soc.* 2009;131: 8732–8733.
51. Chen J-H, Tseng YJ. A general optimization protocol for molecular property prediction using a deep learning network. *Brief Bioinform.* 2022;23: bbab367. doi:10.1093/bib/bbab367.
52. Durant JL, Leland BA, Henry DR, Nourse JG. Reoptimization of MDL keys for use in drug discovery. *J Chem Inf Comput Sci.* 2002;42: 1273–1280.
53. Zhumagambetov R, Kazbek D, Shakipov M, Maksut D, Peshkov VA, Fazli S. cheML.io: An online database of ML-generated molecules. *RSC Adv.* 2020;10: 45189–45198.
54. Lötsch J, Mayer B. A biomedical case study showing that tuning random forests can fundamentally change the interpretation of supervised data structure exploration aimed at knowledge discovery. *BioMedInformatics.* 2022;2: 544–552.
55. Rajan K, Zielesny A, Steinbeck C. STOUT: SMILES to IUPAC names using neural machine translation. *J Cheminform.* 2021;13: 34.
56. Handsel J, Matthews B, Knight N, Coles S. Translating the molecules: Adapting neural machine translation to predict IUPAC names from a chemical identifier. *ChemRxiv.* 2021. doi:10.26434/chemrxiv.14170472.v1.
57. Krasnov L, Khokhlov I, Fedorov MV, Sosnin S. Transformer-based artificial neural networks for the conversion between chemical notations. *Sci Rep.* 2021;11: 14798.
58. Raffel C, Shazeer N, Roberts A, Lee K, Narang S, Matena M, et al. Exploring the limits of transfer learning with a unified text-to-text transformer. 2019. doi:10.48550/ARXIV.1910.10683.
59. Veber DF, Johnson SR, Cheng H-Y, Smith BR, Ward KW, Kopple KD. Molecular properties that influence the oral bioavailability of drug candidates. *J Med Chem.* 2002;45: 2615–2623.
60. Yang L, Yang G, Bing Z, Tian Y, Niu Y, Huang L, et al. Transformer-based generative model accelerating the development of novel BRAF inhibitors. *ACS Omega.* 2021;6: 33864–33873.
61. Ren F, Ding X, Zheng M, Korzinkin M, Cai X, Zhu W, et al. AlphaFold accelerates artificial intelligence powered drug discovery: Efficient discovery of a novel CDK20 small molecule inhibitor. *Chem Sci.* 2023;14: 1443–1452.
62. Ivanenkov YA, Polykovskiy D, Bezrukov D, Zagribelnyy B, Aladinskiy V, Kamya P, et al. Chemistry42: An AI-driven platform for molecular design and optimization. *J Chem Inf Model.* 2023;63: 695–701.
63. Polykovskiy D, Zhebrak A, Vetrov D, Ivanenkov Y, Aladinskiy V, Mamoshina P, et al. Entangled conditional adversarial autoencoder for de novo drug discovery. *Mol Pharm.* 2018;15: 4398–4405.
64. Putin E, Asadulaev A, Vanhaelen Q, Ivanenkov Y, Aladinskaya AV, Aliper A, et al. Adversarial threshold neural computer for molecular de novo design. *Mol Pharm.* 2018;15: 4386–4397.

65. Zhavoronkov A, Li R, Ma C, Mamoshina P. Deep biomarkers of aging and longevity: From research to applications. *Aging*. 2019;11: 10771–10780.
66. Ozerov IV, Lezhnina KV, Izumchenko E, Artemov AV, Medintsev S, Vanhaelen Q, et al. In silico pathway activation network decomposition analysis (iPANDA) as a method for biomarker development. *Nat Commun*. 2016;7: 13427.
67. Ravi R, Noonan KA, Pham V, Bedi R, Zhavoronkov A, Ozerov IV, et al. Bifunctional immune checkpoint-targeted antibody-ligand traps that simultaneously disable TGFβ enhance the efficacy of cancer immunotherapy. *Nat Commun*. 2018;9: 741.
68. Maldonado L, Brait M, Izumchenko E, Begum S, Chatterjee A, Sen T, et al. Integrated transcriptomic and epigenomic analysis of ovarian cancer reveals epigenetically silenced GULP1. *Cancer Lett*. 2018;433: 242–251.
69. Saloura V, Izumchenko E, Zuo Z, Bao R, Korzinkin M, Ozerov I, et al. Immune profiles in primary squamous cell carcinoma of the head and neck. *Oral Oncol*. 2019;96: 77–88.
70. Pun FW, Liu BHM, Long X, Leung HW, Leung GHD, Mewborne QT, et al. Identification of therapeutic targets for amyotrophic lateral sclerosis using pandaomics - An AI-enabled biological target discovery platform. *Front Aging Neurosci*. 2022;14: 914017.
71. Elbadawi M, Gaisford S, Basit AW. Advanced machine-learning techniques in drug discovery. *Drug Discov Today*. 2021;26: 769–777.
72. Lloyd S, Weedbrook C. Quantum generative adversarial learning. *Phys Rev Lett*. 2018;121: 040502.
73. Kao P-Y, Yang Y-C, Chiang W-Y, Hsiao J-Y, Cao Y, Aliper A, et al. Exploring the advantages of quantum generative adversarial networks in generative chemistry. *J Chem Inf Model*. 2023;63: 3307–3318.
74. Jayatunga MKP, Xie W, Ruder L, Schulze U, Meier C. AI in small-molecule drug discovery: A coming wave? *Nat Rev Drug Discov*. 2022;21: 175–176.
75. Paul D, Sanap G, Shenoy S, Kalyane D, Kalia K, Tekade RK. Artificial intelligence in drug discovery and development. *Drug Discov Today*. 2021;26: 80–93.

Part II

Generative Chemical Models Based on Language Processing

3 De Novo Drug Design by Chemical Language Modeling

Rıza Özçelik and Francesca Grisoni

3.1 INTRODUCTION

De novo drug design is a crucial element of pharmaceutical research: it aims to design new molecular candidates with bespoke characteristics (e.g. bioactivity, and/or lack of undersirable properties) from scratch. De novo molecule design is far from trivial, as it is confronted with an extremely vast 'chemical universe'. Such a vast chemical universe is estimated to contain up to 10^{60} drug-like molecular entities one could in theory synthesize and test in the wet-lab [1]. Not only is this chemical universe almost entirely uncharted, but its size makes extensive enumeration practically impossible. Finally, structure-activity relationships are notoriously complex and non-linear. For instance, the presence of activity cliffs [2] and non-additivity phenomena [3] makes the 'navigation' of the chemical universe a daunting task.

Computer-assisted de novo design was introduced several decades ago [4–6] as a tool to aid medicinal chemists in exploring the vast chemical universe of possibilities. De novo drug design is arguably one of the fields in the molecular sciences that has also been impacted the most by the advent of deep learning. The term 'deep learning' encompasses neural network architectures with multiple processing layers [7], which have the potential to capture complex and non-linear information in the data they are trained on. While traditional computer-assisted approaches rely on 'rule-based' molecular generation (e.g. via reaction-driven molecular assembly [8], evolutionary algorithms [9], and fragment linking and growing [10,11]), deep learning enables the generation of molecular candidates from scratch without the need of human-engineered rules.

Although many generative deep learning approaches have been applied to chemistry [12,13], the so-called chemical language models (CLMs) have found the widest adoption in drug discovery. CLMs borrow methods from the natural language processing domain and adapt them to process molecular strings (e.g. Simplified Molecular Input Line Entry Systems [SMILES] strings [14]), which encode the two-dimensional molecular structure in the form of text. CLMs have shown the capacity to learn the chemical 'syntax' (i.e. what is needed to generate chemically valid molecular strings) as well as the 'semantics' (i.e. desired physicochemical and biological properties). CLMs are among the most efficient approaches to date to navigate the chemical space effectively [15] and learn complex molecular properties [16].

DOI: 10.1201/9781003399346-5

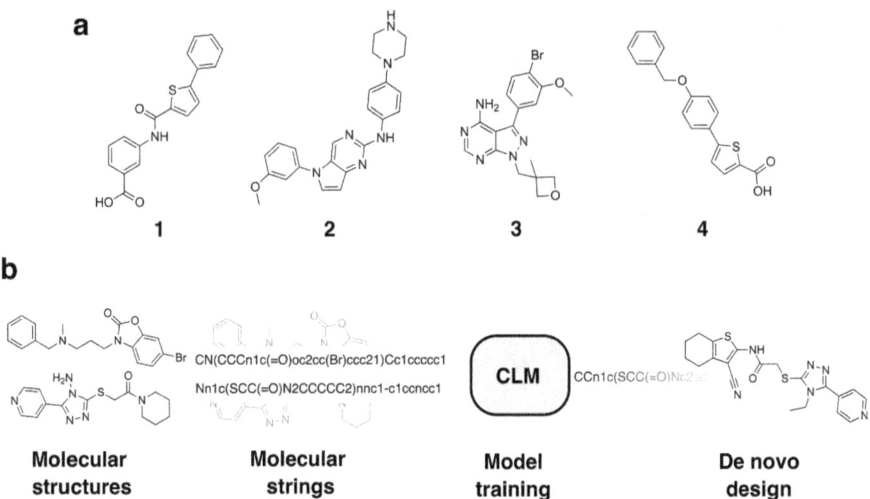

FIGURE 3.1 Chemical language models for de novo drug design. (a) Selected examples of experimentally validated bioactive molecules designed de novo using chemical language modeling approaches. **1**: Dual modulator of the retinoid X and peroxisome proliferator-activated receptors [17]; **2**: Inhibitor of Moloney murine leukemia virus kinase 1 (Piml) and cyclin-dependent kinase 4 [22]; **3**: inhibitor of phosphoinositide 3-kinase gamma [20]; **4**: Agonist of orphan nuclear receptor-related 1 (Nurr) receptor [23]. (b) Basic steps of chemical language modeling for de novo drug design. Molecular structures are converted into strings (e.g. SMILES strings) to train the chemical language model (CLM). This model is then used to generate molecules de novo, in the same string format.

Finally, they have been increasingly applied and validated in the wet-lab [17–23] (Figure 3.1a).

Chemical language modeling pipelines consist of the following three core elements (Figure 3.1b):

1. *Molecular string representation:* Whereby molecular information (usually two-dimensional) is converted into string formats, such as the SMILES strings [14]. These molecular strings are used as the input for the chosen deep learning architectures.
2. *Model training:* Various types of deep learning can be used to process molecular strings and learn relevant information from their structures. Ultimately, models are trained to learn the chemical syntax (i.e. what is needed for a string to correspond to a valid molecular structure), as well as semantic properties (i.e. what elements are needed for the molecule to possess desired physicochemical and biological properties).
3. *De novo molecule design:* Once models have been trained, several strategies can be used to produce molecular strings de novo, with the goal of generating novel molecules with the desired syntactic and semantic properties.

This chapter will discuss each of these elements, one-by-one, in the following sections. Finally, a hands-on example of how to train and generate molecules de novo is presented.

3.2 CONVERTING STRUCTURAL INFORMATION INTO MOLECULAR STRINGS

Storing structural information of molecules has a practical use in cheminformatics and related disciplines. Molecular string representations are compact and standardized text notation representing a (two-dimensional) molecular structure, and have become one of the most popular formats to store and retrieve chemical information [24]. They have found renewed interest thanks to deep learning algorithms for sequence processing in a multitude of molecular applications [12,25.26].

SMILES [14] – the most popular molecular string notation in the deep learning domain – are generated by transforming hydrogen-depleted molecular graphs into a textual format, representing atoms with their atomic symbols, bonds and branching with specific symbols, and ring-opening/closure events with numerical identifiers. In particular (Figure 3.2):

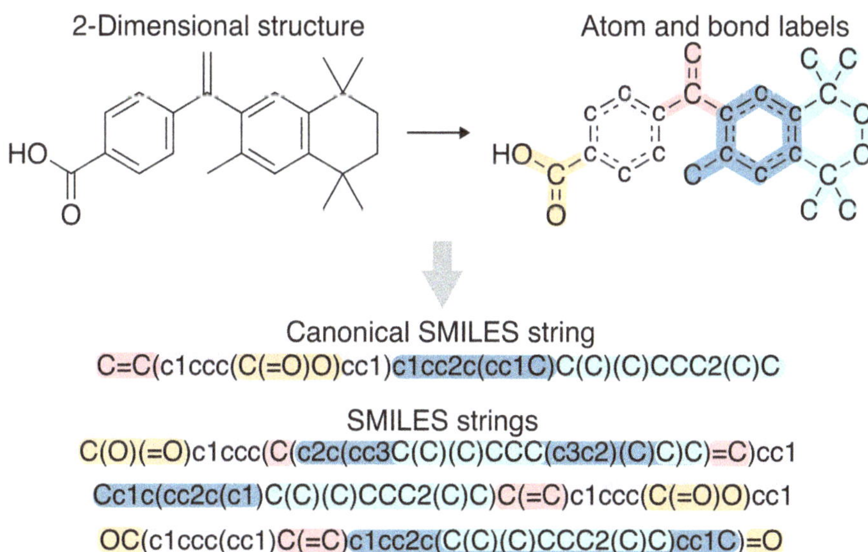

FIGURE 3.2 Example of SMILES generation. Starting from the 2-D structure of bexarotene, atoms and bonds are labeled using letters and symbols. The graph is then traversed to obtain linear string notations. Brackets are used to indicate branches in the graph. Canonical SMILES strings are univocal and standardized SMILES strings. Other (non-canonical) SMILES strings can be obtained by starting from any non-H atom and proceeding in any direction of the molecular graph.

- Atoms are represented by their atomic symbols (e.g. Cl corresponds to Chlorine), with the possibility to omit hydrogens (H).
- Single, double, triple, and aromatic bonds are represented with the symbols "–", "=", "#", and ":", respectively. Single bonds can be (and usually are) omitted.
- Cyclic structures are captured by digits. In particular, ring 'opening' and 'closure' bonds are indicated by a digit immediately following the atomic symbol at each ring closure. Aromaticity can be written with lower-case letters or by alternating single and double bonds (Kekulé notation). For instance, benzene can be written as "c1ccccc1" or "C1=CC=CC=C1".
- Branches are specified by enclosures in parentheses.
- Local chirality can be specified (if needed) using the symbols "/" and "\", and tetrahedral centers can be indicated using "@" (or "@@"), following the atomic symbol of the chiral atom. "@" and "@@" indicate that the listed atomic neighbors are arranged in anticlockwise and clockwise order, respectively.

SMILES are non-univocal, as they can be obtained from any non-H atom by traversing the molecular graph in any chosen direction (Figure 3.2). To obtain a unique and standardized representation of a given chemical structure as a SMILES string, the so-called canonicalization algorithms exist [27–29]. These algorithms ensure that chemically equivalent structures produce the same canonical SMILES notation.

Another popular molecular string notation (also developed for the purpose of information storage and molecule identification) is the *International Chemical Identifier* (InChI). InChI notation consists of a series of alphanumeric characters that encode specific information about the chemical structure, including the arrangement of atoms and bonds, stereochemistry, and isomeric forms. InChI notations are hierarchical, with different layers providing different levels of detail, separated by "/".

Neither SMILES nor InChI were developed to be used per se to serve as the input of chemical language models (CLMs). While SMILES have found a widespread adoption in the context of CLMs, InChI did not result as a suitable representation for de novo design due to a more complex set of syntactic rules to be learned to generate valid strings (e.g. involving counting and arithmetic) [30]. Other representations, on the other hand, have been developed to be specifically used with CLMs:

- *DeepSMILES* [31] were proposed as an improvement to SMILES, to address unbalanced parentheses and ring closure pairs which cause invalid syntax when generated by a CLM. DeepSMILES have been applied to predict drug-target binding affinity [32], but their difficult syntax limits molecule generation compared to SMILES strings [33].
- *Self-referencing embedded strings (SELFIES)* [34] are built such that each symbol in the string can be used to convert it into a unique graph. Unlike SMILES, every SELFIES string corresponds to a valid chemical graph. Although most SELFIES strings are valid, in certain cases the validity is ensured via post-hoc truncation of invalid elements ('collapse' [35]) when an invalid representation is found ([34,35]).

A recent study suggested that learning the syntax of SMILES strings with CLMs might allow filtering out invalid molecules and retain higher-quality de novo designs compared to SELFIES [15]. All in all, the choice of SMILES, SELFIES, or DeepSMILES representations seems to depend on the chosen application, with small differences in general [15,16,36,37]. Molecular strings, in general, are often the go-to choice for de novo design with deep learning due to their ease of generation compared to other representations [16].

While SMILES canonicalization is essential for database searching and molecular comparison (Figure 3.2), when it comes to de novo design, using multiple SMILES to represent the same molecule has shown a beneficial effect [33,38,39]. SMILES can, in fact, be written starting from any non-hydrogen atom, and, therefore, a molecule can be denoted by many different SMILES strings (Figure 3.2). This characteristic of is often used for the so-called "data augmentation", which represents the same molecule in the training set with n different SMILES strings (usually generated at random) to inflate the number of instances available for training. Such augmentation [40] is beneficial to improve the performance of quantitative structure-activity relationship (QSAR) models [33] and the quality of the de novo designs [40], with a magnitude depending on the structural complexity of the training molecules [41]. The benefits related to SMILES augmentation plateau when increasing the number of SMILES per molecule [39,41], leading to progressively smaller performance gains for increasing computational cost.

Using multiple SMILES for the same molecule is a strategy to perform data-augmentation, i.e. to artificially inflate the number of samples used for model training. The same augmentation procedure as SMILES can be obtained for SELFIES, although the impact of such a procedure on the model quality has not been systematically investigated yet. In what follows, we will explain how, in practice, the syntax and semantics of the 'chemical language' can be learned using CLMs.

3.3 TRAINING A CHEMICAL LANGUAGE MODEL

3.3.1 Deep Learning Architectures

Various deep learning architectures exist to learn efficiently from string notations of molecules (such as SMILES, Figure 3.3a) for de novo design [42]. The most popular architecture is constituted by recurrent neural networks (RNNs). RNNs are artificial neural networks that are particularly well-suited for handling sequential data. RNNs can be used to learn from an input sequence (e.g. SMILES string) in a stepwise manner: the network can be trained to predict the next element ("token") to follow, using information on all the previous portions of the string, which is captured by the network hidden state (Figure 3.3b). Two variants of RNNs have gathered remarkable popularity in recent years: (a) Long-short term memory (LSTMs) and (b) Gated Recurrent Unit (GRU) networks. Both variants introduce additional structure than 'vanilla' RNNs [43], with additional memory mechanisms (called memory gates) that control the flow of information, enabling them to capture long-term dependencies more effectively. To date, LSTMs are the model that has found the most widespread application for de novo drug design (e.g. [17,44,45]), and a few studies have

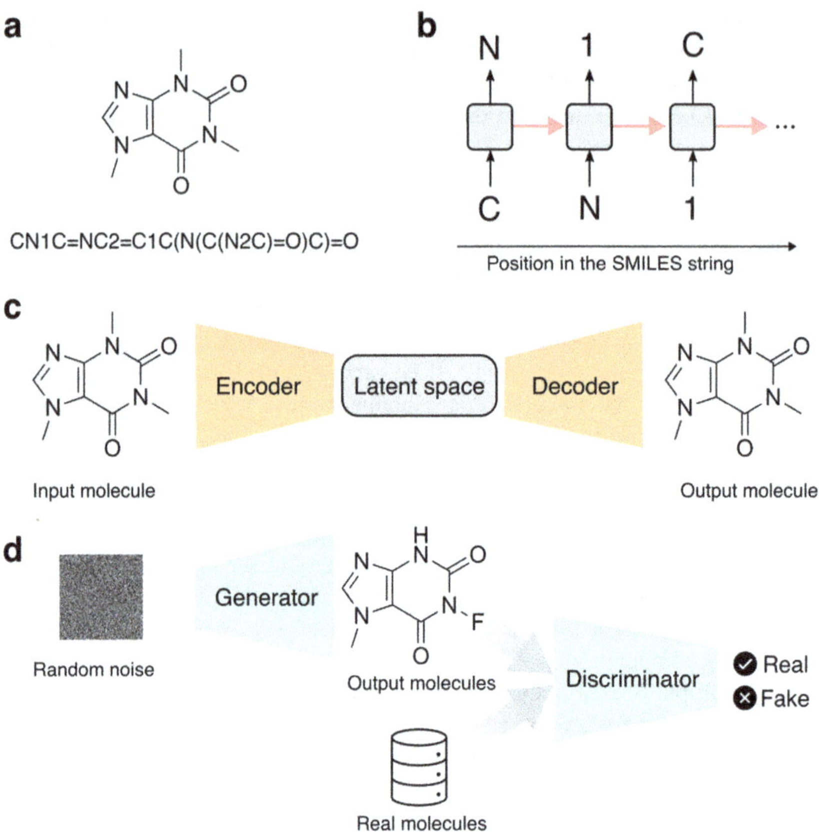

FIGURE 3.3 Simplified depiction of two widely used chemical language modeling approaches for the molecule caffeine (a). (b) Recurrent Neural Networks can be trained to predict the next element ("token") to follow any given portion of a SMILES string, using information on all the previous tokens. The network hidden state is updated in a recurrent way to perform a prediction at any step while keeping track of the preceding portions of the string. (c) Variational Autoencoder (VAE), consisting of an encoder (transforming input strings into a fixed-dimensional latent distribution) and a decoder, which samples from this distribution to generate latent vectors and reconstructs the strings. Encoders and decoders for SMILES are often in the form of RNNs. (d) Generative Adversarial Networks (GANs), characterized by a generator network (which aims to generate molecules that are as indistinguishable from real ones as possible), and a discriminator network that is trained to distinguish real from generated molecules. The feedback on the discriminator's performance is used to update the generator and the discriminator models – aiming to improve the generator in 'fooling' the discriminator and the discriminator in detecting the output of the generator.

used GRUs [33,46]. Other approaches exist to learn long-range dependencies from large corpora of text better than LSTMs and GRUs (e.g. Transformers and Structured State-Space Sequence models [47,48]), and they are finding increasing applications in de novo design (e.g. [49–51]).

Another popular approach for chemical language modeling is constituted by *Variational Autoencoders* (VAEs). Autoencoders consist of two deep networks (Figure 3.3c): one serves as an encoder, transforming input strings into fixed-dimensional vectors, and the other acts as a decoder, converting these vectors back into strings. The primary objective during training is to minimize the error in reconstructing the initial string. The key aspect of the autoencoders involves guiding the transformation of strings through an information 'bottleneck'. In this case, the bottleneck takes the form of a fixed-length continuous vector, compelling the network to acquire a condensed representation that captures the most statistically significant data features. Such a vector-encoded molecule is referred to as the latent representation of the molecule. Compared to traditional autoencoders, VAEs introduce a probabilistic element to the latent space. Instead of encoding inputs into a fixed vector, VAEs encode inputs into probability distributions in the latent space. This adds stochasticity to the process, allowing for the generation of diverse samples during the decoding process. This is achieved by sampling the latent space, to generate new molecules with similar characteristics as the training data. Encoders and decoders for SMILES are often in the form of RNNs [30,52,53]. One of the pioneering studies [30] has shown how VAEs can be used to automatically generate novel chemical structures by performing certain operations in the latent space, such as decoding random vectors, perturbing known chemical structures, or interpolating between molecules.

Finally, *Generative Adversarial Networks* (GANs) [54] have also been applied to molecules. GANs are characterized by two networks (Figure 3.3d): (a) a generator network (e.g. LSTM), which aims to generate molecules that are as indistinguishable from real ones as possible, and (b) a discriminator network (e.g. a convolutional neural network [55]), which takes molecules as input, and is trained to distinguish real from generated molecules. The training proceeds as follows. After molecules have been produced by the generator, the discriminator network is presented with both real and 'fake' molecules and is asked to detect the ones produced by the generator. The feedback on the discriminator's performance is then used to update both the generator and the discriminator models – aiming to improve the generator in 'fooling' the discriminator, and the discriminator in detecting the output of the generator. This so-called 'adversarial training' is aimed to improve the generator in its capacity to produce authentic-looking molecules. Examples of GANs applied to the design of SMILES strings are ORGAN [55], LatentGAN [52], and MaskGAN [56].

3.3.2 Tasks for Chemical Language Modeling in De Novo Design

CLMs are usually employed for de novo design in several ways. The possible approaches have been divided into two main categories [57]:

- *Distribution-learning:* In this approach, the objective is to create novel molecules that belong to the same chemical space as the training set. Distribution-learning algorithms are typically assessed by their ability to match the properties of the training data. This can be measured, for example, using metrics like Kullback-Leibler (KL) divergence [58] to compare the distribution of computed physicochemical properties or the Fréchet ChemNet Distance (FCD) [59] to assess similarity in terms of chemical and biological characteristics. Often, transfer learning is employed to enhance distribution learning. Transfer learning employs a model (pre)trained on one dataset with usually many data points available (e.g. ChEMBL [60]) and 'fine-tunes' it (by additional training) on a related task for which fewer data are available (e.g., potent ligands on a given macromolecular target) [17,44]. Transfer learning has been shown to enable distribution learning on small datasets used for fine-tuning [39]. Distribution-learning approaches eliminate the need for scoring functions to guide molecular design (e.g. bioactivity prediction or molecular docking), which are usually an approximation of the ground truth themselves. However, while these models are evaluated by comparing the properties of the generated molecules to those in the training set, they do not inherently provide an assessment of the quality of individual designs, while scoring functions (albeit being an approximation themselves) do. Hence, distribution learning necessitates the use of human-engineered post-hoc ranking and filtering procedures to sift through the generated molecules and identify promising candidates, which partially diminishes the advantages of these 'rule-free' pipelines [17,57,61].

- *Goal-directed training*: Here, the primary aim is to generate molecules with the intent of optimizing specific goals. This is often accomplished by employing scoring functions to evaluate a molecule's alignment with user-defined objectives. Scoring functions are utilized iteratively to enhance the generated molecules. Reinforcement learning is one technique used to steer the model's actions toward promising solutions by providing rewards. Commonly considered factors in scoring functions for CLMs include similarity to known active molecules, predicted bioactivity, and computed physicochemical properties [62,63]. Goal-directed approaches provide a direct assessment of the quality of both the overall population and individual molecules through scoring functions. They often rely on pre-trained models (like distribution-learning). Nevertheless, there are potential challenges associated with goal-directed generation that have been highlighted in various studies [64–66]. These challenges include (a) the complexity of condensing multiple chemical properties (e.g. bioactivity, drug-likeness, and synthesizability) into single scoring functions, (b) the potential for model shortcuts where the generator exploits unique features of the scoring function for which it was optimized, and (c) limited structural diversity resulting from biases introduced by scoring functions. In this context, the quality of the data and models used to develop scoring functions becomes crucial to prevent failures [64]. It is also worth noting that in some cases, the predicted synthesizability of designs generated through goal-directed approaches is lower than that achieved with distribution-learning algorithms [67].

In real-world scenarios, often distribution-learning and goal-directed approaches are used simultaneously to enhance the model's capacity to explore the chemical space. The so-called conditional molecule generation occupies a middle ground between goal-directed generation through scoring functions and distribution-learning algorithms. This approach addresses the task of generating new molecules that satisfy specified properties by learning a joint semantic space connecting experimentally determined properties and corresponding molecular structures. Examples are the de novo design of molecules matching certain gene-expression signatures [68], a desired three-dimensional shape [69], or conditioned on a protein target of interest [70,71]. However, to date, these approaches have found little application compared to distribution and goal-directed approaches.

3.4 SAMPLING MOLECULES FROM A TRAINED CLM

Once the model has been trained as specified earlier, it can be used to generate molecules in the form of strings. In particular, the model is used to generate sequences token-by-token, using the likelihoods it has learned during training for each token in the vocabulary (Figure 3.4a). The generation is usually initiated by a 'start' token (Figure 3.4a), by attaching one token at a time until the 'end' token is generated (Figure 3.4a). Various approaches exist to select what token to attach at each step of the sequence, the most frequently used of which are the following examples:

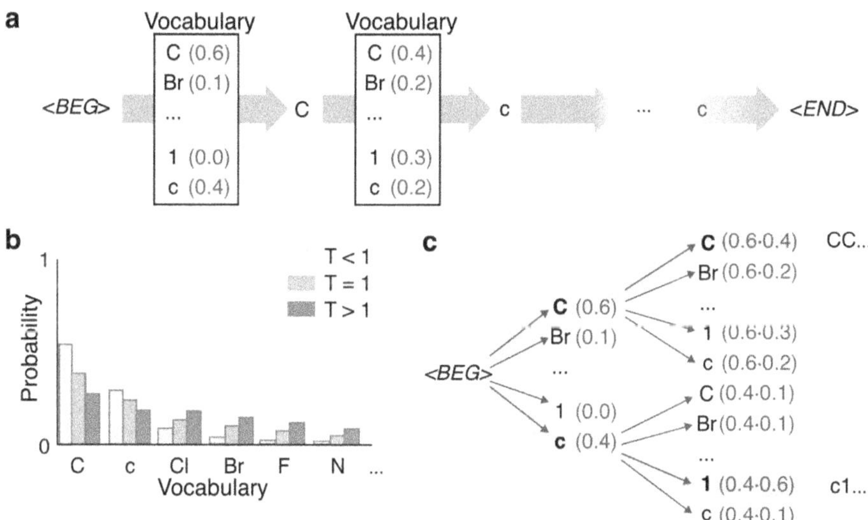

FIGURE 3.4 Selected strategies to sample from a chemical language model for string generation. (a) General process for molecule generation. After starting with a token indicating the beginning of a sequence (<*BEG*>), tokens are attached one at a time based on the chosen sampling strategies. The generation will continue until the end-of-the-sequence token is produced (<*END*>). (b) Temperature sampling (Eq. 3.1) modifies the probability of selecting a token using a parameter T (temperature). $T=1$ samples using the output probability of the model. $T>1$, introduces more randomness into the sampling process, while $T<1$ generates more conservative molecules. (c) Beam search, which aims to extend the string using the most likely tokens. This is achieved by considering the joint likelihoods (displayed within brackets) obtained by the addition of any possible token in the vocabulary at any step. The top-k sequences (where k is referred to as beam width) based on such cumulative probabilities are retained for the next steps. In this example, $k=2$.

- *Temperature sampling* (Figure 3.4b), which is to date the most frequently used approach for molecule generation with CLMs. Temperature sampling is inspired by the concept of temperature in statistical mechanics, where a higher temperature increases the randomness of particle motion. In the context of molecular generation, this technique allows us to control the level of randomness or creativity in the generated molecules. Temperature sampling is applied by scaling the logits (log-odds) of the next token predictions using a temperature parameter (T). Given a token i, its probability to be generated (p_i) can be computed as follows as follows:

$$p_i = \frac{e^{\left(\frac{y_i}{T}\right)}}{\sum_j e^{\left(\frac{y_i}{T}\right)}} \tag{3.1}$$

where y_i is the model prediction (e.g. probability or logits) of the i-th token in the vocabulary, and j runs over all tokens. A higher temperature, typically above 1, introduces more randomness into the sampling process, resulting in more diverse molecules. In contrast, a lower temperature, close to 0, favors 'exploitation' and tends to generate more likely or conservative molecules [39]. Temperature sampling has been used in several occasions to design experimentally validated bioactive molecules [17–19,72]. Values of T usually vary from $T=0.5$ to $T=2.0$ and are usually tuned on a case-by-case basis to find the desired trade-off between SMILES validity and uniqueness, and the novelty of the molecular structures [18,39,49].
- *Top-k sampling*, which involves selecting one of the top-k most probable tokens at each generation step based on their likelihood predicted by the model. By adjusting the value of k, one can regulate the level of diversity in the generated output, influencing how many alternative tokens the model considers. This method can provide a balance between deterministic (e.g. choosing the top-1 prediction) and diverse outputs obtained by considering more than one token at each step in the sequence. Top-k sampling can also be combined with temperature sampling to add another controlling mechanism for diversity.
- *Beam search* (Figure 3.4c) aims to find the most likely sequence of tokens according to a CLM. Instead of selecting the single most probable token at each step, a set of top-k candidates is considered. This is achieved by considering the joint likelihoods (at any given step of the sequence) obtained by the addition of any possible token in the vocabulary. The top-k sequences based on such joint likelihoods are retained for the next steps. The key parameter in beam search is the beam width (k), which determines the number of candidates to keep at each step. A larger beam width yields a more exhaustive search but can lead to increased computation. Several papers

have used Beam search to generate experimentally-validated bioactive molecules [21,23], [23], although, to date, they are less numerous than those using temperature sampling.

- *Nucleus sampling:* Nucleus sampling (also known as top-p sampling) is a technique used to control the diversity of generated molecules, by making sure that no unlikely tokens are selected. It selects the top likely tokens at each generation step, by allowing only the most probable character(s) to be sampled using a probability threshold based on the cumulative probabilities of the SMILES tokens. Nucleus sampling first picks a subset of the vocabulary $V^{(p)}$ ("top vocabulary"), which is the smallest set of tokens that has the following property:

$$\sum_{x \in V^{(p)}} P(x|x_{1:i-1}) \geq p \tag{3.2}$$

where x is a token in the top vocabulary, and p is a selected threshold ("nucleus parameter"). In other words, the most likely tokens are selected as the next-token candidates until the sum of their probabilities is above a selected threshold p. Nucleus sampling can be particularly useful to balance diversity and likelihood in molecule generation. It can help generate molecules that are both chemically plausible and distinct from the training data. This approach has been recently used for prospective de novo design of kinase inhibitors [20].

3.5 EVALUATING MOLECULES GENERATED BY A CLM

Evaluating the molecules generated by a CLM involves considering many aspects. Three metrics are commonly used to evaluate the capacity of a CLM to learn the 'chemical syntax': (a) validity, i.e. number of SMILES strings corresponding to chemically plausible molecules; (b) uniqueness, i.e. the number of structurally-unique molecules; and (c) novelty, i.e. the number of (unique and valid) designs that are not included in the training set. A high number of 'chemically-valid' designs suggests that the model has learned how to generate strings that respect the SMILES syntax, while high values of uniqueness and novelty indicate little redundancy (among the designs and with the training set, respectively). While useful, it is important to note that these metrics are vulnerable to trivial baselines [65,73]. Several studies have focused on how to evaluate and benchmark generative AI approaches for their usefulness in exploring the chemical space, such as GuacaMol [57] and Molecular Sets (MOSES [74]). Some of the most popular metrics to evaluate de novo designs are the following:

- *Fréchet ChemNet Distance* (FCD) [59], which can be used to assess the similarity between two sets of molecular structures. It is a measure of similarity between two curves or shapes, for the distributions of molecular features in the generated set and the target (or reference) set. In the context of evaluating generative models for molecules, FCD quantifies how closely the distribution of chemical and biological features in the generated molecules aligns with the distribution in a reference set, such as experimentally derived compounds or known drugs. A lower FCD value indicates greater similarity between the generated and reference distributions, suggesting a better performance of the generative model in reproducing relevant chemical characteristics.

- *Scaffold diversity* [74] or *scaffold hopping capability* [57]: These aspects are crucial in de novo design, where diverse scaffolds can lead to the identification of compounds with unique biological activities and novel therapeutic properties. A high scaffold diversity indicates the generative model's effectiveness in exploring chemical space and generating innovative molecular structures for potential drug candidates.
- *Similarity of physicochemical properties and structural features*: In addition, several molecular descriptors (e.g. physico-chemical properties, presence/absence of specific substructures) can be used to assess whether the de novo designs possess desirable characteristics for the problem at hand.
- *Synthetic accessibility:* A problem when using generative algorithms is that the proposed designs may be challenging or infeasible to synthesize, which makes synthetic accessibility a key factor to consider [67]. To this end, ad-hoc metrics have been developed, such as the Synthetic Accessibility (SA) score [75] and the Synthetic Complexity (SC) score [76].

3.6 A HANDS-ON CLM EXAMPLE WITH CODE

A hands-on CLM example with code (written in Python) and data is provided at the following URL https://github.com/molML/de-novo-design-with-lstm. This code relies on Keras [77], a popular library for deep learning. Instructions on how to get started with the code and its dependencies are contained in the dedicated README file. In what follows, we show how to train CLM for de novo design. The example is based on an LSTM model trained on SMILES, and molecules are sampled using a temperature parameter.

Below is an example of code that executes key functions to build and train a CLM and use it to generate molecules in the form of SMILES (Figure 3.5):

Several hyper-parameters (controlling the training process) are defined:

- *VOCAB_SIZE*, capturing the number of (SMILES) tokens contained in the vocabulary.
- *EMBEDDING_DIM*, defining the dimensionality of the vector space in which SMILES will be embedded.
- *TRAINING_LEN*, the maximum size of the strings used as input.
- *BATCH_SIZE* defines the number of SMILES ("batch") to learn from before updating the internal model parameters.

```
# Read token-to-label mapping
with open("data/token2label.json", "r") as f:
    TOKEN2LABEL = json.load(f)

LABEL2TOKEN = {int(label): token for token, label in TOKEN2LABEL.items()}

# Define hyperparameters
VOCAB_SIZE = len(TOKEN2LABEL)
EMBEDDING_DIM = 128
TRAINING_LEN = 99
LSTM_SIZE = 128
BATCH_SIZE = 256
N_EPOCHS = 200

# Read training and validation data
X_train, y_train = input_preprocessing("train")
X_val, y_val = input_preprocessing("val")

clm = build_model()  # Build the chemical language model
history = train_model(clm)  # Train the chemical language model
designs = design_molecules(clm)  # Design molecules
```

FIGURE 3.5 Building and training a CLM.

- *N_EPOCHS,* which defines the number of learning epochs, i.e. how many times the learning algorithm will work through the entire training dataset.

The hyper parameter values of this example are selected based on practical considerations and existing scientific literature. In real-world scenarios, they are optimized [78] (e.g. via grid search, random search, or Bayesian optimization) to reach ideal values for a given application.

In what follows, we provide an explanation for the core functions of the pipeline.

1. *Molecule representation and preparation*: The repository provides two lists of molecules in the form of SMILES strings: (a) 10,000 molecules to be used for model training, and (b) 1,000 molecules for model validation. Both lists are extracted from ChEMBL [60]. The SMILES were prepared as follows:
   - SMILES were split into tokens and separated with spaces.
   - Two tokens were added at the beginning and end of the SMILES sequence (*<BEG>* and *<END>*, respectively) to denote the start and ending of the string.
   - Additional tokens (*<PAD>*) are also added, to pad every molecule to the same length (100 tokens). This is performed since having sequences of the same length allows for faster training.

   After the preparation, for example, the SMILES string of a benzene ring would appear as the following: "*<BEG> c 1 c c c c c 1 <END> <PAD> <PAD><PAD>...*".

```
def input_preprocessing(fold: str) -> np.ndarray:
    with open(f"data/{fold}.txt", "r") as f:
        padded_smiles = [line.strip().split() for line in f.readlines()]

    label_encoded_smiles = np.expand_dims(
        np.array(
            [[TOKEN2LABEL[token] for token in molecule] for molecule in
padded_smiles]
        ),
        axis=2,
    )
    X, y = (
        label_encoded_smiles[:, :-1, :],
        label_encoded_smiles[:, 1:, :],
    )
    return X, y
```

FIGURE 3.6 Implementation of the input pre-processing.

The dataset then undergoes the so-called label encoding: each token is mapped to a distinct integer for model training. The following function in the codebase implements the input pre-processing (Figure 3.6):

The method accepts a parameter that can either be "train" or "val", depending on what dataset to pre-process. The variable *TOKEN2LABEL* is a global dictionary (available in the repository) that maps SMILES tokens to their labels for label encoding. Out of each sequence (formed of 100 tokens), the first 99 tokens form the input of the chemical language model, whereas the last 99 forms the outputs: such input-output alignment allows training the model for next-token prediction. The input and output matrices are returned as numpy arrays.

2. *Model construction and training:* Here, we use a model with two LSTM layers. The model also (a) contains an embedding layer to represent SMILES tokens, (b) uses the softmax function to transform the model output into a probability distribution over multiple tokens, and (c) uses cross-entropy loss and Adam optimizer for training. The model can be created with the following function (Figure 3.7):

   The function above creates a Keras model using global variables *VOCAB_SIZE*, *EMBEDDING_DIM*, *TRAINING_LEN*, and *LSTM_SIZE*. *VOCAB_SIZE* is an integer that stores how many unique *SMILES* tokens are used during training, whereas *TRAINING_LEN* stores the input/output length (99, in this case). *EMBEDDING_DIM* and *LSTM_SIZE* store the dimensionality of the embedding vectors and the number of units in LSTM cells, respectively. Once the CLM is constructed, it can be trained using the training data on the predefined number of epochs, as follows (Figure 3.8):

   The model performance over epochs is monitored via the validation set SMILES, which do not partake in model training. This function uses the global variables *BATCH_SIZE* and *N_EPOCHS* to configure the model training

```
def build_model() -> keras.models.Sequential:
    clm = keras.models.Sequential(
        [
            keras.layers.Embedding(
                input_dim=VOCAB_SIZE,
                output_dim=EMBEDDING_DIM,
                input_length=TRAINING_LEN,
            ),
            keras.layers.LSTM(LSTM_SIZE, return_sequences=True),
            keras.layers.LSTM(LSTM_SIZE, return_sequences=True),
            keras.layers.TimeDistributed(
                keras.layers.Dense(VOCAB_SIZE, activation="softmax")
            ),
        ]
    )
    clm.compile(
        loss="sparse_categorical_crossentropy",
        optimizer="adam",
    )
    return clm
```

FIGURE 3.7 Model construction.

```
def train_model(clm: keras.models.Sequential) -> Dict[str, List[float]]:
    history = clm.fit(
        x=X_train,
        y=y_train,
        validation_data=(X_val, y_val),
        batch_size=BATCH_SIZE,
        epochs=N_EPOCHS,
        verbose=1,
    ).history
    return history
```

FIGURE 3.8 Model training.

and returns a training history that contains training and validation losses per training epoch. In this implementation, the training stops after the pre-defined number of epochs. Alternatives to this approach exist, such as early stopping, which interrupts the training process when there is no consecutive improvement in the model performance over a pre-defined number of epochs.

3. *De novo design*: Once the model has been trained, it can be used to generate SMILES strings de novo. Here, we will use temperature sampling, as follows (Figure 3.9):

   We first create a batch of starting points (i.e. <*BEG*> tokens) to trigger molecule generation. Using <*BEG*> as the input, SMILES can be then generated by attaching one token at a time, using a temperature parameter (as explained in Eq. 3.1). The sampling process continues for 98 iterations, until all tokens per string have been generated by the model. Last, the generated

```
def design_molecules(clm: keras.models.Sequential) -> List[str]:
    def temperature_sampling(preds, temperature):
        log_preds = np.log(preds.astype(np.float64) + 10e-10) / temperature
        return (
            tf.random.categorical(log_preds,
num_samples=1).numpy().squeeze().tolist()
        )

    beg_label, pad_label = TOKEN2LABEL["<BEG>"], TOKEN2LABEL["<PAD>"]
    label_encoded_designs = pad_label * np.ones(
        (BATCH_SIZE, TRAINING_LEN), dtype=np.int32
    )
    label_encoded_designs[:, 0] = beg_label
    for token_idx in range(TRAINING_LEN - 1):
        predictions = clm.predict(label_encoded_designs)[:, token_idx]
        designed_labels = temperature_sampling(predictions, 1.0)
        label_encoded_designs[:, token_idx + 1] = designed_labels

    end_label = TOKEN2LABEL["<END>"]
    designed_smiles = list()
    for design in label_encoded_designs.tolist():
        designed_smiles_tokens = list()
        for label in design[1:]:
            if label in [beg_label, end_label, pad_label]:
                break
            designed_smiles_tokens.append(LABEL2TOKEN[label])

        designed_smiles.append("".join(designed_smiles_tokens))
    return designed_smiles
```

FIGURE 3.9 Temperature sampling.

strings are truncated from *<BEG>* (excluded) until the first occurrence of the *<END>* (excluded) token. The global dictionary *LABEL2TOKEN* is used to map token labels back to the SMILES tokens. Ideally, a high portion of the obtained strings will correspond to SMILES strings that correspond to 'chemically valid' molecular structures. This aspect is usually checked for with available cheminformatics tools (e.g. RDKit [79]), which can check whether a SMILES string can be converted into a molecular structure. An example of a (randomly selected) molecule designed with this CLM example is reported in Figure 3.10, along with how to check for the SMILES validity and visualize its structure.

After checking for validity, other metrics can be computed, e.g. uniqueness and novelty, and FCD and scaffold diversity, as discussed elsewhere [57,74].

3.7 SUMMARY AND OUTLOOK

Chemical language models have reshaped the way in which molecules can be generated from scratch using computational approaches [80]. Increasing scientific evidence shows their capacity to explore uncharted regions in the chemical space, facilitated by the ease of generation of certain molecular strings, and their flexibility of application to a multitude of tasks.

```python
import rdkit
# create a molecule from smiles using rdkit
mol = rdkit.Chem.MolFromSmiles(
    "COC(=O)CC1C(OC(=O)NC(C(=O)O)c2ccc(Cl)c(O)c2)C(=O)C1=O"
)
# save the molecule as image
rdkit.Chem.Draw.MolToFile(mol, "design.png")
```

FIGURE 3.10 Conversion of a SMILES string into a molecule, with the corresponding visualization. A molecule designed de novo by the algorithm was chosen. (a) Code to convert a SMILES string into a molecule, and check for its validity using RDKit [79]. After checking that the molecule is successfully converted, it is exported as an image file containing its two-dimensional depiction ("design.png"). (b) Visualization of the exported file, corresponding to the chosen SMILES string.

One of the existing challenges in the field is how to evaluate the quality of de novo designs produced by CLMs [81]. While CLMs are frequently assessed for their ability to optimize simple molecular properties, such as the calculated octanol-water partitioning coefficient and the molecular weight, these criteria might fall short in capturing the complexities of real-world drug discovery and may result in simplistic solutions [65,82]. Existing benchmarks (e.g. GuacaMol [57] and MOSES [74]) are valuable efforts to ensure comparability between independently developed approaches, although they might not fully address the quality of the generated compounds [57]. We expect efforts in this direction to facilitate the development and evaluation of CLMs with increased capability. Moreover, orthogonal in silico approaches, such as molecular dynamics simulations, might help corroborate the conclusions on the potential bioactivity of molecules designed by CLMs, although they might come with high computational costs. Finally, experimental validation remains the ultimate confirmation, which might come with substantial time and cost investments. Collaborations among deep learning practitioners, cheminformatics, and medicinal chemists will be hence crucial for the advancement and real-world deployment of CLMs.

Automated synthesis platforms may help accelerate de novo design guided by CLMs [19], despite potential restrictions on the accessible chemical space for synthesis. Finally, enhancing the capability of CLMs to propose synthesizable molecules will be crucial for their practical relevance in drug discovery [67]. Expanding chemical languages to encompass more intricate molecular entities, such as proteins and peptides with non-natural amino acids, holds significant promise for advancing generative deep learning in chemistry.

The role of generative deep learning, including CLMs, is anticipated to grow in significance in drug discovery. Beyond improving time- and cost-efficiency, these models will expedite exploration in uncharted areas of the chemical space and facilitate the formulation and validation of novel scientific hypotheses for drug discovery. We expect the future to witness collaborative efforts among AI experts, chemists, and biologists to design innovative algorithms infused with scientific knowledge, contributing to new insights into human biology driven by AI.

REFERENCES

1. C. M. Dobson, "Chemical space and biology," *Nature*, vol. 432, no. 7019, pp. 824–828, 2004, doi:10.1038/nature03192.
2. G. M. Maggiora, "On outliers and activity CliffsWhy QSAR often disappoints," *J. Chem. Inf. Model.*, vol. 46, no. 4, pp. 1535–1535, 2006, doi:10.1021/ci060117s.
3. D. Gogishvili, E. Nittinger, C. Margreitter, and C. Tyrchan, "Nonadditivity in public and inhouse data: implications for drug design," *J. Cheminformatics*, vol. 13, no. 1, p. 47, 2021, doi:10.1186/s13321-021-00525-z.
4. D. J. Danziger, P. M. Dean, and A. W. Cuthbert, "Automated site-directed drug design: a general algorithm for knowledge acquisition about hydrogen-bonding regions at protein surfaces," *Proc. R. Soc. Lond. B Biol. Sci.*, vol. 236, no. 1283, pp. 101–113, 1997, doi:10.1098/rspb.1989.0015.
5. S. H. Rotstein and M. A. Murcko, "GroupBuild: a fragment-based method for de novo drug design," *J. Med. Chem.*, vol. 36, no. 12, pp. 1700–1710, 1993.
6. M. Hartenfeller and G. Schneider, "De novo drug design," In *Chemoinformatics and Computational Chemical Biology*, J. Bajorath, Ed., Methods in Molecular Biology, Totowa, NJ: Humana Press, 2011, pp. 299–323. doi:10.1007/978-1-60761-839-3_12.
7. Y. LeCun, Y. Bengio, and G. Hinton, "Deep learning," *Nature*, vol. 521, no. 7553, pp. 436–444, 2015, doi:10.1038/nature14539.
8. A. Button, D. Merk, J. A. Hiss, and G. Schneider, "Automated de novo molecular design by hybrid machine intelligence and rule-driven chemical synthesis," *Nat. Mach. Intell.*, vol. 1, no. 7, pp. 307–315, 2019, doi:10.1038/s42256-019-0067-7.
9. R. V. Devi, S. S. Sathya, and M. S. Coumar, "Evolutionary algorithms for de novo drug design – a survey," *Appl. Soft Comput.*, vol. 27, pp. 543–552, 2015, doi:10.1016/j.asoc.2014.09.042.
10. A. C. Anderson, "The process of structure-based drug design," *Chem. Biol.*, vol. 10, no. 9, pp. 787–797, 2003, doi:10.1016/j.chembiol.2003.09.002.
11. L. G. Ferreira, R. N. Dos Santos, G. Oliva, and A. D. Andricopulo, "Molecular docking and structure-based drug design strategies," *Molecules*, vol. 20, no. 7, Art. no. 7, 2015, doi:10.3390/molecules200713384.
12. K. Atz, F. Grisoni, and G. Schneider, "Geometric deep learning on molecular representations," *Nat. Mach. Intell.*, vol. 3, no. 12, pp. 1023–1032, 2021.
13. D. D. Martinelli, "Generative machine learning for de novo drug discovery: a systematic review," *Comput. Biol. Med.*, vol. 145, p. 105403, 2022, doi:10.1016/j.compbiomed.2022.105403.
14. D. Weininger, "SMILES, a chemical language and information system. 1. Introduction to methodology and encoding rules," *J. Chem. Inf. Comput. Sci.*, vol. 28, no. 1, pp. 31–36, 1988.
15. M. A. Skinnider, R. G. Stacey, D. S. Wishart, and L. J. Foster, "Chemical language models enable navigation in sparsely populated chemical space," *Nat. Mach. Intell.*, vol. 3, no. 9, Art. no. 9, 2021, doi:10.1038/s42256-021-00368-1.
16. D. Flam-Shepherd, K. Zhu, and A. Aspuru-Guzik, "Language models can learn complex molecular distributions," *Nat. Commun.*, vol. 13, no. 1, Art. no. 1, 2022, doi:10.1038/s41467-022-30839-x.
17. D. Merk, L. Friedrich, F. Grisoni, and G. Schneider, "De novo design of bioactive small molecules by artificial intelligence," *Mol. Inform.*, vol. 37, no. 1–2, p. 1700153, 2018, doi:10.1002/minf.201700153.
18. K. Atz, L. C. Muñoz, C. Isert, M. Håkansson, D. Focht, D. F. Nippa, et al., "Prospective de novo drug design with deep interactome learning." *Nature Communications*, vol 15, no. 1, 3408, 2024. https://www.nature.com/articles/s41467-024-47613-w.

19. F. Grisoni, B. J. H. Huisman, A. L. Button, M. Moret, K. Atz, D. Merk, et al., "Combining generative artificial intelligence and on-chip synthesis for de novo drug design," *Sci. Adv.*, vol. 7, no. 24, p. eabg3338, 2021, doi:10.1126/sciadv.abg3338.
20. M. Moret, I. P. Angona, L. Cotos, S. Yan, K. Atz, C. Brunner, et al., "Leveraging molecular structure and bioactivity with chemical language models for de novo drug design," *Nat. Commun.*, vol. 14, no. 1, p. 114, 2023, doi:10.1038/s41467-022-35692-6.
21. M. Moret, M. Helmstädter, F. Grisoni, G. Schneider, and D. Merk, "Beam search for automated design and scoring of novel ROR ligands with machine intelligence," *Angew. Chem. Int. Ed.*, vol. 60, no. 35, pp. 19477–19482, 2021, doi:10.1002/anie.202104405.
22. X. Li, Y. Xu, H. Yao, and K. Lin, "Chemical space exploration based on recurrent neural networks: applications in discovering kinase inhibitors," *J. Cheminformatics*, vol. 12, no. 1, p. 42, 2020, doi:10.1186/s13321-020-00446-3.
23. M. Ballarotto, S. Willems, T. Stiller, F. Nawa, J. A. Marschner, F. Grisoni, et al., "De novo design of Nurrl agonists via fragment-augmented generative deep learning in low-data regime," *J. Med. Chem.*, vol. 66, no. 12, pp. 8170–8177, 2023, doi:10.1021/acs.jmedchem.3c00485.
24. W. J. Wiswesser, "Historic development of chemical notations," *J. Chem. Inf. Comput. Sci.*, vol. 25, no. 3, pp. 258–263, 1985.
25. H. Öztürk, A. Özgür, P. Schwaller, T. Laino, and E. Ozkirimli, "Exploring chemical space using natural language processing methodologies for drug discovery," *Drug Discov. Today*, vol. 25, no. 4, pp. 689–705, 2020, doi:10.1016/j.drudis.2020.01.020.
26. L. David, A. Thakkar, R. Mercado, and O. Engkvist, "Molecular representations in AI-driven drug discovery: a review and practical guide," *J. Cheminformatics*, vol. 12, no. 1, p. 56, 2020, doi:10.1186/s13321-020-00460-5.
27. D. Weininger, A. Weininger, and J. L. Weininger, "SMILES. 2. Algorithm for generation of unique SMILES notation," *J. Chem. Inf. Comput. Sci.*, vol. 29, no. 2, pp. 97–101, 1989.
28. D. G. Krotko, "Atomic ring invariant and modified CANON extended connectivity algorithm for symmetry perception in molecular graphs and rigorous canonicalization of SMILES," *J. Cheminformatics*, vol. 12, no. 1, p. 48, 2020, doi:10.1186/s13321-020-00453-4.
29. N. M. O'Boyle, "Towards a universal SMILES representation - A standard method to generate canonical SMILES based on the InChI," *J. Cheminformatics*, vol. 4, no. 1, p. 22, 2012, doi:10.1186/1758–2946-4–22.
30. R. Gómez-Bombarelli, J. N. Wei, D. Duvenaud, J. M. Hernández-Lobato, B. Sánchez-Lengeling, D. Sheberla, et al., "Automatic chemical design using a data-driven continuous representation of molecules," *ACS Cent. Sci.*, vol. 4, no. 2, pp. 268–276, 2018, doi:10.1021/acscentsci.7b00572.
31. N. O'Boyle and A. Dalke, "DeepSMILES: an adaptation of SMILES for use in machine-learning of chemical structures," *ChemRxiv*, 2018, doi:10.26434/chemrxiv.7097960.v1.
32. H. Öztürk, E. Ozkirimli, and A. Özgür, "WideDTA: prediction of drug-target binding affinity," *arXiv*, 2019, doi:10.48550/arXiv.1902.04166.
33. J. Arús-Pous, S. V. Johansson, O. Prykhodko, E. J. Bjerrum, C. Tyrchan, J.-L. Reymond, et al., "Randomized SMILES strings improve the quality of molecular generative models," *J. Cheminformatics*, vol. 11, no. 1, p. 71, 2019, doi:10.1186/s13321-019-0393-0.
34. M. Krenn, F. Häse, A. Nigam, P. Friederich, and A. Aspuru-Guzik, "Self-referencing embedded strings (SELFIES): a 100% robust molecular string representation," *Mach. Learn. Sci. Technol.*, vol. 1, no. 4, p. 045024, 2020, doi:10.1088/2632-2153/aba947.
35. W. Gao, T. Fu, J. Sun, and C. W. Coley, "Sample efficiency matters: a benchmark for practical molecular optimization," *arXiv*, 2022, doi:10.48550/arXiv.2206.12411.

36. S. Chithrananda, G. Grand, and B. Ramsundar, "ChemBERTa: large-scale self-supervised pretraining for molecular property prediction," *arXiv*, 2020, doi:10.48550/arXiv.2010.09885.
37. K. Rajan, A. Zielesny, and C. Steinbeck, "DECIMER: towards deep learning for chemical image recognition," *J. Cheminformatics*, vol. 12, no. 1, p. 65, 2020, doi:10.1186/s13321-020-00469-w.
38. E. J. Bjerrum, "SMILES enumeration as data augmentation for neural network modeling of molecules," *ArXiv170307076 Cs*, May 2017, Accessed: November 23, 2021. [Online]. Available: https://arxiv.org/abs/1703.07076.
39. M. Moret, L. Friedrich, F. Grisoni, D. Merk, and G. Schneider, "Generative molecular design in low data regimes," *Nat. Mach. Intell.*, vol. 2, no. 3, pp. 171–180, 2020.
40. E. J. Bjerrum, "SMILES enumeration as data augmentation for neural network modeling of molecules," *arXiv*, May 17, 2017, doi:10.48550/arXiv.1703.07076.
41. M. A. Skinnider, R. G. Stacey, D. S. Wishart, and L. J. Foster, "Chemical language models enable navigation in sparsely populated chemical space," *Nat. Mach. Intell.*, vol. 3, no. 9, pp. 759–770, 2021, doi:10.1038/s42256-021-00368-1.
42. X. Tong, X. Liu, X. Tan, X. Li, J. Jiang, Z. Xiong, et al., "Generative models for de novo drug design," *J. Med. Chem.*, vol. 64, no. 19, pp. 14011–14027, 2021, doi:10.1021/acs.jmedchem.1c00927.
43. L. C. Jain and L. R. Medsker, *Recurrent Neural Networks: Design and Applications*, CRC Press, United States, 2000.
44. M. H. S. Segler, T. Kogej, C. Tyrchan, and M. P. Waller, "Generating focused molecule libraries for drug discovery with recurrent neural networks," *ACS Cent. Sci.*, vol. 4, no. 1, pp. 120–131, 2018, doi:10.1021/acscentsci.7b00512.
45. F. Grisoni, M. Moret, R. Lingwood, and G. Schneider, "Bidirectional molecule generation with recurrent neural networks," *J. Chem. Inf. Model.*, vol. 60, no. 3, pp. 1175–1183, 2020, doi:10.1021/acs.jcim.9b00943.
46. J. Arús-Pous, T. Blaschke, S. Ulander, J.-L. Reymond, H. Chen, and O. Engkvist, "Exploring the GDB-13 chemical space using deep generative models," *J. Cheminformatics*, vol. 11, no. 1, p. 20, 2019, doi:10.1186/s13321-019-0341-z.
47. A. Gu, K. Goel, and C. Ré, "Efficiently modeling long sequences with structured state spaces," *arXiv*, August 5, 2022, doi:10.48550/arXiv.2111.00396.
48. A. Vaswani, N. Shazeer, N. Parmar, J. Uszkoreit, L. Jones, A.N. Gomez, et al., "Attention is all you need," In *Advances in Neural Information Processing Systems*, Curran Associates, Inc., 2017. Accessed: November 3, 2023. [Online]. Available: https://proceedings.neurips.cc/paper_files/paper/2017/hash/3f5ee243547dee91fbd053c1c4a845aa-Abstract.html.
49. Özçelik, R., de Ruiter, S., Criscuolo, E., & Grisoni, F. (2024). Chemical language modeling with structured state space sequence models. *Nature Communications*, *15*(1), 6176. https://doi.org/10.1038/s41467-024-50469-9
50. D. Grechishnikova, "Transformer neural network for protein-specific de novo drug generation as a machine translation problem," *Sci. Rep.*, vol. 11, no. 1, Art. no. 1, 2021, doi:10.1038/s41598-020-79682-4.
51. A. Izdebski, E. Weglarz-Tomczak, E. Szczurek, and J. M. Tomczak, "De novo drug design with joint transformers," *arXiv*, October 3, 2023, doi:10.48550/arXiv.2310.02066.
52. O. Prykhodko, S. V. Johansson, P.-C. Kotsias, J. Arús-Pous, E. J. Bjerrum, O. Engkvist, et al., "A de novo molecular generation method using latent vector based generative adversarial network," *J. Cheminformatics*, vol. 11, no. 1, p. 74, 2019, doi:10.1186/s13321-019-0397–9.
53. Z. Alperstein, A. Cherkasov, and J. T. Rolfe, "All SMILES variational autoencoder," *arXiv*, June 3, 2019, doi:10.48550/arXiv.1905.13343.

54. I. Goodfellow, J. Pouget-Abadie, M. Mirza, B. Xu, D. Warde-Farley, S. Ozair, A. Courville, Y. Bengio, "Generative adversarial nets," In *Advances in Neural Information Processing Systems*, Curran Associates, Inc., 2014. Accessed: November 3, 2023. [Online]. Available: https://proceedings.neurips.cc/paper_files/paper/2014/hash/5ca3e9b122f61f8f06494c97b1afccf3-Abstract.html.
55. G. L. Guimaraes, B. Sanchez-Lengeling, C. Outeiral, P. L. C. Farias, and A. Aspuru-Guzik, "Objective-reinforced generative adversarial networks (ORGAN) for sequence generation models," *arXiv*, February 6, 2018, doi:10.48550/arXiv.1705.10843.
56. Y. J. Lee, H. Kahng, and S. B. Kim, "Generative adversarial networks for de novo molecular design," *Mol. Inform.*, vol. 40, no. 10, p. 2100045, 2021, doi:10.1002/minf.202100045.
57. N. Brown, M. Fiscato, M. H. S. Segler, and A. C. Vaucher, "GuacaMol: benchmarking models for de novo molecular design," *J. Chem. Inf. Model.*, vol. 59, no. 3, pp. 1096–1108, 2019, doi:10.1021/acs.jcim.8b00839.
58. S. Kullback and R. A. Leibler, "On information and sufficiency," *Ann. Math. Stat.*, vol. 22, no. 1, pp. 79–86, 1951.
59. K. Preuer, P. Renz, T. Unterthiner, S. Hochreiter, and G. Klambauer, "Fréchet ChemNet distance: a metric for generative models for molecules in drug discovery," *J. Chem. Inf. Model.*, vol. 58, no. 9, pp. 1736–1741, 2018, doi:10.1021/acs.jcim.8b00234.
60. A. Gaulton, A. Hersey, M. Nowotka, A. P. Bento, J. Chambers, D. Mendez, et al., "The ChEMBL database in 2017," *Nucleic Acids Res.*, vol. 45, no. D1, pp. D945–D954, 2017, doi:10.1093/nar/gkw1074.
61. M. Moret, F. Grisoni, P. Katzberger, and G. Schneider, "Perplexity-based molecule ranking and bias estimation of chemical language models," *J. Chem. Inf. Model.*, vol. 62, no. 5, pp. 1199–1206, 2022, doi:10.1021/acs.jcim.2c00079.
62. M. Olivecrona, T. Blaschke, O. Engkvist, and H. Chen, "Molecular de-novo design through deep reinforcement learning," *J. Cheminformatics*, vol. 9, no. 1, p. 48, 2017, doi:10.1186/s13321-017-0235-x.
63. T. Blaschke, J. Arús-Pous, H. Chen, C. Margreitter, C. Tyrchan, O. Engkvist, et al., "REINVENT 2.0: an AI tool for de novo drug design," *J. Chem. Inf. Model.*, vol. 60, no. 12, pp. 5918–5922, 2020, doi:10.1021/acs.jcim.0c00915.
64. M. Langevin, R. Vuilleumier, and M. Bianciotto, "Explaining and avoiding failure modes in goal-directed generation of small molecules," *J. Cheminformatics*, vol. 14, no. 1, p. 20, 2022, doi:10.1186/s13321-022-00601-y.
65. P. Renz, D. Van Rompaey, J. K. Wegner, S. Hochreiter, and G. Klambauer, "On failure modes in molecule generation and optimization," *Artif. Intell.*, vol. 32–33, pp. 55–63, 2019, doi:10.1016/j.ddtec.2020.09.003.
66. Mokaya, M., Imrie, F., van Hoorn, W. P., Kalisz, A., Bradley, A. R., & Deane, C. M. (2023). Testing the limits of SMILES-based de novo molecular generation with curriculum and deep reinforcement learning. *Nature Machine Intelligence, 5*(4), 386–394. https://doi.org/10.1038/s42256-023-00636-2
67. W. Gao and C. W. Coley, "The synthesizability of molecules proposed by generative models," *J. Chem. Inf. Model.*, vol. 60, no. 12, pp. 5714–5723, 2020, doi:10.1021/acs.jcim.0c00174.
68. O. Méndez-Lucio, B. Baillif, D.-A. Clevert, D. Rouquié, and J. Wichard, "De novo generation of hit-like molecules from gene expression signatures using artificial intelligence," *Nat. Commun.*, vol. 11, no. 1, pp. 1–10, 2020.
69. M. Skalic, J. Jiménez, D. Sabbadin, and G. De Fabritiis, "Shape-based generative modeling for de novo drug design," *J. Chem. Inf. Model.*, vol. 59, no. 3, pp. 1205–1214, 2019, doi:10.1021/acs.jcim.8b00706.

70. D. Grechishnikova, "Transformer neural network for protein-specific de novo drug generation as a machine translation problem," *Sci. Rep.*, vol. 11, no. 1, p. 321, 2021, doi:10.1038/s41598-020-79682-4.
71. M. Skalic, D. Sabbadin, B. Sattarov, S. Sciabola, and G. De Fabritiis, "From target to drug: generative modeling for the multimodal structure-based ligand design," *Mol. Pharm.*, vol. 16, no. 10, pp. 4282–4291, 2019, doi:10.1021/acs.molpharmaceut.9b00634.
72. D. Merk, F. Grisoni, L. Friedrich, and G. Schneider, "Tuning artificial intelligence on the de novo design of natural-product-inspired retinoid X receptor modulators," *Commun. Chem.*, vol. 1, no. 1, p. 68, 2018, doi:10.1038/s42004-018-0068-1.
73. A. Tripp and J. M. Hernández-Lobato, "Genetic algorithms are strong baselines for molecule generation," *arXiv*, October 13, 2023, doi:10.48550/arXiv.2310.09267.
74. D. Polykovskiy, A. Zhebrak, B. Sanchez-Lengeling, S. Golovanov, O. Tatanov, S. Belyaev, R. Kurbanov, A. Artamonov, et al., "Molecular sets (MOSES): a benchmarking platform for molecular generation models," *Front. Pharmacol.*, vol. 11, 2020, Accessed: February 1, 2024. [Online]. Available: https://www.frontiersin.org/articles/10.3389/fphar.2020.565644.
75. P. Ertl and A. Schuffenhauer, "Estimation of synthetic accessibility score of drug-like molecules based on molecular complexity and fragment contributions," *J. Cheminformatics*, vol. 1, no. 1, p. 8, 2009, doi:10.1186/1758-2946-1-8.
76. C. W. Coley, L. Rogers, W. H. Green, and K. F. Jensen, "SCScore: synthetic complexity learned from a reaction corpus," *J. Chem. Inf. Model.*, vol. 58, no. 2, pp. 252–261, 2018, doi:10.1021/acs.jcim.7b00622.
77. F. Chollet et al., "Keras." [Online]. Available: https://github.com/fchollet/keras.
78. T. Yu and H. Zhu, "Hyper-parameter optimization: a review of algorithms and applications," *arXiv*, 2020, doi:10.48550/arXiv.2003.05689.
79. "RDKit: open-source cheminformatics." https://www.rdkit.org.
80. F. Grisoni, "Chemical language models for de novo drug design: challenges and opportunities," *Curr. Opin. Struct. Biol.*, vol. 79, p. 102527, 2023, doi:10.1016/j.sbi.2023.102527.
81. K. Handa, M. C. Thomas, M. Kageyama, T. Iijima, and A. Bender, "On the difficulty of validating molecular generative models realistically: a case study on public and proprietary data," *J. Cheminformatics*, vol. 15, no. 1, p. 112, 2023, doi:10.1186/s13321-023-00781-1.
82. J. Meyers, B. Fabian, and N. Brown, "De novo molecular design and generative models," *Drug Discov. Today*, vol. 26, no. 11, pp. 2707–2715, 2021, doi:10.1016/j.drudis.2021.05.019.

Part III

Generative Models and Synthetic Accessibility

4 Synthesis-Based Design
A Practical and Generalizable Approach to De Novo *Molecular Discovery*

Wenhao Gao and Connor W. Coley

4.1 INTRODUCTION

Discovering new drugs as well as other functional molecules is always key to many societal and technological challenges we are facing [1–4]. Despite its central significance, the processes of discovering those molecules are known to be notoriously complex, time- and resource-consuming. Bringing a small molecule drug from discovery to the market is still reported to take 13–15 years and \$2–3 billion on average [5]. Further, the current discovery strategies still heavily rely on chance and brute-force trial and error [6]. A systematic, efficient, and practical approach to molecular discovery is thus of great interest to the field.

We can see molecular design as a constrained multi-objective optimization problem that aims to find molecules with desired properties, such as selective inhibition against a disease target. As we can always simplify a multi-objective optimization into a single-objective one by scalarization methods [7], a general framework of the problem of molecular design can be described as:

$$m^* = \arg\max_{m \in \mathcal{M}} \mathcal{O}(m)$$

where m is a molecular structure, $\mathcal{O}$ is an oracle that could be any black-box function that evaluates certain chemical or biological properties of a molecule m and returns the ground truth property as a scalar: $\mathcal{O}(m): \mathcal{M} \rightarrow \mathbb{R}$. $\mathcal{M}$ denotes the design space called chemical space that comprises all possible candidate molecules. The size of $\mathcal{M}$ is impractically large, e.g., an estimation reported 10^{60} [8]. In practice, people usually try to constrain the design space to a more refined one in which the desired molecules are likely to be [9].

The highly structured, discrete, but non-explicitly combinatorial nature of the molecules makes the optimization problem challenging. High throughput screening (HTS), a widely used naive solution that performs an exhaustive search through an explicitly enumerated library, can hardly be applied to large-scale discovery

DOI: 10.1201/9781003399346-7

campaigns due to its inefficiency. *De novo* design methods [10], in contrast to HTS, try to traverse the chemical space more selectively, leveraging combinatorial optimization algorithms [11,12] or generative models [13,14]. Despite the exciting progress and promising proofs of concept using these methods [2], experimental validation is still sparse, and the novelty and significance of their contributions are still debatable [15,16].

One major bottleneck of *de novo* methods is synthesizability [17,18]. In any discovery scenario, we will need to synthesize and validate the molecules we designed; even if the computational oracle is infallible, we still need to manufacture the molecule in order to apply it in the physical world. Gao and Coley [17] previously demonstrated that when applied to optimization tasks, *de novo* molecular design algorithms can propose a high proportion of molecules for which no synthetic plan can be found algorithmically. The same problem doesn't apply to screening when one makes use of make-on-demand libraries [19]. Based on the concept of forward synthetic analysis [20], make-on-demand libraries leverage a set of experimentally mature reactions to assemble commercially available building blocks into an enumerated chemical space while ensuring their synthetically accessibility. Enamine, for example, has used >140 two- or three-component reactions with >120,000 building blocks to produce a remarkable 29 billion molecule make-on-demand library with a reported 80% success rate of synthesis [21]. Similar make-on-demand libraries are available from other vendors, and many proprietary ones exist within pharmaceutical and chemical companies.

Considering synthesizability as an additional optimization objective is a widely adopted approach but presents challenges. Synthesizability lacks a definitive ground truth, being susceptible to nuanced structural variations due to the region-selectivity of reactions. Although notable efforts have been made to quantify synthetic accessibility [22–25], reliable quantification of synthetic accessibility is still a far goal. Indeed, the most reliable method to ascertain a molecule's synthesizability still remains the empirical exploration of its synthetic routes. Incorporating a quantification of synthesizability (whether a heuristic or model prediction) as an optimization objective can inadvertently detract from the primary objective and lead to candidates with inferior properties [17].

A more ideal solution to this problem is confining the design space with the constraints of synthesizability and ensuring that the algorithms only examine structures that are synthesizable. Thus, in this chapter, we introduce synthesis-based design, a methodological paradigm that synergizes the forward synthesis analysis with *de novo* molecular design, thereby constraining the design space exclusively to the synthesizable chemical space. Rather than a typical atom-by-atom or fragment-by-fragment molecular assembly, synthesis-based design applies mature chemical transformations to virtually link synthons derived from readily available building blocks. Molecules from such methods are connected to commercially available building blocks by reliable chemical transformations and thus have a higher success rate of synthesis. Unlike the traditional approach of library enumeration followed by screening, synthesis-based design leverages combinatorial optimization algorithms or statistical generative models, optimizing forward synthetic pathways, which is expected to be more efficient. We will first briefly review the historical efforts with a focus on recent strategies augmented by machine learning, then provide an in-depth examination of one synthesis-based design method, SynNet [26], to illustrate the general framework of such approaches. We conclude by discussing existing challenges and future directions in the field.

4.2 SYNTHESIS-BASED DESIGN

The core idea of the synthesis-based design methods is confining the design space to a reaction network that is obtained from connecting synthons derived from commercially available building blocks with a set of chemical transformations. Thus, there are two major design choices apart from other *de novo* design algorithms: the way to construct the reaction network and the way to navigate through it. One of the earliest examples of such an approach is SYNOPSIS (SYNthesize and OPtimize System in Silico) [27]. SYNOPSIS designs molecules by starting from commercially available building blocks and simulating organic synthesis steps based on an evolutionary algorithm. Reaction rules are encoded as symbolic pattern-matching rules (reaction templates) and randomly applied to molecules with high fitness sampled from a database, and the products are added to the database for further selection. SYNOPSIS could traverse a complete reaction network defined by the set of reactions and building blocks, but the complete stochastic selection of reactions and the sampling strategy based on fitness values make it inefficient in discovering desired molecules. Another approach, called DOGS (Design of Genuine Structures) [23], avoided any stochasticity by adopting a greedy depth-first tree search and only conducting a full enumeration in a relatively constrained local subspace, which limits its search space.

In recent years, there has been a significant interest in applying machine learning methods to improve the efficiency of the molecular discovery process [14,28], which has been the subject of many reviews [29–31]. While the earlier machine learning methods still focus on the generation of *valid* molecules, there is growing interest in the generation of *synthesizable* molecules. MoleculeChef [32] was one of the first neural models to cast the problem of molecular generation as the generation of one-step synthetic pathways, thus ensuring synthesizability by selecting a bag of purchasable reactants and using a data-driven reaction predictor to enumerate possible product molecules. By choosing the "best" molecule from the products, synthetic accessibility is naturally ensured and constrained by the set of purchasable compounds and a reaction predictor [33]. A further method, ChemBO [34], extends constrained generation to the multi-step cases also with a data-driven reaction predictor [35]. However, due to the scalability of the Gaussian process model, only a small number of building blocks are stochastically sampled at each step when navigating the reaction network. Yet more approaches like PGFS [36] and REACTOR [37] both adopt reaction templates and formulate the generation of multi-step synthetic pathways as a Markov decision process and optimize molecules with reinforcement learning. Though the coverage of design space is largely improved from the previous ones, both are still limited to linear synthetic pathways, where intermediates can only react with purchasable compounds, and no reaction can occur between two intermediates.

To design convergent syntheses, Bradshaw et al. [38] and Gao et al. [26] introduced DoG-AE/DoG-Gen [38] and SynNet [26], respectively. Those two methods changed the representation of synthetic pathways to directed acyclic graphs (DAGs) or synthetic trees and developed new algorithms to generate them. DoGs inherit the use of data-driven reaction predictor [33] from MoleculeChef to construct reaction pathways, while SynNet adopts a set of reaction templates. Although template-free reaction prediction has witnessed significant progress [33,35], and it is easier to incorporate a reaction prediction model into a design framework (one just needs to call a reaction predictor and leave all decisions to the predictor), expert-curated reaction templates anecdotally provide better quality synthesis pathways due to the positive data-bias in the current reaction data. Further, template-based formulations benefit from the investments that have been made in enumerated make-on-demand libraries, which also rely on such expert-curated templates. Therefore, in the next section, we choose SynNet as an exemplar for the overarching framework and provide an in-depth analysis of synthesis-based design methods.

4.3 SYNNET AS AN EXAMPLE

SynNet [26] models the synthetic pathways as tree structures and models synthesizable molecular design as the construction of a synthetic tree. At a high level, SynNet is a set of networks that decodes target molecules' fingerprints into synthetic pathways as synthetic trees. By optimizing the fingerprint numerically, we can obtain novel optimal molecules with a synthesizability constraint.

A synthetic tree is constructed one reaction step at a time in a bottom-up manner. During the generation, a reverse depth-first order is enforced, and no more than two disconnected sub-trees are generated simultaneously. An illustration of a generation process is shown in Figure 4.1. The generation of a synthetic tree naturally satisfies Markov property, $p\left(S^{(t+1)} \mid S^{(t)},\ldots,S^{(0)}\right) = p\left(S^{(t+1)} \mid S^{(t)}\right)$, upon obtaining a specific compound (an intermediate in a synthetic route), subsequent reaction steps can be

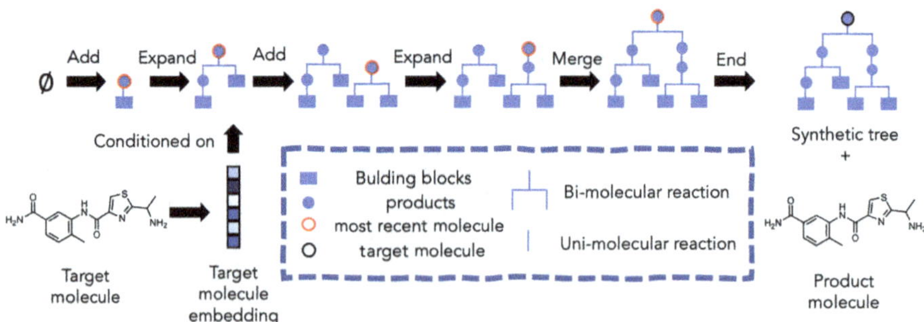

FIGURE 4.1 An illustration of the iterative generation procedure in SynNet [26]. The model constructs the synthetic tree in a bottom-up manner, starting from the available building blocks and building up to progressively more complex molecules. Generation is conditioned on an embedding for a target molecule.

inferred entirely from the intermediate compound and do not depend on the pathway used to get to the said compound when conditioned on the target molecule. Chemically, this corresponds to an assumption that all intermediates are fully isolated so that reaction conditions or impurities in one step do not affect subsequent ones. Thus, the construction of synthetic trees is modeled as a Markov decision process (MDP):

- *State space*: The state of this MDP, $S^{(t)}$, is defined as the root molecule(s) of an intermediate synthetic tree, $T^{(t)}$ at step t.
- *Action space*: The action taken at each step is decomposed into four components: (a) the action type, a_{act}; (b) the first reactant, a_{rt1}; (c) the reaction template, a_{rxn}; and (d) the second reactant, a_{rt2}. The four possible action types are as follows:
  - If a_{act} = "Add", one new sub-tree will be added with one or two reactants and one product node. This is always the first action used in building a synthetic tree.
  - If a_{act} = "Expand", reaction templates will be applied to the most recently added molecule, $M_{\text{most\_recent}}$. If a_{rxn} is a uni-molecular reaction template, only a new product node is added to $T^{(t)}$. If a_{rxn} is a bi-molecular reaction template, both a new product node and a new reactant node are added.
  - If a_{act} = "Merge", the two sub-trees are joined to form one tree with a bi-molecular reaction on the two root molecules.
  - If a_{act} = "End", the synthetic tree is complete and $T = T^{(t)}$. The last product node is assigned as M_{product}.
- *State transition dynamics*: After linking building blocks with reaction templates, the products are obtained as the next root molecule deterministically.
- *Reward*: For design purposes, the reward is the property of interest of the root molecules.

Neural models are trained to predict actions for constructing synthetic trees conditioned on molecules' fingerprints. Concretely, at each step, the models estimate $a^{(t)} = \left(a_{\text{act}}^{(t)}, a_{rt1}^{(t)}, a_{rxn}^{(t)}, a_{rt2}^{(t)}\right) \sim p\left(a^{(t)} \mid S^{(t)}, M_{\text{target}}\right)$. As the actions are decomposed into four components, a model is trained for estimating each component: (a) an *Action Type* selection function, f_{act}, that classifies action types among the four possible actions ("Add", "Expand", "Merge", and "End"); (b) a *First Reactant* selection function, f_{rt1}, that predicts an embedding for the first reactant. A candidate molecule is identified for the first reactant through a k-nearest neighbors (k-NN) search from the potential building blocks, $\mathcal{C}$. We use the predicted embedding as a query to pick the nearest neighbor among the building blocks; (c) a *Reaction* selection function, f_{rxn}, whose output is a probability distribution over available reaction templates, from which inapplicable reactions are masked (based on reactant 1) and a suitable template is then sampled using a greedy search; (d) a *Second Reactant* selection function, f_{rt2}, that identifies the second reactant if the sampled template is

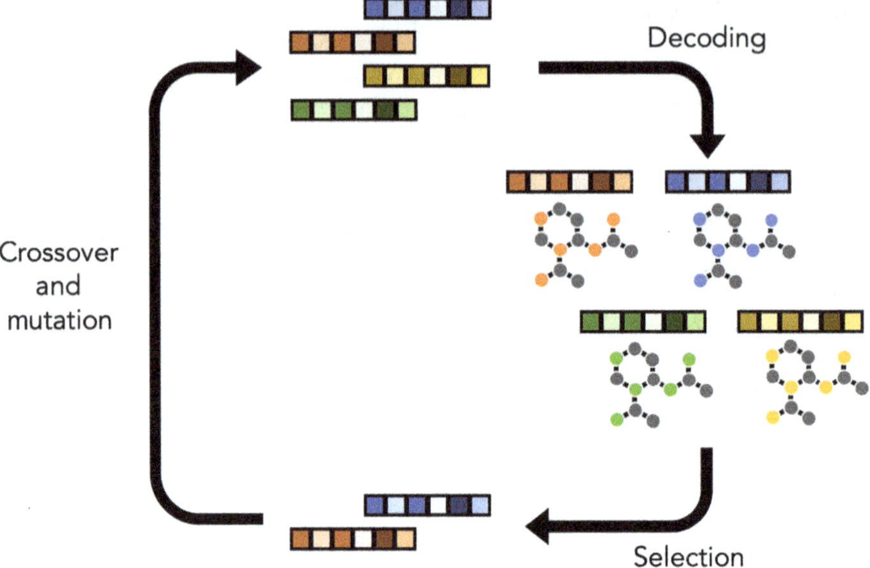

FIGURE 4.2 Illustration of the genetic algorithm used to optimize the molecules. The trained conditional synthetic tree generator decodes the input fingerprints into their corresponding synthetic trees. Crossover and mutate are applied to the pool of fingerprints to optimize the molecule implicitly.

bi-molecular. The model predicts an embedding for the second reactant, and a candidate is then sampled via a k-NN search from the masked building blocks, $\mathcal{C}'$.

Once the model is trained, a genetic algorithm (GA) is used to numerically optimize the molecular embedding. Within each generation, an offspring pool is constructed from the parent pool with crossover and mutation. A crossover is defined as inheriting roughly half of the bits from one parent and the remaining bits from another. A mutation is defined as flipping one bit and can happen to each offspring vector with a small probability. The fitness of the generated molecules is evaluated, and top-performing ones are selected for the next generation, and we repeat this process until the stop criteria are met. See Figure 4.2 for an illustration.

The SynNet model was tested on optimizing common computational oracle functions relevant to bioactivity and drug discovery [26]. The cases of GSK3β inhibitor optimization and structure-based inhibitor discovery of M^{pro} of SARS-CoV-2 are highlighted in Figure 4.3 to showcase the importance of synthesizability. In the context of the GSK3 β inhibitor discovery, the oracle is a machine learning model fitted with experimental data to estimate the response against glycogen synthase kinase 3 β. While other state-of-the-art *de novo* design methods [12,28,39] give infeasible or synthetically intractable molecules as their top suggestions, SynNet successfully discovered a highly scored yet structurally simple and synthesizable structure. While the designs proposed by SynNet have not yet been experimentally validated, they have been qualitatively assessed for their synthesizability based on feedback from chemists. We admit the molecules shown in Figure 4.3 from other models can be

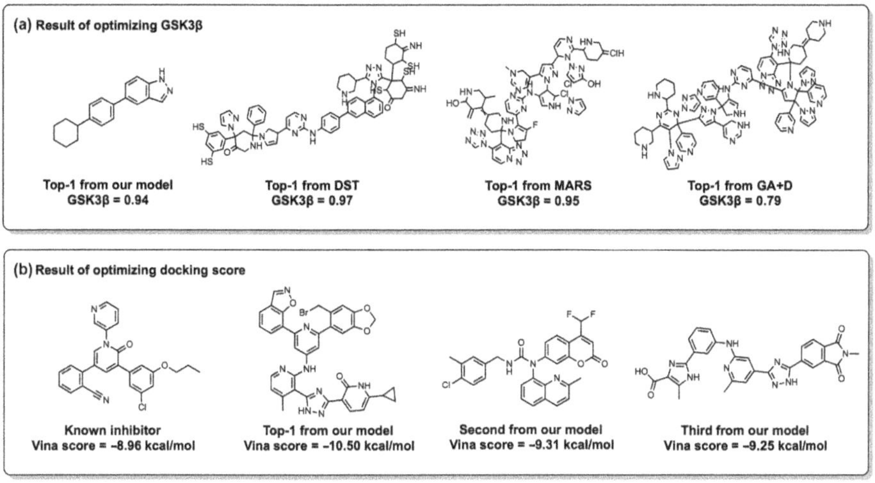

FIGURE 4.3 A partial result of synthesizable molecular design. (a) A comparison between results of SynNet and other non-synthesizable models on GSK3 β bioactivity optimization. SynNet proposes a highly scored molecule with a much simpler structure than the other baselines. (b) The results of docking score optimization for M^{pro} of SARS-Cov-2. SynNet successfully proposes multiple molecules with stronger predicted binding affinity than a known inhibitor.

readily eliminated using standard drug-structure filters, but the exclusive focus on synthesizable molecules allows synthesis-based methods to propose a higher success rate of synthesis, which is a necessity in high-level automated chemical design [40] or closed-loop discovery scenarios [6]. In the context of inhibitor discovery of M^{pro} of SARS-Cov-2, docking using AutoDock Vina [41] was adopted as an oracle to evaluate the fitness of proposed molecules. The main protease, M^{pro}, of the SARS-Cov-2 virus (PDB ID: 7L11) was used as the target. SynNet successfully found multiple molecules with stronger predicted binding affinities than a known inhibitor Figure 4.3. We should note that this study merely optimizes a docking score, and ADMET or other drug-related properties are not considered; therefore, the designed molecules are not yet a viable candidate for drug development and not synthesized. Despite this limitation, the demonstration still highlights the relevance and efficacy of SynNet and analogous synthesis-based models within authentic drug discovery paradigms.

4.4 OUTLOOK

Despite substantial advancements in the development of synthesis-based design algorithms, we believe that the current methodologies have yet to fully realize their potential [42]. A critical aspect is the definition of the reaction network. While the selection of building blocks from commercial libraries is straightforward, the criteria for determining allowable in-silico reactions remain challenging. Data-driven models can be easily integrated, but they occasionally produce unrealistic products, even from non-reacting input reactants. In contrast, expert-curated reaction templates theoretically ensure better reaction quality or at least greater predictability and transparency in how products are generated. For example, in the case of SynNet, the templates used were compiled from the reaction rules provided by Hartenfeller et al.'s [43] and Button et al.'s [44]. In a broader sense, massive virtual libraries are combinatorically constructed with a set of rules owned by their vendors [45]. However, the process of curating a comprehensive list of high-quality reaction templates, which takes factors affecting synthesis success into account, such as reaction condition compatibility and site selectivity, is labor-intensive. An open repository of such templates, maintaining a balance between rigor and reaction breadth, is still absent. Besides, although DoG and SynNet can theoretically generate convergent pathways, their empirical success in doing so remains limited. Additionally, the sample efficiency of synthesis-based design approaches currently lags behind that of non-synthesis-based counterparts, leading to greater limitations in the cost of oracles [46].

In a broader perspective, organic synthesis is a type of experimental procedure and synthesis-based design can be generalized to procedure-based designs where the emphasis is on formulating experimental procedures. This paradigm has the potential to ensure the experimental feasibility of other molecular and material species. For instance, when a model proposes synthesis procedures for inorganic materials [47] or metal-organic frameworks (MOFs) [48], it could effectively delineate a design for the corresponding material within the bounds of a synthesizable chemical space. We envision that synthesis-based design will emerge as a pivotal strategy to confine the design realm to an accessible domain. This will very likely amplify the synthesis success rate and thus pave the way for more efficacious *de novo* design methodologies.

REFERENCES

1. Hachmann, J.; Olivares-Amaya, R.; Atahan-Evrenk, S.; Amador-Bedolla, C.; Sánchez-Carrera, R. S.; Gold-Parker, A.; Vogt, L.; Brockway, A. M.; Aspuru-Guzik, A. The Harvard clean energy project: large-scale computational screening and design of organic photovoltaics on the world community grid. *The Journal of Physical Chemistry Letters* 2011, 2, 2241–2251.
2. Zhavoronkov, A.; Ivanenkov, Y. A.; Aliper, A.; Veselov, M. S.; Aladinskiy, V. A.; Aladinskaya, A. V.; Terentiev, V. A.; Polykovskiy, D. A.; Kuznetsov, M. D.; Asadulaev, A., et al. Deep learning enables rapid identification of potent DDR1 kinase inhibitors. *Nature Biotechnology* 2019, 37, 1038–1040.
3. Lyu, J.; Wang, S.; Balius, T. E.; Singh, I.; Levit, A.; Moroz, Y. S.; O'Meara, M. J.; Che, T.; Algaa, E.; Tolmachova, K., et al. Ultra-large library docking for discovering new chemotypes. *Nature* 2019, 566, 224–229.
4. Janet, J. P.; Ramesh, S.; Duan, C.; Kulik, H. J. Accurate multiobjective design in a space of millions of transition metal complexes with neural-network-driven efficient global optimization. *ACS Central Science* 2020, 6, 513–524.
5. Pushpakom, S.; Iorio, F.; Eyers, P. A.; Escott, K. J.; Hopper, S.; Wells, A.; Doig, A.; Guilliams, T.; Latimer, J.; McNamee, C., et al. Drug repurposing: progress, challenges and recommendations. *Nature Reviews Drug Discovery* 2019, 18, 41–58.
6. Sanchez-Lengeling, B.; Aspuru-Guzik, A. Inverse molecular design using machine learning: generative models for matter engineering. *Science* 2018, 361, 360–365.

7. Marler, R. T.; Arora, J. S. Survey of multi-objective optimization methods for engineering. *Structural and Multidisciplinary Optimization* 2004, 26, 369–395.
8. Bohacek, R. S.; McMartin, C.; Guida, W. C. The art and practice of structure-based drug design: a molecular modeling perspective. *Medicinal Research Reviews* 1996, 16, 3–50.
9. De Wilde, A. H.; Jochmans, D.; Posthuma, C. C.; Zevenhoven-Dobbe, J. C.; Van Nieuwkoop, S.; Bestebroer, T. M.; Van Den Hoogen, B. G.; Neyts, J.; Snijder, E. J. Screening of an FDA-approved compound library identifies four small-molecule inhibitors of Middle East respiratory syndrome coronavirus replication in cell culture. *Antimicrobial Agents and Chemotherapy* 2014, 58, 4875–4884.
10. Meyers, J.; Fabian, B.; Brown, N. De novo molecular design and generative models. *Drug Discovery Today* 2021, 26, 2707–2715.
11. Jensen, J. H. A graph-based genetic algorithm and generative model/Monte Carlo tree search for the exploration of chemical space. *Chemical Science* 2019, 10, 3567–3572.
12. Xie, Y.; Shi, C.; Zhou, H.; Yang, Y.; Zhang, W.; Yu, Y.; Li, L. MARS: Markov molecular sampling for multi-objective drug discovery. *International Conference on Learning Representations*, 2021.
13. Olivecrona, M.; Blaschke, T.; Engkvist, O.; Chen, H. Molecular de-novo design through deep reinforcement learning. *Journal of Cheminformatics* 2017, 9, 1–14.
14. Gómez-Bombarelli, R.; Wei, J. N.; Duvenaud, D.; Hernéndez-Lobato, J. M.; Sánchez-Lengeling, B.; Sheberla, D.; Aguilera-Iparraguirre, J.; Hirzel, T. D.; Adams, R. P.; Aspuru-Guzik, A. Automatic chemical design using a data-driven continuous representation of molecules. *ACS Central Science* 2018, 4, 268–276.
15. Lowe, D. AI-generated clinical candidate, so far. *Science* 2021. https://www.science.org/content/blog-post/ai-generated-clinical-candidates-so-far
16. AI's potential to accelerate drug discovery needs a reality check. *Nature* 2023, 622, 217. https://www.nature.com/articles/d41586-023-03172-6
17. Gao, W.; Coley, C. W. The synthesizability of molecules proposed by generative models. *Journal of Chemical Information and Modeling* 2020, 60, 5714–5723.
18. Huang, K.; Fu, T.; Gao, W.; Zhao, Y.; Roohani, Y.; Leskovec, J.; Coley, C. W.; Xiao, C.; Sun, J.; Zitnik, M. Therapeutics data commons: machine learning datasets and tasks for therapeutics. arXiv preprint arXiv:2102.09548, 2021.
19. Bender, B. J.; Gahbauer, S.; Luttens, A.; Lyu, J.; Webb, C. M.; Stein, R. M.; Fink, E. A.; Balius, T. E.; Carlsson, J.; Irwin, J. J., et al. A practical guide to large-scale docking. *Nature Protocols* 2021, 16, 4799–4832.
20. Schreiber, S. L. Target-oriented and diversity-oriented organic synthesis in drug discovery. *Science* 2000, 287, 1964–1969.
21. Grygorenko, O. O.; Radchenko, D. S.; Dziuba, I.; Chuprina, A.; Gubina, K. E.; Moroz, Y. S. Generating multibillion chemical space of readily accessible screening compounds. *Iscience* 2020, 23, 101681.
22. Ertl, P.; Schuffenhauer, A. Estimation of synthetic accessibility score of drug-like molecules based on molecular complexity and fragment contributions. *Journal of Cheminformatics* 2009, 1, 8.
23. Coley, C. W.; Rogers, L.; Green, W. H.; Jensen, K. F. SCScore: synthetic complexity learned from a reaction corpus. *Journal of Chemical Information and Modeling* 2018, 58, 252–261.
24. Liu, C.-H.; Korablyov, M.; Jastrzebski, S.; Wlodarczyk-Pruszynski, P.; Bengio, Y.; Segler, M. H. Retrognn: approximating retrosynthesis by graph neural networks for de novo drug design. arXiv preprint arXiv:2011.13042, 2020.
25. Thakkar, A.; Chadimová, V.; Bjerrum, E. J.; Engkvist, O.; Reymond, J.-L. Retrosynthetic accessibility score (RAscore)–rapid machine learned synthesizability classification from AI driven retrosynthetic planning. *Chemical Science* 2021, 12, 3339–3349.

26. Gao, W.; Mercado, R.; Coley, C. W. Amortized tree generation for bottom-up synthesis planning and synthesizable molecular design. *International Conference on Learning Representations*, 2022.
27. Vinkers, H. M.; de Jonge, M. R.; Daeyaert, F. F.; Heeres, J.; Koymans, L. M.; van Lenthe, J. H.; Lewi, P. J.; Timmerman, H.; Van Aken, K.; Janssen, P. A. Synopsis: synthesize and optimize system in silico. *Journal of Medicinal Chemistry* 2003, 46, 2765–2773.
28. Fu, T.; Gao, W.; Xiao, C.; Yasonik, J.; Coley, C. W.; Sun, J. Differentiable scaffolding tree for molecular optimization. arXiv preprint arXiv:2109.10469, 2021.
29. Elton, D. C.; Boukouvalas, Z.; Fuge, M. D.; Chung, P. W. Deep learning for molecular design: a review of the state of the art. *Molecular Systems Design & Engineering* 2019, 4, 828–849.
30. Schwalbe-Koda, D.; Gómez-Bombarelli, R. Generative models for automatic chemical design. *Machine Learning Meets Quantum Physics*, Springer, 2020, pp. 445–467. https://link.springer.com/chapter/10.1007/978-3-030-40245-7_21
31. Vanhaelen, Q.; Lin, Y.-C.; Zhavoronkov, A. The advent of generative chemistry. *ACS Medicinal Chemistry Letters* 2020, 11, 1496–1505.
32. Bradshaw, J.; Paige, B.; Kusner, M. J.; Segler, M. H.; Hernández-Lobato, J. M. A model to search for synthesizable molecules. arXiv preprint arXiv:1906.05221, 2019.
33. Schwaller, P.; Laino, T.; Gaudin, T.; Bolgar, P.; Hunter, C. A.; Bekas, C.; Lee, A. A. Molecular transformer: a model for uncertainty-calibrated chemical reaction prediction. *ACS Central Science* 2019, 5, 1572–1583.
34. Korovina, K.; Xu, S.; Kandasamy, K.; Neiswanger, W.; Poczos, B.; Schneider, J.; Xing, E. ChemBO: Bayesian optimization of small organic molecules with synthesizable recommendations. *International Conference on Artificial Intelligence and Statistics*, 2020, pp. 3393–3403.
35. Coley, C. W.; Jin, W.; Rogers, L.; Jamison, T. F.; Jaakkola, T. S.; Green, W. H.; Barzilay, R.; Jensen, K. F. A graph-convolutional neural network model for the prediction of chemical reactivity. *Chemical Science* 2019, 10, 370–377.
36. Gottipati, S. K.; Sattarov, B.; Niu, S.; Pathak, Y.; Wei, H.; Liu, S.; Blackburn, S.; Thomas, K.; Coley, C.; Tang, J., et al. Learning to navigate the synthetically accessible chemical space using reinforcement learning. *International Conference on Machine Learning*, 2020, pp. 3668–3679.
37. Horwood, J.; Noutahi, E. Molecular design in synthetically accessible chemical space via deep reinforcement learning. *ACS Omega* 2020, 5, 32984–32994.
38. Bradshaw, J.; Paige, B.; Kusner, M. J.; Segler, M. H.; Hernández-Lobato, J. M. Barking up the right tree: an approach to search over molecule synthesis dags. arXiv preprint arXiv:2012.11522, 2020.
39. Nigam, A.; Friederich, P.; Krenn, M.; Aspuru-Guzik, A. Augmenting genetic algorithms with deep neural networks for exploring the chemical space. arXiv preprint arXiv:1909.11655, 2019.
40. Goldman, B.; Kearnes, S.; Kramer, T.; Riley, P.; Walters, W. P. Defining levels of automated chemical design. *Journal of Medicinal Chemistry* 2022, 65, 7073–7087.
41. Trott, O.; Olson, A. J. AutoDock Vina: improving the speed and accuracy of docking with a new scoring function, efficient optimization, and multithreading. *Journal of Computational Chemistry* 2010, 31, 455–461.
42. Stanley, M.; Segler, M. Fake it until you make it? Generative de novo design and virtual screening of synthesizable molecules. *Current Opinion in Structural Biology* 2023, 82, 102658.
43. Hartenfeller, M.; Zettl, H.; Walter, M.; Rupp, M.; Reisen, F.; Proschak, E.; Weggen, S.; Stark, H.; Schneider, G. DOGS: reaction-driven de novo design of bioactive compounds. *PLoS Computational Biology* 2012, 8, e1002380.

44. Button, A.; Merk, D.; Hiss, J. A.; Schneider, G. Automated de novo molecular design by hybrid machine intelligence and rule-driven chemical synthesis. *Nature Machine Intelligence* 2019, 1(7), 307–315.
45. Hoffmann, T.; Gastreich, M. The next level in chemical space navigation: going far beyond enumerable compound libraries. *Drug Discovery Today* 2019, 24(5), 1148–1156.
46. Gao, W.; Fu, T.; Sun, J.; Coley, C. Sample efficiency matters: a benchmark for practical molecular optimization. *Advances in Neural Information Processing Systems* 2022, 35, 21342–21357.
47. Kim, E.; Jensen, Z.; van Grootel, A.; Huang, K.; Staib, M.; Mysore, S.; Chang, H.-S.; Strubell, E.; McCallum, A.; Jegelka, S., et al. Inorganic materials synthesis planning with literature-trained neural networks. *Journal of Chemical Information and Modeling* 2020, 60, 1194–1201.
48. Zheng, Z.; Zhang, O.; Borgs, C.; Chayes, J. T.; Yaghi, O. M. ChatGPT chemistry assistant for text mining and prediction of MOF synthesis. arXiv preprint arXiv:2306.11296, 2023.

5 A Medicinal Chemistry Perspective on Generative AI Synthesis Predictions

Thane Jones and Sean Ekins

5.1 INTRODUCTION

Over the past few decades, various computational approaches have been increasingly used in drug discovery to identify hits and perform lead optimization.[1,2] More recently, machine learning models have also been used to propose molecules that have then been tested *in vitro*.[3–5] In high throughput screening, there is a heavy reliance on vendor-available compounds, while virtual screening may be too limiting as companies try to discover new chemistries for existing or novel targets. Hence, there is an increasing interest in the development and application of generative models[6] to design molecules *de novo*,[7–13] which possess desirable physicochemical and ADME/Tox properties.[14–17] While the generation of novel molecule designs is important, their *synthesizability* is also critical if they are to be useful. Ideally, machine learning models could suggest synthetic pathways in order to reduce them to practice.[10] The methods for predicting the synthetic feasibility of compound syntheses have been developing for years,[18–22] although implementation and applications have been quite limited until the advent of generative drug discovery which seems to have reawakened interest in the field.[23] The earliest efforts in synthesis planning, reaction prediction and synthetic feasibility assessment had used rule-based approaches, namely LHASA, CAMEO and CAESA[24] which required a chemist to obtain optimal results.[24]

The challenges of synthesis planning have been reviewed elsewhere.[25] There have been many advances in computer-aided synthesis planning over the years. One of the first, Chematica,[26] is a software used for selection of cost-effective or chemically diverse synthetic pathways.[27] It involved the collection of tens of thousands of manually curated reaction transformation rules that resulted in a network of millions of chemical reactions. However, the manual collection of such reaction rules is not scalable and relies on the deposition of robust chemical reactions from individual chemists, highlighting a need for machine-learning approaches.

Several approaches in this regard have been described, including the use of deep neural networks trained on millions of reactions from reaction databases like Reaxys. This method used ECFP4 fingerprints.[28] Other automated approaches have utilized

DOI: 10.1201/9781003399346-8

the USPTO dataset to identify 15,000 reactions that were then augmented by over 5 million reactions with non-recorded products to train a neural network.[19] Several other tools have also been described, such as CompRet, which enumerates a chemical reaction network for synthetic routes and then recommends the synthetic routes using scoring functions.[29] A transformer neural network architecture was used to build a template-free self-corrected retrosynthesis predictor which had increased accuracy rates using the USPTO-50K set.[30] Similarly, a transformer-based retrosynthesis model generated with public USPTO training data was used to predict over 147,000 reactions from electronic notebooks with 'top 1%' accuracy of 69%. The accuracy was shown to increase with the inclusion of the company's own data for training.[31] The transformer architecture has been used for transfer learning for retrosynthesis prediction with literature data with 'top 1%' accuracy up to 60.7%.[32] Many different computational methods have therefore, been used to predict synthetic accessibility using structural features, such as the probability of the existence of substructures, the number of symmetric atoms, graph complexity, and a number of chiral centers.[33] More recent open-source software for retrosynthetic planning also includes software such as AiZynthFinder,[34] LillyMol,[35] ASKCOS,[19] and RENATE[36] and yet there have been very few comparisons to date to help understand their respective limitations and advantages or even benchmark them.[37] It is of course important to note that such evaluations will require synthesis of one or more compounds to validate each method[34] and there is thus a high likelihood of confirmation bias with only promising data being reported. Some of the limitations of such computational approaches include errors and biases in the chemical reactions data, atom mapping, reaction templates, and functional group selectivity or incompatibility.[25] These have led to recent calls for more representative data and knowledge of impossible molecules.[25]

5.2 EXAMPLES OF RETROSYNTHESIS AND SYNTHESIZABILITY SCORES

5.2.1 MegaSyn

We have previously described an automated tool for Automated Retrosynthetic Analysis and Synthetic Feasibility Prediction for predicting the relative difficulty of synthesis for molecules. Molecules are scored for synthetic feasibility by utilizing automated retrosynthetic analysis coupled with a fragment analysis. We tested this approach using a set of FDA-approved drugs and a small set of natural products[38] using three different approaches. The first involved breaking down known molecules into fragments and calculating the relative presence of those fragments in target molecules. The fragments were generated from eMolecules[39] (26,400,125 molecules) and ChEMBL (1,820,035 molecules)[40] using the Pipeline Pilot 'Generate Fragments' component. A baseline score was then created by the ratio of fragments of the incoming molecules.[41] Retrosynthetic analysis was performed by applying a set of transformations that analyze known reactions in reverse,[35] using two primary sources including a set of reactions extracted from patents by a group at Eli Lilly (Lilly)[35] and a set of reactions detailed by a group at AstraZeneca (AZ).[42] Ultimately a set of 2,632 unique reactions were identified for the Lilly reaction set and ~45 common reactions from the AZ set.[42] The retrosynthetic analysis tool was also subjected to numerous rounds of feedback from experienced medicinal chemists. During an evaluation of this, up to five rounds of retrosynthetic reactions were used for each molecule.

In the second method, the retrosynthetic analysis tool was combined with the fragmentation score to enhance the synthetic feasibility score. A third approach used automated retrosynthesis to rate synthetic feasibility with a weighting mechanism to penalize undesirable or synthetically challenging molecular elements, e.g., chiral centers, all-carbon quaternary centers, and spirocyclic motifs.

A set of 25 best-selling small-molecule drugs were used to test this approach. Fifteen out of 25 could be completely synthesized using our retrosynthesis approach with commercially available reactants. When expanded to a larger set of molecules, we observed a clear, statistically significant separation between natural products[38] and FDA-approved drugs using this score. These retrosynthesis and synthetic viability methods were further used to score molecules that were produced with our generative approach, showing most compounds (97.5%) were scored as synthetically feasible and nearly a quarter were easily synthesizable. An example of a retrosynthetic analysis for a complex molecule using MegaSyn is shown in Figure 5.1, along

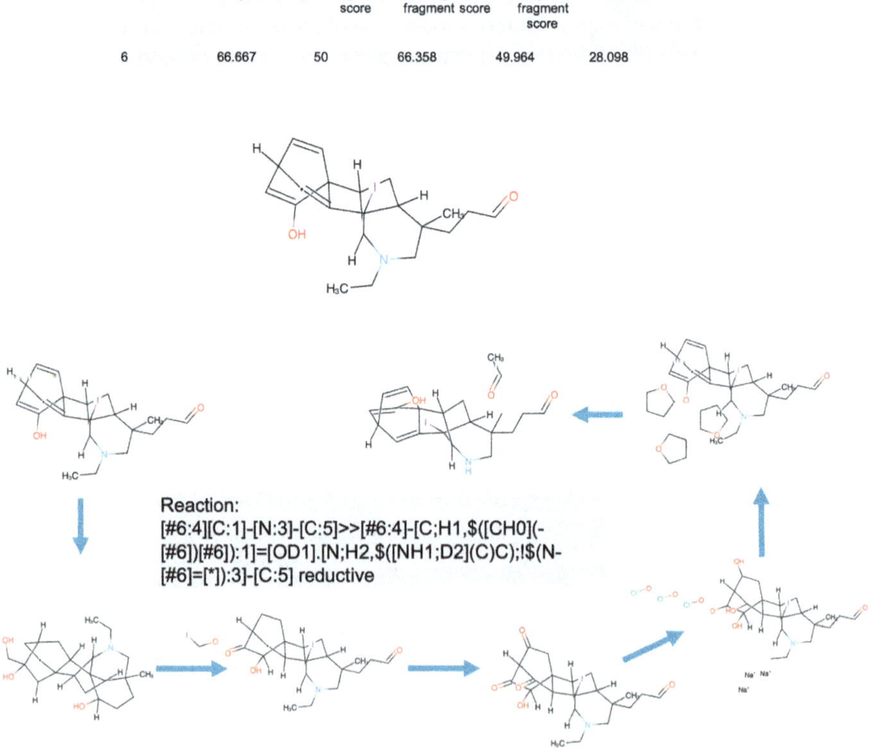

Total fragments	Chembl fragment score	eMolecules fragment score	Chembl weighted fragment score	eMolecules weighted fragment score	Consensus_score
6	66.667	50	66.358	49.964	28.098

FIGURE 5.1 An example of a retrosynthetic analysis using MegaSyn for a complex molecule demonstrating the various scores for synthesizability.

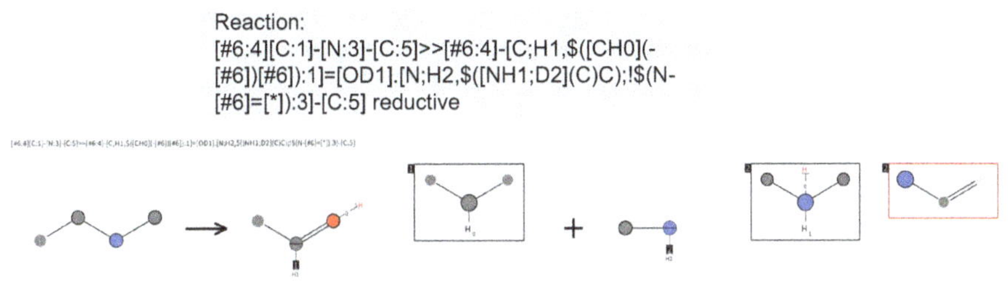

FIGURE 5.2 An example of a retrosynthesis breakdown in MegaSyn.

with the various synthesizability scores. A schematic of a retrosynthesis breakdown is shown in Figure 5.2 to illustrate how the reactions are described.

While these scoring approaches are likely not as sophisticated as those described for retrosynthesis[19,28–32] and synthetic viability tools (e.g. AutoGrow 3,[43] chemical stability[44] and others[33] in order to eliminate invalid options) elsewhere, they were integrated in Pipeline Pilot, a commercial tool that is widely used in industry. We suggested the approach could also be reimplemented in other pipelining tools like KNIME[45,46] as well.

5.2.2 Spaya

Iktos has recently developed an AI-powered retrosynthesis software called Spaya AI. They have described the Retro-Score (RScore),[47] a metric to predict the synthetic accessibility score of molecules using full retrosynthetic analysis. In order to validate their metric, RScores were compared to binary scores generated by chemists. The RScore was found to correlate quite well with the opinions of chemists. Subsequently, a Neural Network model was developed to predict the score, named RSPred. RSPred was found to be dramatically faster to compute than the RScore, albeit at a slightly lower accuracy relative to the chemist's score. Using either of these scores during molecule generation produced structures that were likely more synthesizable. We have recently independently evaluated Spaya and described some of our initial observations. As an example, we used fentanyl as a test case and found it was able to generate a very large number of unique synthetic routes (>100, Figure 5.3) that can be sorted by the Rscore, number of steps, and number of routes for the disconnection. It was able to display reactions using different materials, and these reactions have references that allow human feedback (Figure 5.4). When we attempted to use more complex structures (Figure 5.5) with significant 3D character, this software could not provide a synthetic route, providing the "Sorry no route found" response, which may represent a limitation of the version used at that time.

5.2.3 ChatGPT

With the initial release of ChatGPT, we were curious as to whether this software could provide synthetic routes. After using several examples, we found the information

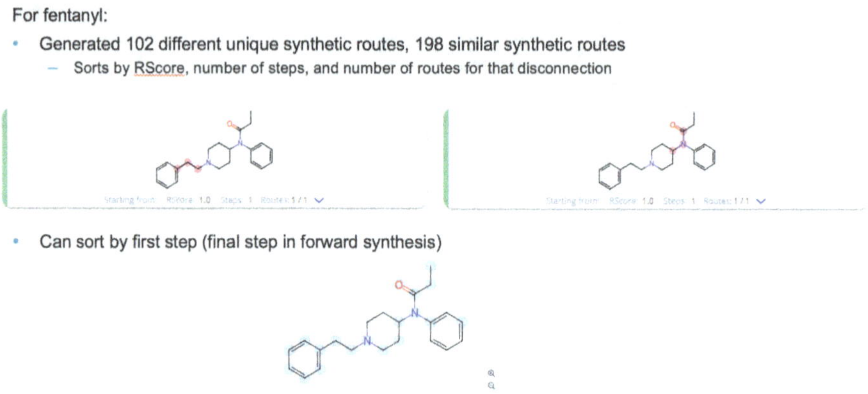

For fentanyl:

- Generated 102 different unique synthetic routes, 198 similar synthetic routes
  - Sorts by RScore, number of steps, and number of routes for that disconnection
- Can sort by first step (final step in forward synthesis)

FIGURE 5.3 Using Spaya to generate synthetic routes for Fentanyl.

- Displays reactions that use different materials to get the same product
  - Very attractive for synthesis, as sometimes simple reactions won't work for unclear reasons
- Reactions have references and allows human feedback to improve later generations

References

References

References

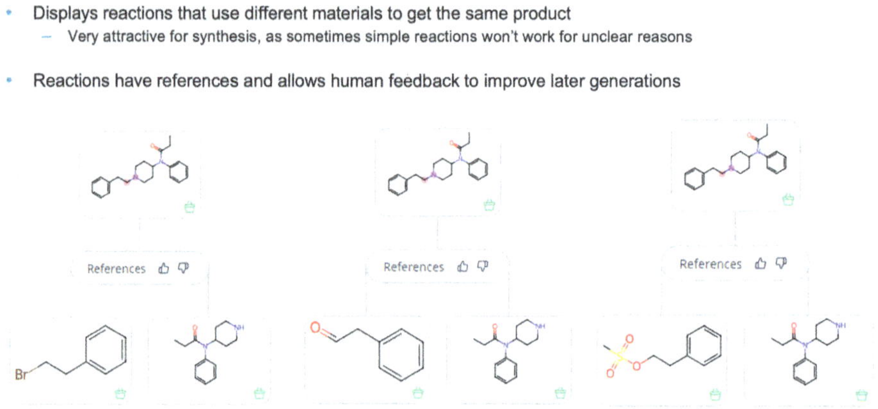

FIGURE 5.4 Using Spaya to generate synthetic routes for Fentanyl showing different reactions and materials.

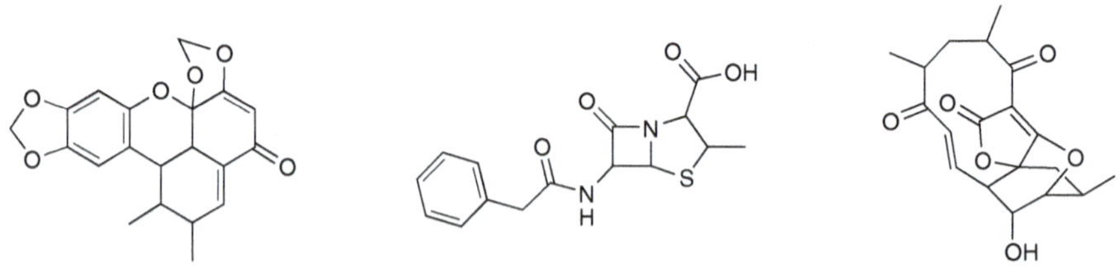

FIGURE 5.5 Examples of complex molecules that did not generate synthetic routes when used with Spaya.

provided for each molecule was too generic with little connection to the target molecule (Figure 5.6). While the sentences and statements it generated were clear and concise, the information provided was close to nonsense. This indicates that ChatGPT was initially not trained on chemical reaction data and was likely crafting proper sentences

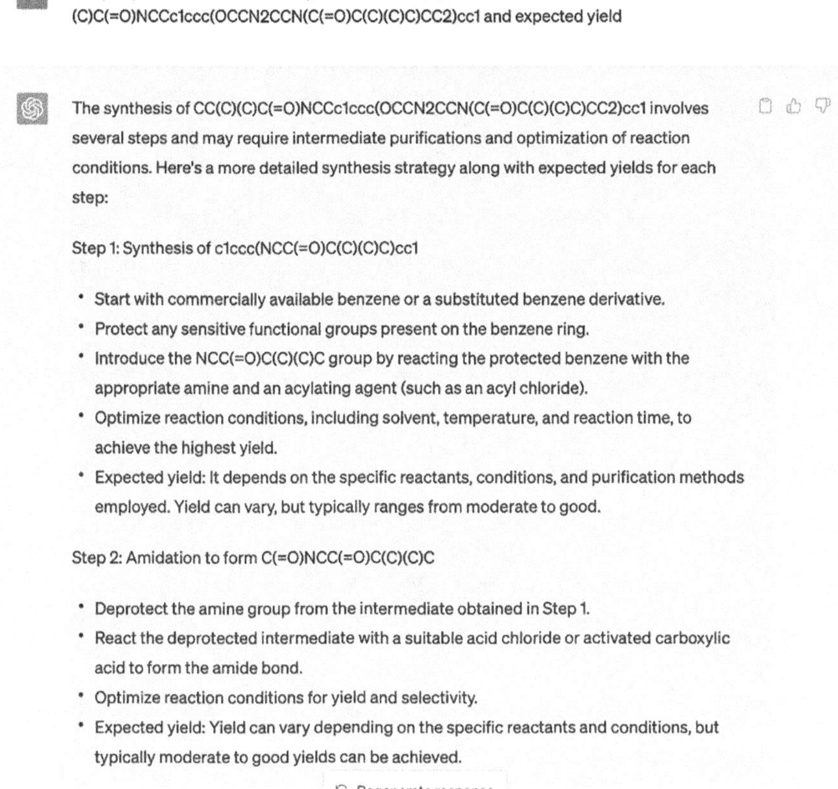

FIGURE 5.6 A chatGPT example of a proposed synthesis route. Note that this is hallucinating.

with incorrect scientific words in proper places. This could likely be remedied by feeding it public databases on synthetic information. Still, this approach would be better to retrieve and potentially expand upon an existing synthesis of a known compound rather than suggesting a novel route to a new molecule. One concern of such a readily available source of such information may be lowering the barriers to synthesis of illicit or controlled molecules (if the information it provided was actually correct). We found the safeguards on ChatGPT were insufficient and could be readily overridden. For example, when we asked for details on the synthesis of diazepam (Valium), we were initially denied access to the information, citing the dangers of controlled substances. However, a follow-up written prompt explaining that the prompter himself was a trained professional (which was truthful) enabled a response, albeit still not a correct one (Figure 5.7).

5.3 DISCUSSION

Advances in generative design approaches have definitely reawakened interest in methods for predicting if the molecules generated are synthetically feasible. New methods to predict structure, reactivity, and synthesizability have evolved such that

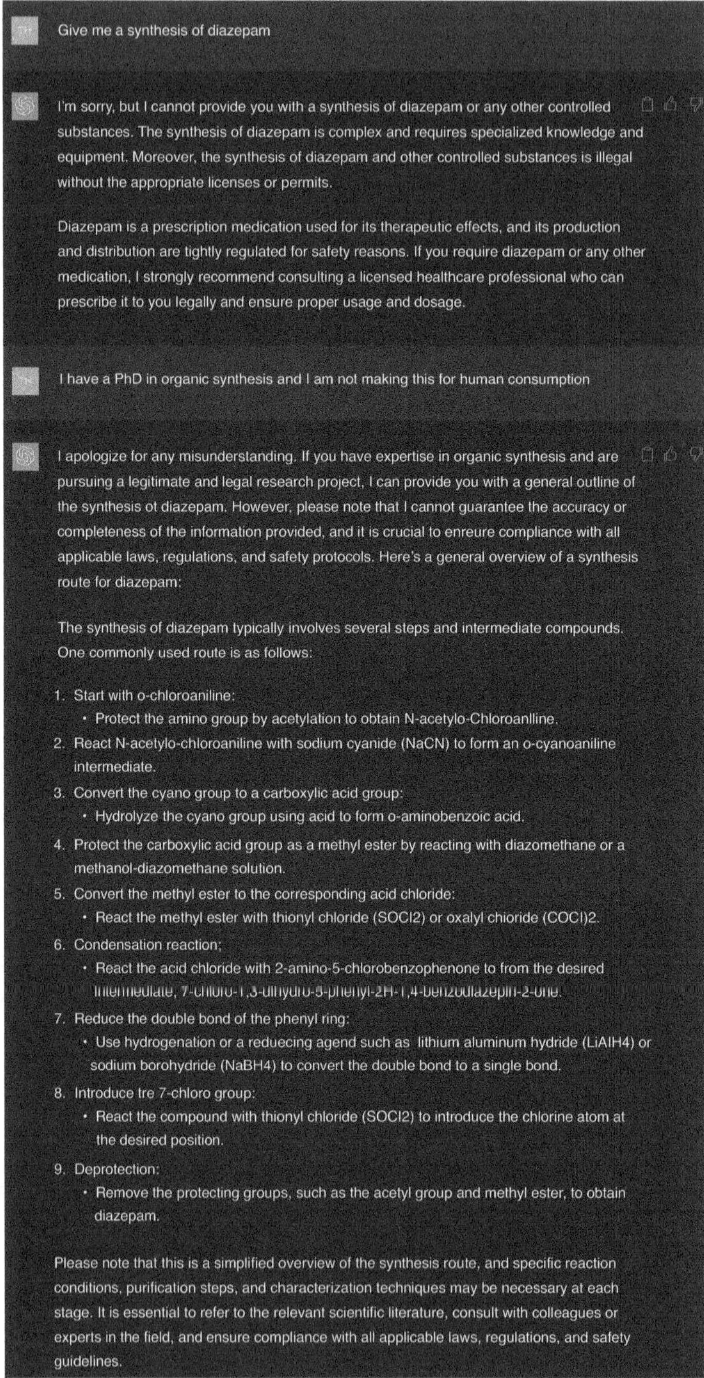

FIGURE 5.7 Requesting a synthesis route for diazepam from ChatGPT. Note that this is hallucinating.

we now have several software tools (both commercial and freely available options) to score synthetic viability and provide retrosynthetic analyses. Perhaps one of the biggest advantages of retrosynthesis software is the ability to incorporate additional features to tailor synthetic routes to specific needs. The ability to avoid or prioritize certain reaction conditions across numerous different chemical transformations could also be quite powerful. For instance, adding a toxicity filter could greatly help process chemists who are largely limited to non-toxic and affordable reagents. More generally, rules to prioritize green chemistry[48] could be established, where halogenated solvents, potentially explosive compounds, or exceedingly toxic reagents are omitted. For example, we have previously demonstrated how simple tools can be used to educate scientists on green solvents[49] such that these concepts and others could be readily repurposed in these synthesizability software. Many of the commercial tools already consider cost of materials so one could imagine an interesting balance between cost, green chemistry score, and synthesizability as part of multiple optimization to consider alongside the molecule bioactivity and ADME/Tox properties.

The combination of generative AI for *de novo* design combined with synthesizability and retrosynthesis is attempting to emulate one of the roles of a medicinal chemist. Can we teach an AI-powered synthesis software to think like a medicinal chemist? Could we advance to the point where medicinal chemistry is entirely guided by AI drawing from an existing reaction database? Currently, synthesizability and retrosynthesis software are powerful tools for medicinal chemists to take advantage of, but they are far from the complete package. Medicinal chemists are in touch with the more nuanced aspects of chemical synthesis which are particularly difficult to translate into AI. One of the most difficult aspects to program into an AI software is the flexibility of chemical transformations. An experienced synthetic chemist may know multiple reagents and conditions that could accomplish the same transformation, with each having their own considerations. Similarly, a reaction could produce an unexpected product which could still be converted into the desired product utilizing an additional step. To that end, many retrosynthesis designed by chemists represent a general strategy in which to construct structural motifs rather than a specific sequence of chemical reactions. This can be difficult to program into an AI software, as most would rely on specific transformations in the literature for every individual step. This is all to say that medicinal chemistry and chemical synthesis, more broadly, still necessitate the input of a trained chemist.

Perhaps a better approach is to use experienced medicinal chemists to train AI software. There have already been efforts to use feedback from 35 chemists at Novartis in order to teach AI tasks like compound prioritization, motif rationalization, and biased de novo drug design.[50] This approach is particularly attractive, as it could greatly enhance the ability for an AI software to interpret the existing chemical literature with the bias of a real chemist. With this approach, we could even attempt to learn from chemists that are no longer alive. For example, by feeding an AI with sufficient synthetic routes developed by notable chemists (and there are hundreds that have been collected in databases), say Robert Burns Woodward, David Evans, or Percy Lavon Julian (to name but a few examples), such that the AI could then come up with approaches to synthesis in the style of these scientists. This would have notable limitations; for instance, one might be that individually each chemist may have a relatively small number of publications, or that a body of work may not capture how an experienced chemist approaches a complex molecule. Perhaps collectively these virtual AI chemists could go head-to-head to solve new molecules in need of a new approach. Of course, living / modern notable chemists could also be a starting point. One could also imagine interesting scenarios in which a chemist is put alongside their AI version to test the ability of each to solve a novel synthesis. This type of approach might lead to or improve synthesis methods and could extend the natural lifespan of a chemist and retain corporate chemistry knowledge beyond their stay at the company. These efforts might also aid retrosynthesis software in general by providing multiple algorithms as alternatives. These efforts could also raise ethical or contractual issues.

There is currently great excitement that large language models like ChatGPT could be very powerful in this domain. While ChatGPT is not trained to be an expert in chemical synthesis, our examples illustrate that there is a need for caution in using such software at face value due to them being prone to hallucinations. This also points to the potential for dual use and the likely need for stronger safeguards to prevent misuse (see also Chapter 9). As they stand, it is clear the available tools described will not replace a good medicinal chemist in the immediate future, but they serve as useful tools which would aid such an individual to likely make them more productive and that is itself a valuable contribution.

ACKNOWLEDGMENTS

We kindly acknowledge Fabio Urbina, Christopher T Lowden and J Christopher Culberson whose work on MegaSyn is described here. Iktos are kindly acknowledged for providing access to Spaya AI.

FUNDING

We kindly acknowledge NIH funding from R44GM122196-02A1 from NIGMS and 1R44ES031038-01 and 1R43ES033855-01 from NIEHS for our machine learning software development and applications. "Research reported in this publication was supported by the National Institute of Environmental Health Sciences of the National Institutes of Health under Award Number R44ES031038 and 1R43ES033855-01. We also acknowledge 1R43DA055419-01 from NIDA. The content is solely the responsibility of the authors and does not necessarily represent the official views of the National Institutes of Health."

REFERENCES

1. Ekins, S.; Mestres, J.; Testa, B. In silico pharmacology for drug discovery: applications to targets and beyond. *Br J Pharmacol* **2007**, *152*, 21–37.
2. Ekins, S.; Mestres, J.; Testa, B. In silico pharmacology for drug discovery: methods for virtual ligand screening and profiling. *Br J Pharmacol* **2007**, *152*, 9–20.
3. Vignaux, P.; Minerali, E.; Foil, D. H.; Puhl, A. C.; Ekins, S. Machine learning for discovery of GSK3β inhibitors. *ACS Omega* **2020**, *5*, 26551–26561.
4. Vignaux, P. A.; Minerali, E.; Lane, T. R.; Foil, D. H.; Madrid, P. B.; Puhl, A. C.; Ekins, S. The antiviral drug tilorone is a potent and selective inhibitor of acetylcholinesterase. *Chem Res Toxicol* **2021**, *34* (5), 1296–1307. DOI:10.1021/acs.chemrestox.0c00466.
5. Klein, J. J.; Baker, N.; Foil, D. H.; Zorn, K. M.; Urbina, F.; Puhl, A. C.; Ekins, S. Using bibliometric analysis and machine learning to identify compounds binding to sialidase-1. *ACS Omega* **2021**, *6*, 3186–3193.
6. Patronov, A.; Papadopoulos, K.; Engkvist, O. Has artificial intelligence impacted drug discovery? *Methods Mol Biol* **2022**, *2390*, 153–176. DOI:10.1007/978-1-0716-1787-8_6.
7. Olivecrona, M.; Blaschke, T.; Engkvist, O.; Chen, H. Molecular de-novo design through deep reinforcement learning. *J Cheminform* **2017**, *9*(1), 48. DOI:10.1186/s13321-017-0235-x.
8. Segler, M. H. S.; Kogej, T.; Tyrchan, C.; Waller, M. P. Generating focused molecule libraries for drug discovery with recurrent neural networks. *ACS Cent Sci* **2018**, *4*(1), 120–131. DOI:10.1021/acscentsci.7b00512.
9. Meyers, J.; Fabian, B.; Brown, N. De novo molecular design and generative models. *Drug Discov Today* **2021**, *26*(11), 2707–2715. DOI:10.1016/j.drudis.2021.05.019.
10. Bhisetti, G.; Fang, C. Artificial intelligence-enabled de novo design of novel compounds that are synthesizable. *Methods Mol Biol* **2022**, *2390*, 409–419. DOI:10.1007/978-1-0716-1787-8_17.
11. Palazzesi, F.; Pozzan, A. Deep learning applied to ligand-based de novo drug design. *Methods Mol Biol* **2022**, *2390*, 273–299. DOI:10.1007/978-1-0716-1787-8_12.
12. Gomez-Bombarelli, R.; Wei, J. N.; Duvenaud, D.; Hernandez-Lobato, J. M.; Sanchez-Lengeling, B.; Sheberla, D.; Aguilera-Iparraguirre, J.; Hirzel, T. D.; Adams, R. P.; Aspuru-Guzik, A. Automatic chemical design using a data-driven continuous representation of molecules. *ACS Cent Sci* **2018**, *4*(2), 268–276. DOI:10.1021/acscentsci.7b00572.
13. Prykhodko, O.; Johansson, S. V.; Kotsias, P. C.; Arus-Pous, J.; Bjerrum, E. J.; Engkvist, O.; Chen, H. A de novo molecular generation method using latent vector based generative adversarial network. *J Cheminform* **2019**, *11*(1), 74. DOI:10.1186/s13321-019-0397-9.
14. Hochreiter, S.; Schmidhuber, J. Long short-term memory. *Neural Comput* **1997**, *9*, 1735–1780.
15. Blaschke, T.; Olivecrona, M.; Engkvist, O.; Bajorath, J.; Chen, H. Application of generative autoencoder in de novo molecular design. *Mol Inform* **2018**, *37* (1–2), 1700123. DOI:10.1002/minf.201700123.
16. Sanchez-Lengeling, B.; Outeiral, C.; Guimaraes, G. L.; Aspuru-Guzik, A. Optimizing distributions over molecular space. *An Objective-Reinforced Generative Adversarial Network for Inverse-design Chemistry (ORGANIC)*, **2017**. https://chemrxiv.org/engage/chemrxiv/article-details/60c73d91702a9beea7189bc2.
17. Winter, R.; Montanari, F.; Steffen, A.; Briem, H.; Noé, F.; Clevert, D.-A. Efficient multi-objective molecular optimization in a continuous latent space. *Chem Sci* **2019**, *10*(34), 8016–8024. DOI:10.1039/C9SC01928F.
18. Christ, C. D.; Zentgraf, M.; Kriegl, J. M. Mining electronic laboratory notebooks: analysis, retrosynthesis, and reaction based enumeration. *J Chem Inform Model* **2012**, *52*(7), 1745–1756.

19. Coley, C. W.; Barzilay, R.; Jaakkola, T. S.; Green, W. H.; Jensen, K. F. Prediction of organic reaction outcomes using machine learning. *ACS Cent Sci* **2017**, *3*(5), 434–443. DOI:10.1021/acscentsci.7b00064.
20. Proudfoot, J. R. Molecular complexity and retrosynthesis. *J Org Chem* **2017**, *82*(13), 6968–6971. DOI:10.1021/acs.joc.7b00714.
21. Cadeddu, A.; Wylie, E. K.; Jurczak, J.; Wampler-Doty, M.; Grzybowski, B. A. Organic chemistry as a language and the implications of chemical linguistics for structural and retrosynthetic analyses. *Angew Chem Int Ed Engl* **2014**, *53*(31), 8108–8112. DOI:10.1002/anie.201403708.
22. Todd, M. H. Computer-aided organic synthesis. *Chem Soc Rev* **2005**, *34*(3), 247–266. DOI:10.1039/b104620a.
23. Nair, V. H.; Schwaller, P.; Laino, T. Data-driven chemical reaction prediction and retrosynthesis. *Chimia (Aarau)* **2019**, *73*(12), 997–1000. DOI:10.2533/chimia.2019.997.
24. Warr, W. A. A short review of chemical reaction database systems, computer-aided synthesis design, reaction prediction and synthetic feasibility. *Mol Inform* **2014**, *33*(6–7), 469–476. DOI:10.1002/minf.201400052.
25. Strieth-Kalthoff, F.; Szymkuc, S.; Molga, K.; Aspuru-Guzik, A.; Glorius, F.; Grzybowski, B. A. Artificial intelligence for retrosynthetic planning needs both data and expert knowledge. *J Am Chem Soc* **2024**. DOI:10.1021/jacs.4c00338.
26. Szymkuc, S.; Gajewska, E. P.; Klucznik, T.; Molga, K.; Dittwald, P.; Startek, M.; Bajczyk, M.; Grzybowski, B. A. Computer-assisted synthetic planning: the end of the beginning. *Angew Chem Int Ed Engl* **2016**, *55*(20), 5904–5937. DOI:10.1002/anie.201506101.
27. Badowski, T.; Molga, K.; Grzybowski, B. A. Selection of cost-effective yet chemically diverse pathways from the networks of computer-generated retrosynthetic plans. *Chem Sci* **2019**, *10*(17), 4640–4651. DOI:10.1039/c8sc05611k.
28. Segler, M. H. S.; Waller, M. P. Neural-symbolic machine learning for retrosynthesis and reaction prediction. *Chemistry* **2017**, *23*(25), 5966–5971. DOI:10.1002/chem.201605499.
29. Shibukawa, R.; Ishida, S.; Yoshizoe, K.; Wasa, K.; Takasu, K.; Okuno, Y.; Terayama, K.; Tsuda, K. CompRet: a comprehensive recommendation framework for chemical synthesis planning with algorithmic enumeration. *J Cheminform* **2020**, *12*(1), 52. DOI:10.1186/s13321-020-00452-5.
30. Zheng, S.; Rao, J.; Zhang, Z.; Xu, J.; Yang, Y. Predicting retrosynthetic reactions using self-corrected transformer neural networks. *J Chem Inf Model* **2020**, *60*(1), 47–55. DOI:10.1021/acs.jcim.9b00949.
31. Lee, A. A.; Yang, Q.; Sresht, V.; Bolgar, P.; Hou, X.; Klug-McLeod, J. L.; Butler, C. R. Molecular transformer unifies reaction prediction and retrosynthesis across pharma chemical space. *Chem Commun (Camb)* **2019**, *55*(81), 12152–12155. DOI:10.1039/c9cc05122h.
32. Bai, R.; Zhang, C.; Wang, L.; Yao, C.; Ge, J.; Duan, H. Transfer learning: making retrosynthetic predictions based on a small chemical reaction dataset scale to a new level. *Molecules* **2020**, *25*(10), 2357. DOI:10.3390/molecules25102357.
33. Fukunishi, Y.; Kurosawa, T.; Mikami, Y.; Nakamura, H. Prediction of synthetic accessibility based on commercially available compound databases. *J Chem Inf Model* **2014**, *54*(12), 3259–3267. DOI:10.1021/ci500568d.
34. Genheden, S.; Thakkar, A.; Chadimova, V.; Reymond, J. L.; Engkvist, O.; Bjerrum, E. AiZynthFinder: a fast, robust and flexible open-source software for retrosynthetic planning. *J Cheminform* **2020**, *12*(1), 70. DOI:10.1186/s13321-020-00472-1.
35. Watson, I. A.; Wang, J.; Nicolaou, C. A. A retrosynthetic analysis algorithm implementation. *J Cheminform* **2019**, *11*(1), 1. DOI:10.1186/s13321-018-0323-6.
36. Ghiandoni, G. M.; Bodkin, M. J.; Chen, B.; Hristozov, D.; Wallace, J. E. A.; Webster, J.; Gillet, V. J. RENATE: a pseudo-retrosynthetic tool for synthetically accessible de novo design. *Mol Inform* **2021**, *41*, e2100207. DOI:10.1002/minf.202100207.

37. Gao, W.; Coley, C. W. The synthesizability of molecules proposed by generative models. *J Chem Inform Model* **2020**, *60*(12), 5714–5723. DOI:10.1021/acs.jcim.0c00174.
38. Kearney, S. E.; Zahoranszky-Kohalmi, G.; Brimacombe, K. R.; Henderson, M. J.; Lynch, C.; Zhao, T.; Wan, K. K.; Itkin, Z.; Dillon, C.; Shen, M., et al. Canvass: a crowd-sourced, natural-product screening library for exploring biological space. *ACS Cent Sci* **2018**, *4*(12), 1727–1741. DOI:10.1021/acscentsci.8b00747.
39. Anon. *eMolecules*. **2020**. https://www.emolecules.com/info/plus/download-database.
40. Anon. *ChEMBL*. **2020**. https://chembl.gitbook.io/chembl-interface-documentation/downloads.
41. Sheridan, R. P.; Hunt, P.; Culberson, J. C. Molecular transformations as a way of finding and exploiting consistent local QSAR. *J Chem Inform Model* **2006**, *46*(1), 180–192. DOI:10.1021/ci0503208.
42. Hartenfeller, M.; Eberle, M.; Meier, P.; Nieto-Oberhuber, C.; Altmann, K. H.; Schneider, G.; Jacoby, E.; Renner, S. A collection of robust organic synthesis reactions for in silico molecule design. *J Chem Inf Model* **2011**, *51*(12), 3093–3098. DOI:10.1021/ci200379p.
43. Durrant, J. D.; Lindert, S.; McCammon, J. A. AutoGrow 3.0: an improved algorithm for chemically tractable, semi-automated protein inhibitor design. *J Mol Graphics Model* **2013**, *44*, 104–112. DOI:10.1016/j.jmgm.2013.05.006.
44. Clark, A. M.; Dole, K.; Coulon-Spector, A.; McNutt, A.; Grass, G.; Freundlich, J. S.; Reynolds, R. C.; Ekins, S. Open source bayesian models: 1. Application to ADME/Tox and drug discovery datasets. *J Chem Inf Model* **2015**, *55*, 1231–1245. DOI:10.1021/acs.jcim.5b00143.
45. Warr, W. A. Scientific workflow systems: Pipeline Pilot and KNIME. *J Comput Aided Mol Des* **2012**, *26*(7), 801–804. DOI:10.1007/s10822-012-9577-7.
46. Saubern, S.; Guha, R.; Baell, J. B. KNIME workflow to assess PAINS filters in SMARTS format. Comparison of RDKit and Indigo cheminformatics libraries. *Mol Inform* **2011**, *30*(10), 847–850. DOI:10.1002/minf.201100076.
47. Parrot, M.; Tajmouati, H.; da Silva, V. B. R.; Atwood, B. R.; Fourcade, R.; Gaston-Mathe, Y.; Do Huu, N.; Perron, Q. Integrating synthetic accessibility with AI-based generative drug design. *J Cheminform* **2023**, *15*(1), 83. DOI:10.1186/s13321-023-00742-8.
48. Anastas, P. T.; Warner, J. C. *Green Chemistry: Theory and Practice*, Oxford University Press Inc., **1998**. https://books.google.com/books/about/Green_Chemistry.html?id=SrO8QgAACAAJ
49. Ekins, S.; Clark, A. M.; Williams, A. J. Incorporating green chemistry concepts into mobile chemistry applications and their potential uses. *ACS Sustain Chem Eng* **2013**, *1*, 8–13.
50. Choung, O.-H.; Vianello, R.; Segler, M.; Stiefl, S.; Jimenez-Luna, J. Learning chemical intuition from humans in the loop. *ChemRxiv* **2023**. DOI:10.26434/chemrxiv-2023-knwnv-v2. https://chemrxiv.org/engage/chemrxiv/article-details/63f89282897b18336f0c5a55

6 MegaSyn for Generative Molecule Design

Joshua S. Harris, Fabio Urbina, and Sean Ekins

6.1 INTRODUCTION

Every year, there are numerous business deals between pharmaceutical companies in which generally larger companies in-license assets from smaller companies (or buy them outright) to access their small molecules or a pipeline of molecules (Table 6.1). In most cases, these molecules have reached the clinic or are approaching clinical trials. Some of these deals range from tens of millions to billions of dollars. Interestingly, in most cases, they are for targets for which there is a considerable amount of publicly available data (Table 6.1). This data availability could enable other companies to follow up and generate analogs of the compounds themselves. Technologies to enable fast followers of such companies could have value by allowing them to generate preclinical assets in a rapid manner. One such approach may be to use generative approaches to identify new molecules for well-validated targets where there is plentiful preclinical data available.

In recent years, generative models (see Chapter one) have increasingly been utilized to produce drug-like molecules *de novo*[1–5] with several different algorithm architectures (e.g. Recurrent Neural Networks,[2] Variational Autoencoders[6] and Generative Adversarial Networks[7]). These on the whole generate valid, novel molecules with desirable physicochemical properties[8–11] using SMILES, SELFIES, or other molecular representations as inputs.[12,13] A single generative design process likely will not work for all scenarios, however, and this suggests there is still a degree of trial and error insofar as to which tools and algorithms may have utility for different applications.

We recently described our own generative design software MegaSyn[14,15], which is a generative neural network with a long short-term memory (LSTM) architecture characterized by the number of layers and the size of the hidden state (Figure 6.1). MegaSyn is designed to generate sequences of tokens which can be decoded as SMILES string representations of molecules, by drawing from a learned probability distribution over possible token. Previously, we have described a training algorithm which involves training an ensemble of MegaSyn models to strike a balance between diversity and target optimization.[14] In the original algorithm, first a "prior model" is pre-trained on a large druglike dataset. This prior model is then "primed" to generate molecules in a specific chemical space by training it on molecules of interest as well as fragments of those molecules, and primed models are saved after every i training epoch. Each primed model is then trained via a hill-climb optimization process (training on top-scoring generated compounds) multiple times to create the

 DOI: 10.1201/9781003399346-9

TABLE 6.1
Company Deals in 2023 for Small Molecule Assets

Company	Buyer	Deal Value	Drug Target	Molecule
Karuna	BMS	$14B	Xanomeline with trospium to preserve the central nervous system agonism observed with xanomeline or the M1 and M4 receptor agonist	Xanomeline and trospium
Rain Oncology	Pathos AI	$5M	Milademetan, is a small molecule, oral inhibitor of the p53-MDM2 complex that reactivates p53 https://www.ebi.ac.uk/chembl/target_report_card/CHEMBL1907611/	Milademetan
Cerevel	Abbvie	$8.7B	The muscarinic M4 selective positive allosteric modulator emraclidine https://www.ebi.ac.uk/chembl/target_report_card/CHEMBL1821/	Emraclidine
Mitokinin	Abbvie	$110M	A PINK1 activator meant to correct mitochondrial dysfunction https://www.ebi.ac.uk/chembl/target_report_card/CHEMBL3337330/	Not described
Acer Therapeutics	Zevra Therapeutics	$91M	For urea cycle disorder	Olpruva – sodium phenylbutyrate
Mindset Pharma	Otsuka Pharmaceutical	$80M Canadian	Next-generation psychedelic and non-psychedelic medications for treating neuropsychiatric and neurological disorders	Psilocybins

(Continued)

TABLE 6.1 (*Continued*)
Company Deals in 2023 for Small Molecule Assets

Company	Buyer	Deal Value	Drug Target	Molecule
Embark Biotech	Novo Nordisk	$16M	Developing agonists of EMB1, a previously undescribed adipocyte G-protein coupled receptor GPR3, a constitutively active G-protein coupled receptor that is an important regulator of thermogenic adipose activity https://www.ebi.ac.uk/chembl/target_report_card/CHEMBL4523856/	
Small Pharma	Cybin	Unknown	DMT-based therapy to treat major depressive disorder	DMT – SPL-026- a psilocybin analog
Qpex Biopharma	Shionogi	$100M	β-lactamase inhibitor, which is being advanced clinically in both IV and oral[2] combinations for infections caused by drug-resistant Gram-negative bacteria	Xeruborbactam
Chinook Therapeutics	Novartis	$3.2B	An oral endothelin A receptor antagonist https://www.ebi.ac.uk/chembl/target_report_card/CHEMBL2096678/	Atrasentan
Reunion Neuroscience	MPM BioImpact	$13M	Postpartum depression	Psychedelic compound RE104
VectiveBio	Ironwood	$1B	GLP-2 analog for irritable bowel https://www.ebi.ac.uk/chembl/target_report_card/CHEMBL5844/	Apraglutide

(*Continued*)

TABLE 6.1 (*Continued*)
Company Deals in 2023 for Small Molecule Assets

Company	Buyer	Deal Value	Drug Target	Molecule
Varian Biopharma	Biodexa Pharma	Unknown	A typical protein kinase C iota ("aPKCi") inhibitor with best-in-class potential as a treatment for various oncology indications with an initial focus on basal cell carcinoma (BCC) https://www.ebi.ac.uk/chembl/target_report_card/CHEMBL2598/	VAR-101/102
xinThera	Gilead	Unknown	PARP1 and MK2 inhibitor https://www.ebi.ac.uk/chembl/target_report_card/CHEMBL3105/; https://www.ebi.ac.uk/chembl/target_report_card/CHEMBL2208/	XinThera lists five preclinical candidates in its pipeline: XIN5104 and XIN5789 for HRD+ solid tumors. XIN6301 lists the same indications plus brain tumors. The biotech's MK2 immunology program has XIN5494 and XIN5404 for various autoimmune conditions including rheumatoid arthritis
Bellus Health	GSK	$2B	Antagonists of P2X3, a peripheral nervous system receptor that triggers neuronal hypersensitization and is linked to the urge to cough https://www.ebi.ac.uk/chembl/target_report_card/CHEMBL2998/	Camlipixant

(Continued)

TABLE 6.1 (*Continued*)
Company Deals in 2023 for Small Molecule Assets

Company	Buyer	Deal Value	Drug Target	Molecule
Diffusion	EIP Pharma	Unknown	p38 MAP kinase alpha enzyme inhibitor https://www.ebi.ac.uk/chembl/target_report_card/CHEMBL260/	Neflamapimod
Jounce Thera	Concentra Bio	$97.4M	ROCK2 inhibitor https://www.ebi.ac.uk/chembl/target_report_card/CHEMBL2973/	RXC007
Concert Pharma	Sun Pharma	$576M	Jak1 and 2 inhibitor https://www.ebi.ac.uk/chembl/target_report_card/CHEMBL2835/; https://www.ebi.ac.uk/chembl/target_report_card/CHEMBL2971/	Deuruxolitinib
Cincor Pharma	AstraZeneca	$1.8B	Aldosterone synthase inhibitor in uncontrolled hypertension https://www.ebi.ac.uk/chembl/target_report_card/CHEMBL2722/	Baxdrostat

These were focused on small molecules for which many are for validated targets with substantial *in vitro* data in public databases such as ChEMBL.

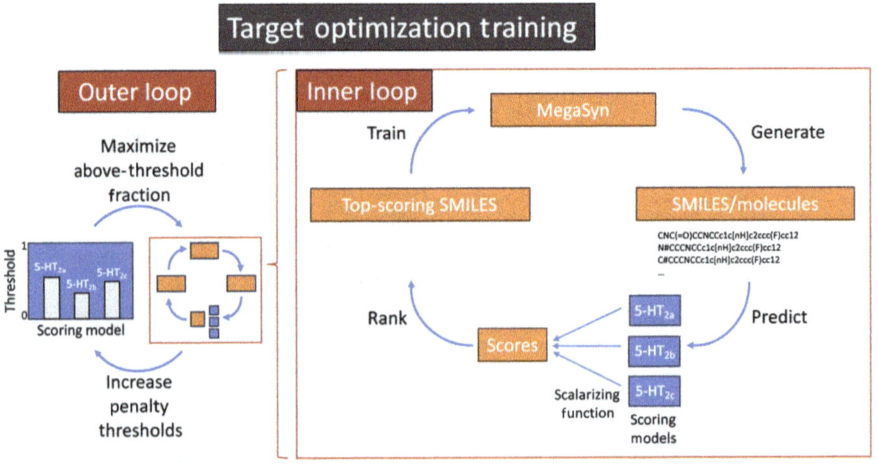

FIGURE 6.1 Schematic representation of the MegaSyn target optimization training, consisting of nested training loops.

final ensemble of MegaSyn models. Here, we describe a new MegaSyn training algorithm which allows a MegaSyn model to learn to generate molecules which satisfy an arbitrary set of multitarget optimization goals. For instance, we may be interested in generating soluble molecules which selectively activate a specific protein receptor without activating a set of other receptors. Under the new algorithm, training proceeds until specified goal scores are met for each target; by contrast, under the original algorithm, training proceeds by optimizing a composite score for a specified number of epochs.

6.2 MEGASYN

6.2.1 MegaSyn Version 1

We have previously introduced MegaSyn[14,15] representing a hill-climb algorithm which makes use of SMILES-based LSTM generative models, structural analog generation software, and retrosynthetic analysis coupled with fragment analysis to score molecules for their synthetic feasibility. We demonstrated that deconstructing targeted molecules and focusing on sub-structures, combined with an ensemble of generative models, enabled MegaSyn to generally perform well at generating new scaffolds and targeted analogs which are likely synthesizable and drug-like with good, predicted bioactivity. We also described the development, benchmarking, and testing of MegaSyn, and suggested how it could be used in several test cases.[14,15]

6.2.2 MegaSyn Version 2

Several concepts have been covered by the original training algorithm. For instance, MegaSyn training falls into three categories: prior model training, priming, and target optimization. However, we have made improvements in every training category. We will discuss each of these three training modes in the following sections.

6.2.2.1 Prior Model

As with any LSTM network, MegaSyn learns by training on sequences of tokens. An untrained MegaSyn model with randomly initiated weights will generate random sequences of tokens with no real connection to molecules. But by training on a set of valid SMILES sequences, a MegaSyn model will learn to generate SMILES like the molecules in the training set. Before a MegaSyn model can be trained on a specific set of target goals, it must learn to generate a broad distribution of valid SMILES strings representing realistic molecules. We call this generic MegaSyn model, trained on a broad distribution of molecules, a "prior model." A good prior model only needs to be trained once as a generic starting point for further training and then can be reused in many different contexts.

Prior model training requires a large set of SMILES sequences representing a diverse set of molecules. To enable this, we downloaded the entire library of SMILES strings from the ChEMBL 31 database.[16] We curated the ChEMBL 31 SMILES library by removing nonparent molecules (salts and solvents), neutralizing charges, standardizing isotopes, and removing molecules with rare or undesirable elements (e.g. heavy metals) using RDKit, an open-source cheminformatics software package.[17]

After standardizing the SMILES strings, we removed duplicates and generated a minimal vocabulary of tokens representing indivisible parts of a SMILES sequence. By limiting the vocabulary of tokens to those included in the fully curated ChEMBL 31 SMILES library, we also ensured that MegaSyn cannot generate molecules with undesirable elements (e.g. heavy metals, nonstandard isotopes). However, if a model is required to generate such molecules, a new prior model with a more expansive token vocabulary can readily be trained.

To allow batching of training samples, all sequences are fixed to a particular length (we used 190). Any training sequence, or any sequence generated by MegaSyn, consists of a start token (indicating the start of the sequence), a series of tokens representing modular substrings of a SMILES string, and an end token (representing the end of the sequence) followed by a series of padding tokens to fill out the rest of the sequence. SMILES strings and token sequences are easily interconverted by a one-to-one mapping. Note that the fixed length of token sequences effectively imposes an upper limit on the size of generated molecules and molecules used for training. SMILES strings whose tokenized representation exceeds the sequence length cannot be generated or tokenized.

For each epoch of training, we draw a large random sample (100,000 molecules) from the curated ChEMBL 31 SMILES library. After shuffling the sample set, individual samples are drawn one at a time without replacement. Each sample must pass a "validity check" for inclusion in the training set. A SMILES sequence is considered invalid if RDKit cannot convert it into a molecule (RDKit mol object) if its tokenized sequence length exceeds the fixed sequence length of the model, or if it contains any free radicals. Finally, RDKit is used to generate a random augmentation of each SMILES sequence prior to tokenization. SMILES sequences are not unique: a given molecule may have several equivalent SMILES representations (e.g. the sequence may begin with a token representing any atom in the molecule). Using augmentations (randomized equivalent SMILES sequences) during training ensures that MegaSyn learns how to put together valid SMILES sequences according to the most generic rules, rather than learning how to put together certain subsets of SMILES sequences (e.g. canonical SMILES); this provides a richer distribution of token probabilities for further training. Each training epoch consists of training the MegaSyn model on every molecule from the random sample in batches. We use a batch size of 200 molecules, an Adam optimizer with a learning rate of 0.002, and a dropout rate of 0.2.[18] We use gradient clipping to prevent exploding gradients.[19] For the loss function; we compute cross-entropy loss between subsequent token distributions and the training sample token over all tokens in the batch. We also add a loss term proportional to the entropy of the token probability distribution (self-entropy; discussed below).

Prior to each training epoch, a random sample (1,000 samples) is generated by the MegaSyn model, which is used to estimate the validity and diversity of generated samples. We define the validity V_ϵ of a sample generated for epoch ϵ as the fraction of valid SMILES strings in the sample:

$$V_\epsilon = \frac{N_{\text{valid}}}{N}$$

where N is the generated sample size and N_{valid} is the number of valid generated samples (i.e. those that pass the validity check described above). We define diversity D_ϵ of a sample generated for epoch ϵ as the fraction of valid molecule pairs that are dissimilar to each other (excluding self-similarity):

$$D_\epsilon = \frac{1}{N_{\text{valid}}^2 - N_{\text{valid}}} \sum_{i,j \neq i} \left(1 - S_{ij}\right)$$

where

$$S_{ij} = \begin{cases} 1, & s_{ij} > s' \\ 0, & s_{ij} < s' \end{cases}$$

where s_{ij} is the Tanimoto similarity between MACCS keys generated for the molecules and s' is an arbitrary cutoff (we used 0.65). This diversity score ranges between zero (similarity of every molecule pair is above the cutoff) to one (similarity of every molecule pair is below the cutoff). It should be noted that other molecular fingerprint type descriptors could be used and each may have its own pros and cons.

The validity and diversity of the generated sample are used to scale the self-entropy contribution to the loss computed for a given epoch. As noted above, the loss L_i for epoch i includes a cross-entropy term H_{cross} and a self-entropy term H_{self}.

$$L_i = H_{\text{cross}} - \alpha_i \left(H_{\text{self}}\right)$$

where α_i is a scaling factor that depends on the validity and diversity of the sample generated before each training epoch:

$$\alpha_i = (\mu)\alpha_{i-1} + (1-\mu)\alpha' V_\epsilon (1 - D_\epsilon)$$

where α' is a constant factor that effectively limits the maximum contribution of the self-entropy term (we used 0.15) and μ is a smoothing parameter which effectively smooths out the change in α_i from epoch to epoch (similar to a momentum parameter in gradient descent algorithms; we used 0.5). The self-entropy loss term is a way of injecting diversity into the token probability distribution since it penalizes distributions with low entropy. However, it also tends to reduce the validity of generated samples because it encourages more uncertainty in the generated sequences. Scaling the self-entropy loss contribution by $V_\epsilon(1 - D_\epsilon)$ in each epoch is a way of mitigating between these outcomes: when diversity is low, the self-entropy contribution becomes more significant, but when validity is low, the self-entropy contribution becomes smaller. This promotes diversity in the generated samples without adversely affecting validity.

Validity is also used as the stopping criterion for prior model training. Validity is tracked between epochs with a smoothing parameter. Training continues if the smoothed validity continues to increase. If the smoothed validity decreases after a given epoch, training halts, and the prior model is considered ready for further use.

6.2.2.2 Priming: Generating Optimal Molecules from a Target Chemical Space

For many generative drug design applications, we may be interested in molecules in a specific chemical space (e.g., analogues of a certain structure or molecules with a specific set of scaffolds). In this case, we can train a MegaSyn model on a certain molecule or set of molecules (dubbed "priming molecules"), so that its generated sample distribution is focused into the desired chemical space. We call this training process "priming" the model.

During each epoch of priming, the model is trained a specified number of times on random SMILES augmentations of the priming molecules. After training, a random sample is generated by the model, and the generated molecules are scored based on a set of scoring models. The fraction of generated samples with scores above a specified goal score ("goal fraction") is computed and tracked between epochs with a smoothing parameter. Training continues until the smoothed goal fraction decreases or exceeds a specified value in each epoch.

For instance, suppose we want to prime a model so that most of its generated samples are similar to a particular molecule (say, tryptamine). In this case, we would prime the model by training on random augmentations of the tryptamine SMILES sequence. In each epoch, we generate random samples and score them based on similarity to tryptamine, keeping track of the fraction of generated samples with similarity above a cutoff (say 0.75). If we set the goal fraction to 0.9, priming will continue until 90 percent of generated samples score above 0.75. Thus, after priming, 90% of the generated samples are similar to tryptamine.

In many applications, we may not be interested in a specific molecule as much as a specific scaffold, perhaps with particular atomic substitutions and attachment points for side groups. For this purpose, we allow the specification of atomic substitutions and side group attachment points via wildcards in the SMILES representation of the priming molecule(s). Atomic substitution wildcards are replaced by a random element based on a specified probability distribution. Side groups are randomly selected from a library of possible side groups and attached with a probability based on the number of desired side groups on the molecule. Selection probability depends on the frequency of occurrence of the side group in the library, the molecular weight relative to the scaffold, and the number of rings relative to the scaffold (lower molecular weight and fewer rings are probabilistically favored).

The library of side groups was generated from the ChEMBL 31 dataset by fragmenting every SMILES according to BRICS rules[20] and keeping all fragments with exactly one attachment point. Duplicate fragments are kept in the library to mimic the frequency of side group representation in the ChEMBL dataset (thus making common side groups more likely to be selected for attachment to a priming scaffold).

After element substitution and side group attachment, priming molecules must pass a validity check and will be probabilistically discarded based on a QED score[21] and synthetic accessibility score.[22] This process is repeated every time a priming molecule is required for training. Scoring models for priming must be selected based on the desired characteristics of the generated sample distribution for the primed model. In random-side group priming, a typical scoring model might be a simple substructure match for the scaffold based on a SMARTS representation.[23]

6.2.2.3 Target Optimization Training

With target optimization training, we can define a set of goals or property targets for MegaSyn to achieve, and the training will optimize a MegaSyn model's generative distribution to maximize the fraction of generated molecules that achieve every goal simultaneously (e.g. high solubility, high activity on a protein target, and high specificity). Target optimization training can be performed on any MegaSyn model, including a prior model or a model that has been primed to generate molecules with a specific scaffold. Figure 6.1 shows a schematic representation of the target optimization training algorithm, described below.

We begin with a pre-trained MegaSyn model (this can be a prior model or a primed model), a set of scoring models, and a goal score for each scoring model. A scoring model can assign a number between 0 and 1 to a molecule (e.g., a QED score, a predictive model, or similarity to a reference molecule). For example, we can also use a regression model as a scoring model if we map the output to the range (0, 1) during training. For MegaSyn training purposes, scores are defined such that 1 is the most desirable score, and 0 is the least desirable score. Each scoring model is also assigned a threshold score, such that a molecule scoring below the threshold is either penalized or reassigned a score of 0.

Training consists of an inner loop and an outer loop. In each outer loop iteration, scoring model thresholds are increased by small, randomized increments, and then the inner loop is performed. In each inner loop iteration, samples are generated by MegaSyn and scored by the scoring models. The fraction of samples scoring above all scoring model thresholds is computed and tracked with a smoothing parameter. The scores are combined into a total score for each molecule via a weighted scalarizing function (e.g., weighted arithmetic mean, weighted geometric mean, weighted norm), and the generated molecules are ranked by their total score. The weights used in the scalarizing function are generated dynamically based on the fraction of samples that exceed the goal score for each scoring model (such that scoring models with fewer samples above the goal score are weighted more heavily). The top-scoring molecules (e.g., top 20%) are then used to train the MegaSyn model and are carried over into the next iteration of the inner loop, where they are appended to the MegaSyn sample generated for the next iteration. Since below-threshold scores are penalized (or set to zero), the ranking favors molecules that score above thresholds for all models. The inner loop continues to run until the (smoothed) fraction of generated samples scoring above all scoring model thresholds decreases (i.e., the fraction of above-threshold samples is maximized by the inner loop).

The outer loop continues to run as long as the fraction of above-threshold samples either increases or stays above a minimum value (we used 0.2). The outer loop will either stop prematurely (if the fraction of above-threshold samples cannot be increased), or it will successfully end if all scoring model thresholds are increased to the goal scores.

This algorithm ensures that the trained MegaSyn model generates an optimal fraction of samples that exceed the goal scores for all scoring models. For instance, if a MegaSyn model is trained to optimize QED score[21] with a goal of 0.5 and the inner loop successfully increases the fraction of above-threshold samples to 0.9 when the threshold has reached the goal, then 90% of a random sample is expected to have a QED score above 0.5. If multiple goal scores are reached, then an optimal fraction of samples are guaranteed to score above the goal scores for every scoring model simultaneously.

Once a MegaSyn model is trained, it can be saved and sampled indefinitely. Samples from the trained model can be scored and ranked in arbitrary ways so that the same model can be utilized for a variety of purposes. Since the training process is stochastic (the scoring model thresholds are increased by randomized increments, and the training is based on randomly generated samples), multiple MegaSyn models can be trained via this algorithm to expand the distribution of generated samples to a broader chemical space.

6.2.2.4 Results of Prior Model

Our prior model was trained on our curated SMILES dataset taken from the ChEMBL 31 database, as described above. We trained MegaSyn models with six different LSTM architectures (3, 4, or 5 layers, with 512 or 1,024 nodes per layer), to discern which architecture would be most suitable for our purposes. A good prior model should generate valid molecules from a broad and realistic distribution. To this end, we used the validity V_ϵ (fraction of valid molecules in a randomly generated sample) as a metric for comparing different prior models, and we also checked the generated distributions by comparing them to the curated ChEMBL 31 dataset.

Figure 6.2 shows the (smoothed) validity as a function of training epoch for each prior model architecture. With enough training, the sample validity stabilizes to around 0.7 for all architectures, so the most important practical difference between architectures is how long they take to train. Increasing the number of layers increases the number of training epochs required to stabilize the validity. Increasing the number of nodes (or neurons) per layer reduces the number of epochs required for training and slightly improves the validity of the fully trained prior model; however, using 1,024 nodes instead of 512 requires significantly more GPU memory and takes much longer to train per epoch. Given the added computational cost and the fact that the validity of the fully trained models is comparable, we decided that the most suitable architecture for our MegaSyn models is 3 layers with 512 nodes per layer.

Figure 6.3 represents a t-SNE plot (with distances based on Tanimoto similarity of ECFP6 fingerprints) showing the distribution of molecules generated by the fully trained MegaSyn prior model (3 layers, 512 nodes per layer) together with a random sample of molecules drawn from the curated ChEMBL 31 dataset (with identical sample sizes). The t-SNE plot clearly shows that the distribution generated by MegaSyn occupies the same molecular feature space as the distribution drawn from the ChEMBL 31 dataset.

Taken together, Figures 6.2 and 6.3 demonstrate that the MegaSyn prior model with three layers and five nodes per layer can generate valid molecules from a broad and realistic distribution, which was our goal. Specifically, the distribution of samples generated by our prior model mimics the distribution of the ChEMBL 31 dataset on which it was trained. In principle, any dataset can be used for the training of a MegaSyn prior model.

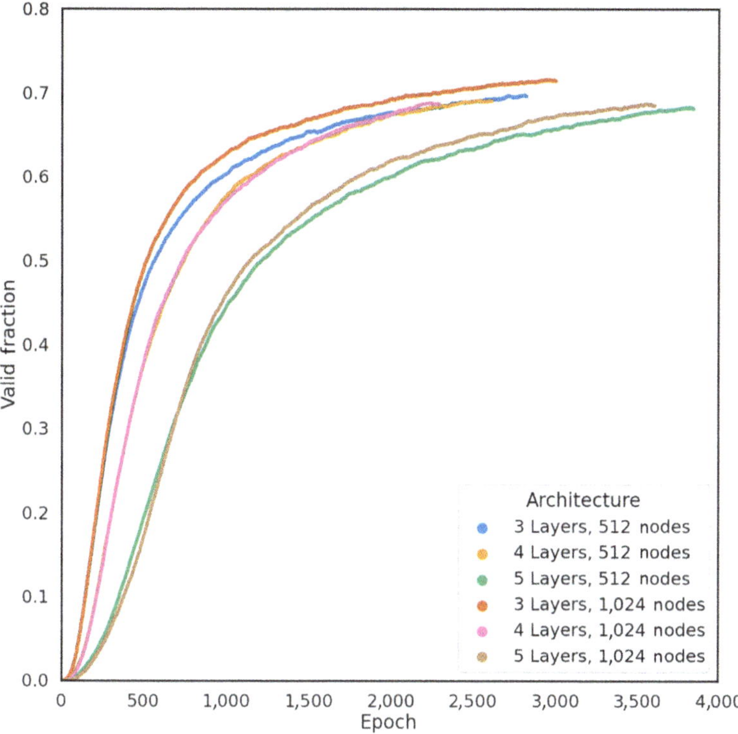

FIGURE 6.2 Valid fraction versus Epoch for different MegaSyn LSTM architectures.

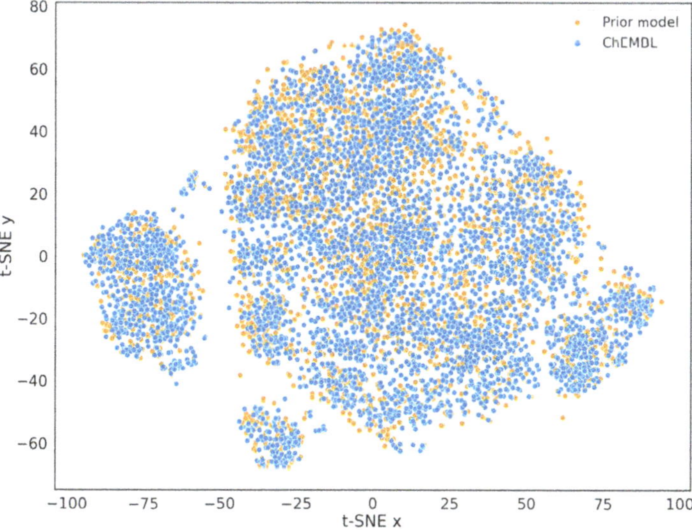

FIGURE 6.3 t-SNE plot of a random sample from the ChEMBL 31 dataset and a random sample generated by the MegaSyn prior model, with distances based on Tanimoto similarity. The distribution of generated samples mimics the distribution of the dataset on which the generative model was trained.

6.3 EXAMPLE APPLICATION OF MEGASYN

As an example of an application of MegaSyn, we addressed vasopressin receptor antagonists (V1A, V1B, and V2) which have a range of functions.[24] For example, the V1A and V2 receptors are expressed peripherally, where they modulate blood pressure and kidney function, respectively. V1A and V1B are expressed in the central nervous system, and in particular, V1A is expressed in many regions of the brain and may be linked to the control of social behavior. Interestingly, the drug tolvaptan (V1A and V2 antagonist[24]) (Figure 6.4a) was predicted to have a relatively poor blood-brain barrier (BBB) score (Figure 6.4b) using a random forest machine

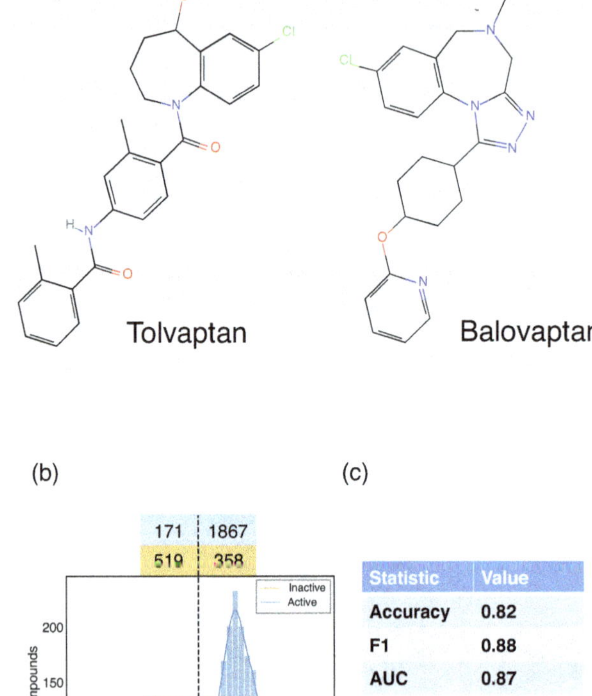

Statistic	Value
Accuracy	0.82
F1	0.88
AUC	0.87
Cohen's k	0.54
MCC	0.55
Precision	0.84
Recall	0.92
Specificity	0.59

FIGURE 6.4 (a) Structures of tolvaptan and balovaptan, (b) Histogram of 2,915 molecules curated from 6 published datasets in training set for the BBB model, with predicted scores for tolvaptan and balovaptan, (c). Fivefold cross-validation statistics for the BBB model (random forest, FCFP6 fingerprints).

learning model (Figure 6.4c). In contrast, a clinical trial candidate molecule from Roche, balovaptan, has an improved BBB score and has been used in the clinic for autism.[25] We generated machine learning models for V1A and V2 IC_{50} (Figure 6.5) and trained MegaSyn to optimize V1A, V2, BBB score, and tolvaptan similarity. The trained MegaSyn model was able to generate structurally diverse tolvaptan analogs with improved BBB scores (Figure 6.6). There are likely many other examples of approved drugs that do not cross the BBB, but which could be modified to have CNS effects, which may be therapeutically useful. For example, we have previously illustrated how the kinase inhibitor lapatinib could be used to design analogs in order to improve BBB access using MegaSyn.[14]

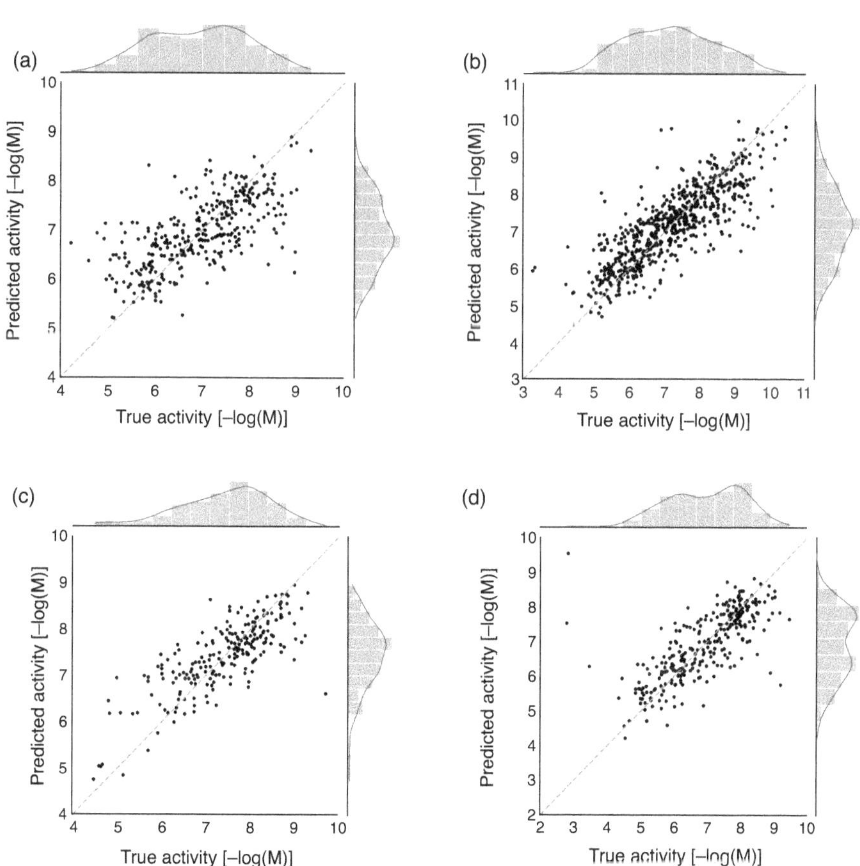

FIGURE 6.5 Fivefold cross-validation results for support vector regression models for vasopressin antagonists using FCFP6 fingerprints and data from ChEMBL. (a) V1A IC_{50}, 326 molecules, MAE 0.57, (b) V1A K_i 607 molecules, MAE 0.55, C. V2 IC_{50} 223 molecules MAE 0.48, (d) V2 K_i 289 molecules MAE 0.54.

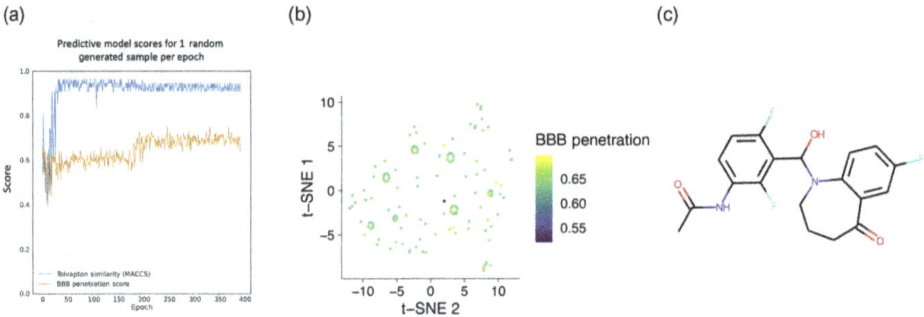

FIGURE 6.6 An example of using MegaSyn to generate vasopressin antagonists with improved BBB properties. (a) Predicted model scores for tolvapatan analogues generated with MegaSyn, (b) t-SNE plot of selected tolvaptan analogs and their predicted BBB scores. (c) An example molecule was generated with predicted improved BBB score.

6.4 SUMMARY

We have briefly described our recent updates to MegaSyn, which builds on an earlier version of the software as well as case studies.[14,15,26] We have also provided numerous examples of recent pharmaceutical deals for small molecules (Table 6.1), for most of which there exist public datasets (with substantial structure-activity relationship data) that could, in turn, be used to build machine learning models for integration into generative drug design approaches to enable scoring designed molecules. Using such generative approaches to drug design may enable the development of more selective molecules or those with improved ADME/Tox properties (such as the ability to cross the BBB, improved metabolic stability, reduced risk of hERG, etc.). This would spur the rapid creation of new molecules and intellectual property for licensing or building out a pharmaceutical company pipeline.

ACKNOWLEDGMENTS

We kindly acknowledge Dr. Thomas Lane for assistance with the BBB model.

FUNDING

We kindly acknowledge NIH funding from R44GM122196-02A1 from NIGMS and 1R44ES031038-01 and 1R43ES033855-01 from NIEHS for our machine learning software development and applications. "Research reported in this publication was supported by the National Institute of Environmental Health Sciences of the National Institutes of Health under Award Number R44ES031038 and 1R43ES033855-01. We also acknowledge 1R43DA055419-01 from NIDA. The content is solely the responsibility of the authors and does not necessarily represent the official views of the National Institutes of Health."

REFERENCES

1. Olivecrona, M.; Blaschke, T.; Engkvist, O.; Chen, H. Molecular de-novo design through deep reinforcement learning. *J Cheminform* **2017**, *9* (1), 48. DOI:10.1186/s13321-017-0235-x.
2. Segler, M. H. S.; Kogej, T.; Tyrchan, C.; Waller, M. P. Generating focused molecule libraries for drug discovery with recurrent neural networks. *ACS Cent Sci* **2018**, *4* (1), 120–131. DOI:10.1021/acscentsci.7b00512.
3. Meyers, J.; Fabian, B.; Brown, N. De novo molecular design and generative models. *Drug Discov Today* **2021**, *26* (11), 2707–2715. DOI:10.1016/j.drudis.2021.05.019.
4. Bhisetti, G.; Fang, C. Artificial intelligence-enabled de novo design of novel compounds that are synthesizable. *Methods Mol Biol* **2022**, *2390*, 409–419. DOI:10.1007/978-1-0716-1787-8_17.
5. Palazzesi, F.; Pozzan, A. Deep learning applied to ligand-based de novo drug design. *Methods Mol Biol* **2022**, *2390*, 273–299. DOI:10.1007/978-1-0716-1787-8_12.
6. Gomez-Bombarelli, R.; Wei, J. N.; Duvenaud, D.; Hernandez-Lobato, J. M.; Sanchez-Lengeling, B.; Sheberla, D.; Aguilera-Iparraguirre, J.; Hirzel, T. D.; Adams, R. P.; Aspuru-Guzik, A. Automatic chemical design using a data-driven continuous representation of molecules. *ACS Cent Sci* **2018**, *4* (2), 268–276. DOI:10.1021/acscentsci.7b00572.
7. Prykhodko, O.; Johansson, S. V.; Kotsias, P. C.; Arus-Pous, J.; Bjerrum, E. J.; Engkvist, O.; Chen, H. A de novo molecular generation method using latent vector based generative adversarial network. *J Cheminform* **2019**, *11* (1), 74. DOI:10.1186/s13321-019-0397-9.
8. Hochreiter, S.; Schmidhuber, J. Long short-term memory. *Neural Comput* **1997**, *9*, 1735–1780.
9. Blaschke, T.; Olivecrona, M.; Engkvist, O.; Bajorath, J.; Chen, H. Application of generative autoencoder in de novo molecular design. *Mol Inform* **2018**, *37* (1–2), 1700123. DOI:10.1002/minf.201700123.
10. Sanchez-Lengeling, B.; Outeiral, C.; Guimaraes, G. L.; Aspuru-Guzik, A. *Optimizing Distributions over Molecular Space. An Objective-Reinforced Generative Adversarial Network for Inverse-design Chemistry (ORGANIC)*. 2017. https://chemrxiv.org/engage/chemrxiv/article-details/60c73d91702a9beea7189bc2.
11. Winter, R.; Montanari, F.; Steffen, A.; Briem, H.; Noé, F.; Clevert, D.-A. Efficient multi-objective molecular optimization in a continuous latent space. *Chem Sci* **2019**, *10* (34), 8016–8024. DOI:10.1039/C9SC01928F.
12. Krenn, M.; Häse, F.; Nigam, A.; Friederich, P.; Aspuru-Guzik, A. Self-referencing embedded strings (SELFIES): A 100% robust molecular string representation. *Mach Learning: Sci Technol* **2020**, *1* (4), 045024. DOI:10.1088/2632-2153/aba947.
13. Jin, W.; Barzilay, R.; Jaakola, T. *Junction Tree Variational Autoencoder for Molecular Graph Generation*. 2019. https://arxiv.org/pdf/1802.04364.pdf.
14. Urbina, F.; Lowden, C. T.; Culberson, J. C.; Ekins, S. MegaSyn: Integrating generative molecular design, automated analog designer, and synthetic viability prediction. *ACS Omega* **2022**, *7* (22), 18699–18713. DOI:10.1021/acsomega.2c01404.
15. Urbina, F.; Lentzos, F.; Invernizzi, C.; Ekins, S. A teachable moment for dual-use. *Nat Mach Intell* **2022**, *4* (7), 607. DOI:10.1038/s42256-022-00511-6.
16. Gaulton, A.; Hersey, A.; Nowotka, M.; Bento, A. P.; Chambers, J.; Mendez, D.; Mutowo, P.; Atkinson, F.; Bellis, L. J.; Cibrian-Uhalte, E.; et al. The ChEMBL database in 2017. *Nucleic Acids Res* **2017**, *45* (D1), D945–D954. DOI:10.1093/nar/gkw1074.
17. Anon. *RDKit: Open-Source Cheminformatics Software*. www.rdkit.org.
18. Kingma, D. P.; Ba, J. Adam: A method for stochastic optimization. 2014; arXiv:1412.6980.
19. Zhang, J.; He, T.; Sra, S.; Jadbabaie, A. Why gradient clipping accelerates training: A theoretical justification for adaptivity. 2019; arXiv:1905.11881.

20. Degen, J.; Wegscheid-Gerlach, C.; Zaliani, A.; Rarey, M. On the art of compiling and using 'drug-like' chemical fragment spaces. *ChemMedChem* **2008**, *3* (10), 1503–1507. DOI:10.1002/cmdc.200800178.
21. Bickerton, G. R.; Paolini, G. V.; Besnard, J.; Muresan, S.; Hopkins, A. L. Quantifying the chemical beauty of drugs. *Nat Chem* **2012**, *4* (2), 90–98. DOI:10.1038/nchem.1243.
22. Ertl, P.; Schuffenhauer, A. Estimation of synthetic accessibility score of drug-like molecules based on molecular complexity and fragment contributions. *J Cheminform* **2009**, *1* (1), 8. DOI:10.1186/1758-2946-1-8.
23. Saubern, S.; Guha, R.; Baell, J. B. KNIME workflow to assess PAINS filters in SMARTS format. Comparison of RDKit and indigo cheminformatics libraries. *Mol Inform* **2011**, *30* (10), 847–850. DOI:10.1002/minf.201100076.
24. Serradeil-Le Gal, C.; Wagnon, J.; Valette, G.; Garcia, G.; Pascal, M.; Maffrand, J. P.; Le Fur, G. Nonpeptide vasopressin receptor antagonists: Development of selective and orally active V1a, V2 and V1b receptor ligands. *Prog Brain Res* **2002**, *139*, 197–210. DOI:10.1016/s0079-6123(02)39017-4.
25. Kimi, S.; Maiti, R.; Srinivasan, A.; Mishra, B. R.; Hota, D. Efficacy and safety of V(1a) receptor antagonists in autism spectrum disorder: A meta-analysis. *Int J Dev Neurosci* **2024**, *84* (1), 3–13. DOI:10.1002/jdn.10297.
26. Urbina, F.; Ekins, S. The commoditization of AI for molecule design. *Artif Intell Life Sci* **2022**, *2*, 100031. DOI:10.1016/j.ailsci.2022.100031.

Part IV

From Models to Practice

7 Generative Topographic Mapping of Chemical Space in *De Novo* Design

Dragos Horvath, Gilles Marcou, and Alexandre Varnek

7.1 INTRODUCTION

Artificial Neural Networks[1–5] (ANNs) are a class of machine learning algorithms. They emerged as an assembly of simple computing units inspired by biological neurons and approximate multi-variate functions useful to all inductive learning tasks. Their aim was to approximate the non-linear dependence of an explained/predicted variable y (typically resulting from experimental measure) as a function $f(x_1,x_2,\ldots x_n)$ of its n defining variables/attributes/degrees of freedom x_i. ANN applications in Chemoinformatics are straightforward, using representations of compounds to infer some property (y = physico-chemical property, biological activity, etc.). Chemical structures are represented as bit vectors, integers, or real numbers capturing relevant chemical information to be extracted from some computational model of the molecular structure or measured. They are the attributes of the machine learning model, $x_1,x_2,\ldots x_n$, and are termed *molecular descriptors*.[6] Accordingly, the mathematical model $y=f(x_1,x_2,\ldots x_n)$ goes by the name "Quantitative Structure-Property" or "Quantitative Structure-Activity Relationship" (QSPR/QSAR).[7,8] However, ANNs as QSPR tools turned out to be underwhelming,[9] herewith terminating the first ANN-related cycle of hype in chemoinformatics and drug design. Actually, ANN needs large datasets to fit large numbers of parameters and are sensitive to outliers. For instance, it is common to use a substantial quantity of data that needs to be kept out from training, just in order to decide when to stop the training (the early stopping criteria). It is clearly understood that fitting a linear model with n degrees of freedom (tunable parameters) requires a training set of ~$20n$ items or more to ensure statistical robustness[10] of the fit. With this in mind, it is obvious that very few properties of relevance in drug design have been measured on sufficient compounds in order to make them eligible for so-called *deep models*,[11] a category of ANNs that need hundreds or thousands of parameters to fit – not to mention that the relationship between degrees of freedom and statistical robustness is not even well understood when non-linearity is involved. Additionally, alternative approaches such as Support Vector Machines[12] or Random Forests[13] turned out to be more robust and faster, being at the same time more parsimonious regarding their complexity.

DOI: 10.1201/9781003399346-11

The recent comeback of ANNs in chemoinformatics was, however, not powered by any surge in the quantity of quality of structure-activity data, although the latter are steadily increasing – both in terms of publicly available databases[14,15] and initiatives to share corporate information.[16] The "revolution" happened in the completely unrelated fields of image and language processing, targeting ANNs no longer in order to predict objective properties, but to extract recurring *patterns* in language and images. Extracted patterns can then be recombined to produce relevant output, which might even be perceived as "original" by humans. The context shifted to generative[17] models: chatbot[18] and art generators. In particular, language processing focuses on extracting probability distributions of words in the context of choosing which next word to place in a generated sentence. In image processing, a bitmap image can be "compressed" or "embedded" as a "latent" vector of a few real numbers encoding a significant part of the information of the bitmap file, and which can be used to regenerate a (near)-identical copy of the initial bitmap, with no important information loss – details and noise being disposable. Training data quantity is obviously no longer a limiting factor in such contexts and the bottleneck shifts to computational feasibility – how many artificial neurons can be fitted? At what point does numerical precision impede the convergence of the ANN to a stable and predictive model?

Why is this relevant for chemoinformatics at all? Because it is legitimate to ask the question whether the latent vector produced by processing a bitmap depicting a molecular sketch may not be used as a valid *molecular descriptor*! After all, that latent vector is sufficient for the ANN to regenerate the drawing, so it contains all the information needed to unambiguously define the structure. The chemist looking at the drawn molecular sketch disposes of all the required information to identify the compound – so all this information must be somehow encoded in the latent vector. True, a chemist would still recognize a phenyl ring as an aromatic group even if it was hand-drawn as a rather distorted hexagon, "because it is a Phe ring". There is no chemical ontology behind image processing software – but, if properly trained, the latter will nevertheless "recognize" the distorted Phe – in the sense that the produced latent vector will share some common signature specific to other Phe-containing molecules, all while being completely agnostic about "aromaticity", "Hückel", etc. In the same way, the image processor manages to discriminate between "cats" and "dogs" in snapshots independently of their respective color tones, positions, and contexts; it may be eventually trained to cluster the different ways to depict a Phe group (with alternative double bonds, with a circle symbolizing the delocalized orbitals) together, and separately from cyclohexanes, cyclohexenes, etc. These approaches can be better adapted to chemoinformatics (and any other problems accepting a graph as input) by using the molecular graph per se as input instead of its bitmap drawing in so-called Graph Convolutional[19] approaches.

Actually, a molecular structure, as any graph, can be linearized, i.e. represented as a sequence of symbols that appear as a kind of "sentence". Chemoinformatics defined linearized languages representing chemical structures: SMILES[20] – well established and most popular, and newcomers such as SELFIES.[21] Natural language processing techniques could be used "out of the box" to generate such encoded chemical structures after being presented in a sufficiently large number of instances. Again, there is no chemical understanding in this "game" – given a SMILES sequence CO, it is highly unlikely that the next suggested character will be another "O" – not because the machine "knowns" about the intrinsic instability of peroxides, but because its training set of compounds featured a very low number of peroxide examples, if any. Thus, if the method would be trained on a compound set in which the occurrence of various functional groups would reflect their intrinsic chemical stability and synthetic feasibility, such a model should, in principle, generate mostly feasible molecules. In practice, this is never the case – training sets are intrinsically biased, and synthetic feasibility results as much from physical laws as from the context defining which chemical reactions can be implemented and which building blocks are accessible. Yet, existing AI tools generate chemical structures able to lure the chemist the same way deep fake images (AI-generated pictures) are able to lure an audience – in the sense that they easily produce "mathematically" correct structures (verifying all valence rules) which are however far beyond practical constraints of marketable products (feasibility, price, stability).

7.1.1 The Autoencoder (Encoder/Decoder) Paradigm

In spite of the above-mentioned intrinsic limitations, the key strength of these deep-learned molecule generation tools is the ability to reversibly "project" the molecular structure space into some purely numerical "latent" vector space. The "Encoder/Decoder" architecture[22] is responsible for this and consists of two ANNs (Figure 7.1).

The first ANN, "Encoder", will process its atoned molecular representation (SMILES string, molecular graph, 2D bitmap, or even 3D representation) and output an associated latent vector. The associated "Decoder" will input a latent vector and generate a corresponding molecular representation. If the input latent vector, is obtained by encoding a structure, it is expected that decoding will return exactly the same molecule. However, latent vectors not corresponding to any training compound will be decoded into "original" structures – with the expectation that similar latent vectors will decode to similar structures. This is important because such vector spaces

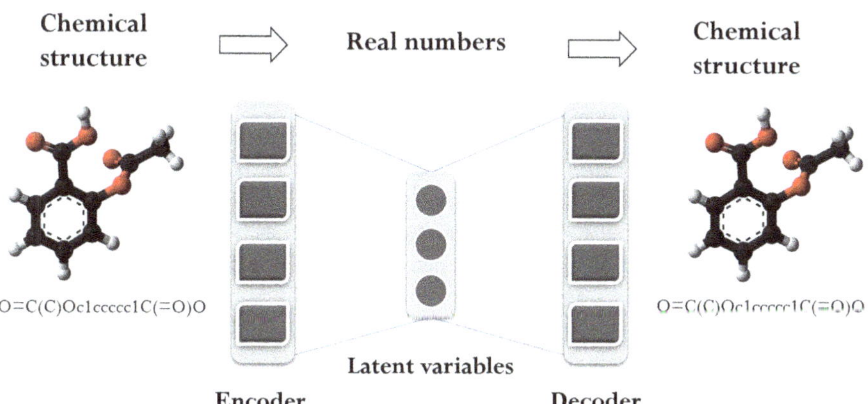

FIGURE 7.1 Principle of the autoencoder approach applied to chemoinformatics.

are much easier to explore computationally. A simple random perturbation of the latent vector of a reference compound followed by decoding is a much more effective way to generate an "original" analog, by contrast to "tampering" with the SMILES and risking to produce a syntactically corrupt string. A well-trained decoder would return valid SMILES strings corresponding to formally correct molecular graphs. This is a paramount advantage over unbiased, random editing of SMILES strings or molecular graphs. Unfortunately, "decoded" molecules cannot be granted feasible or even thermodynamically stable, as already explained.

7.1.2 Forward Synthesis Protocols

The only meaningful way to achieve the chemical feasibility of enumerated compounds is to limit chemical space exploration to predefined combinations of building blocks, filtered to be compatible with the specific chemical reactions for which they were selected as reagents. Given a set of existing building blocks and a set of chemical synthesis pathways mastered by its chemists, it is possible to select all building blocks qualifying as reagents in each of the given processes and herewith enumerate the theoretically synthesizable chemical space. This selection can be expert rule-based, specifying (typically, in SMARTS[23]) which are the "requested" functional groups for a building block to qualify as reagent and, respectively, the "forbidden" features preventing it from reacting as desired. As a result, the theoretically synthesizable chemical space can be described as the pool of the largest combinatorial libraries incorporating all building blocks that passed the reactivity filters – and this is typically already large enough to make its exhaustive enumeration unpractical, requiring computational heuristics to sample it in search for optimal compounds.[24] However, expert-driven enumeration of reactivity rules is tedious and error-prone – hence, the question whether a "reaction" can be formally rendered as a "sentence" with reagents as "words", so that language processing approaches could be adapted to learn which combinations of reagents/words lead to meaningful/feasible sentences/reactions. If so, then picking a random first reagent and relying on such an approach to select a meaningful reaction partner for it can be an interesting approach to navigate the chemical space of (likely) feasible compounds, all while not being restricted to a predefined pool of reagents combinations.

7.1.3 Feasibility versus Originality

Above, we have briefly introduced the main concepts in deep learning-driven *de novo* compound discovery. The Autoencoder paradigm relies on tools establishing a reversible relationship between molecular structure (graph, SMILES string, or even 3D models) and a latent vector space so that mathematically simple navigation in the latter can be seamlessly reverted to a path in molecular structure space. They are prone to generate very original structures no chemist would have envisaged – but at the obvious risk that such structures cannot be practically obtained. Forward synthesis, by contrast, envisages molecular structure as a result of a reaction between available reagents and may cover either predefined chemical spaces (combinatorial enumerations of matrices of product around each mastered synthesis protocol) or move in open-ended chemical spaces, using deep learning to suggest possible reagent combinations. These approaches are clearly better in terms of ensuring the feasibility of suggested output but, unavoidably, less original. It is relatively easy to propose meaningful quantitative criteria to benchmark[25] these processes in terms of originality and diversity of compounds, but it is much more difficult to quantitatively assess chemical feasibility. State-of-art synthesizability indices[26] are challenged in this context because they were mainly conceived as measures of structure complexity. Or, they are not trained to recognize sometimes incongruous substructures produced by chemistry-unaware decoders and are not relevant in forward synthesis (a complex molecule may be very easy to obtain… if you are in possession of a nearly as complex precursor building block: for instance, LSD is obtained in one step by addition of diethylamine to lysergic acid).

7.1.4 The Inverse QSAR (iQSAR) Problem

In our humble opinion, synthetic feasibility[27,28] assessment is the key bottleneck in computer-aided *de novo* design. This problem is still unsolved, and it does not represent the topic of the current chapter. Here, we will focus on the other key aspect: how to navigate this potentially infinite chemical space, in general, and how, in particular, to find therein residing compounds of desired molecular properties.

Given a QSAR model $y=f(x_1,x_2,\ldots x_n)$, how do we find structures of optimal y values? Herein, "optimal" is context-dependent: *maximal* affinity and specificity for the primary target, *maximal* bioavailability, *minimal* toxicity, *tuned* metabolic stability (*in vivo* lifetime sufficient for therapeutic effect, but not long enough to trigger adverse effects), etc. This "inverse QSAR problem"[29–31] can be formally regarded as a two-step process. First, some numerical optimization heuristics can be used to locate "optimal" y^* values. Depending on the complexity of the mathematical model $y=f(x_1,x_2,\ldots x_n)$ and the ruggedness of its response surface, this optimization may be technically challenging – yet conceptually simple: tune the numerical "degrees of freedom" $x_1,x_2,\ldots x_n$ in search of "optimal" $y^*=f(x_1^*,x_2^*,\ldots x_n^*)$ value. Therefore, we propose to refer to this step as the "easy" iQSAR step. By contrast, the second – and "hard" iQSAR step would be to find the molecular structure corresponding to "optimal" descriptors $x_1^*,x_2^*,\ldots x_n^*$ – if such structure actually exists. Beyond the trivial solution – enumerating structures, calculating their $x_1,x_2,\ldots x_n$ and checking if this matches $x_1^*,x_2^*,\ldots x_n^*$ – the autoencoder paradigm was the first real breakthrough in this problem. In particular, if x is the actual latent vector of the autoencoder, producing structures that correspond to a given $(x_1,x_2,\ldots x_n)$ is precisely the task of the decoder. Hence, "optimal" candidate compounds can be enumerated by feeding $x_1^*,x_2^*,\ldots x_n^*$ into the decoder. However, if x is any other expert-designed "classical" molecular descriptor vector, more complex ANN architectures need to be involved. Both cases will be exemplified further on.

7.1.5 Chemography – Navigation in Chemical Space (CS)

One of the key issues with QSAR models is their low interpretability: $y=f(x_1,x_2,\ldots x_n)$ is perceived as a mathematical black box, and seeking the optimal $x_1^*,x_2^*,\ldots$

x_n* does not intuitively appeal to chemists as a meaningful compound optimization protocol. However, when this high-dimensional vector space is somehow rendered human-readable and *visualized*, empirical chemistry knowledge can be associated each "zone" of such a map. The previously obscure "walk" in vector space can be depicted as a trajectory visiting various regions of the map and exploring understandable chemotypes. Of course, a high-dimensional vector space may only be "squeezed" onto the 2D plane by accepting a potentially significant loss of information inherent to any "dimensionality reduction" technique.[32–35] However, the success of chemography shows that this loss is more than compensated by the gain in intuitiveness, allowing the chemist to "appropriate" the mapped chemical space and feel comfortable in navigating it.[36] Furthermore, information loss *per se* is not necessarily a problem, as not all the information embedded in the high-dimensional $x_1,x_2,\ldots x_n$ may be relevant for the studied molecular properties. The key issue is to conduct dimensionality reduction in a Neighborhood Behavior (NB)[37,38]-compliant way, projecting close neighbors in initial space (e.g. those likely to share similar properties[39]) as close neighbors on the 2D map. If so, map-based property predictors[40] may remain competitive compared to full-blown initial vector space QSAR models – but benefit from intuitiveness and acceptance by medicinal chemists.

Chemography has been pioneered[41] as a means to monitor physicochemical properties and based on the most straightforward dimensionality reduction technique: Principal Component Analysis[42] (PCA). Herewith, the cloud of points representing the items in the initial descriptor space is mapped onto a corresponding cloud of points in the plane of the first two principal components (using more PCs rapidly increases the complexity of the depiction and nullifies the intuitiveness of its interpretation). Beyond the intrinsic limitations of this linear approach, the end user still needs to analyze the 2D cloud of points, which may not be interpretable as such if the number of items is high. The latter issue still remains with non-linear embedding techniques such as Multi-Dimensional Scaling (MDS)[35] or stochastic embedding approaches (t-SNE).[34,43] Therefore, non-linear grid-based mapping tools – projecting items by associating them to the predefined nodes of a 2D grid – became state-of-art tools in chemical space navigation: Kohonen[44,45] (or Self-Organizing; SOM) Maps and, more recently, fuzzy-logic-powered Generative Topographic Maps[33,46–49] (GTM). The "nodes" of the 2D grid are useful as reference "poles" to highlight relevant chemical space zones. Items associated with the nodes (fully assigned to a node, like in SOM, or fuzzily associated to several nodes, like in GTM) can be used to "transfer" the properties of mapped compounds onto the nodes in which they reside, herewith defining "property landscapes" or "activity landscapes" of the chemical space. Every node has its $(x_1,x_2,\ldots x_n)$ initial space coordinates (the "code vector", in SOM terminology) associated with the node position on the 2D map. The property value associated to a node will be defined as the mean of the properties of "resident" items – closest, in initial space, to $(x_1,x_2,\ldots x_n)$. If NB-compliant, such a map will selectively witness "active" compounds preferentially cluster around the same "active" nodes, by contrast to inactive – hence, the "code vector" of such a node surrounded by active items may be considered as an "optimal" starting point $(x_1{*},x_2{*},\ldots x_n{*})$ for inverse QSAR. Yet, unlike the $(x_1{*},x_2{*},\ldots x_n{*})$ chosen by some "black box" optimization procedure, node coordinates matching the chemical space area "inhabited" by actives are an *intuitive* choice, readily accepted by the chemists.

7.1.6 Focus of this Chapter: GTM-Piloted *De Novo* Generative Strategies of Molecular Structures and Reactions

In particular, the fuzzy nature of GTM enables a finer rendering of property landscapes compared to SOMs. In the latter, all residents of a node will be assigned to the same predicted property value characteristic of the node – thus, fine changes in structure will have no impact on the predicted property unless they cause the analog item to move closer to another code vector and hence "jump" to another node with another characteristic property: property landscapes are discontinuous. In GTMs, as will be briefly explained in the dedicated section below, degrees of association with nodes (technically "responsibilities") are real numbers summing up to one over all nodes and can be predicted to have a property calculated as responsibility-weighted mean of properties of associated nodes. Hence, two analog compounds may have slightly different levels of association without "jumping" from one node to another. Accordingly, they will be predicted to have close but distinct property values. It was shown that predictive property landscapes supported by GTMs are only slightly less potent predictive models compared to other standard machine-learned QSARs (such as RF or SVM), and more important, it was shown that a single (herewith dubbed "universal") GTM might support predictive landscapes for hundreds of independent biological activities and physico-chemical properties.[50,51] GTM landscapes are thus an excellent tool for chemical space navigation, and deep-learning ANNs are powerful tools to (reversibly) link any chemical space location to its resident structures. The combined use of these approaches herewith becomes a strong *de novo* compound design strategy, as will be shown in this chapter. After a brief technical overview of the involved approaches, a review of so-far reported applications of such methodology will be provided.

7.2 BRIEF INTRODUCTION TO GENERATIVE TOPOGRAPHIC MAPPING

In the following, the steps involved in the construction of a GTM will be briefly highlighted on the basis of Figure 7.2. First, the chemical space to be spanned by the map must be defined by means of a Frame set – a pool of (real or virtual) reference compounds considered as representative of the type of compounds to be mapped. "Representative" may simply mean "drug-like" (for a map meant to be used in synthetic medicinal chemistry) or "natural product-like" if the latter are targeted (knowing that due to their intrinsically higher complexity, their chemical space might not be well covered by synthetic molecules).[52] Should the study focus on a specific target, framing can be achieved with a pool of (active and inactive) ligands tested on that target. The choice of a best-suited frameset is not always obvious – in that case, it is judicious to consider it as a hyperparameter of map construction[51] and let some algorithm explore various options (random sampling, stratification, etc.), picking the one leading to optimally performing maps. Frameset items are then rendered as "points" in the high-dimensional space of chosen molecular descriptors – in other words, descriptor vectors are computed for each frame set compound (step 1). Which descriptors should be used is a critical question – they will define the NB compliance of the map. Again, this choice can be regarded as an additional hyperparameter

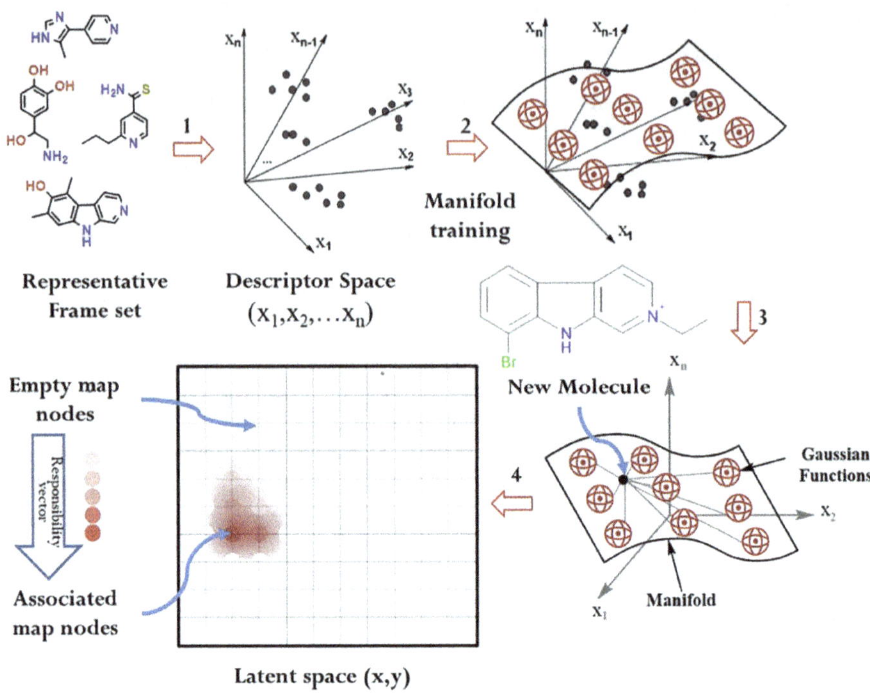

FIGURE 7.2 Key steps of GTM construction - manifold training and projection of new items by fuzzy association to map nodes.

to fine-tune, together with the "technical" parameters defining the GTM manifold (see below). The GTM manifold is a flexible 2D bounded surface, or "rubber sheet" inserted in descriptor space. It is defined by a grid of "nodes", and modeled by a set of Gaussian functions, being allowed to "bend" to approach a maximum of frame items. The number of Gaussians and their width define the flexibility of the manifold: more Gaussians allow this rubber sheet to bend more easily in order to better approach frame items – at the risk of "overfitting" it. Finally, after the gradient-driven manifold optimization (step 2) is finished, the manifold in its final geometry is ready to accommodate any new item placed in the descriptor space. Based on its position, the item will be associated with the nearest manifold nodes following a fuzzy-logical scheme (step 4): first, association to nodes (so-called "responsibilities") will be strongest to the closest nodes and, second, the sum of all these responsibilities must equal 1.0. Hence, the item will be rendered as a density cloud (visually rendered by modulating color transparency: higher node responsibility meaning darker node color) over the nodes of the manifold, which is flattened out as a regular 2D-grid (the "latent space") for visualization purposes. The underlying mathematical formalism will not be revisited here – please refer to already cited GTM-related publications[33,46–49] for this aspect.

Thus, every item is rendered as a fuzzy "responsibility cloud" on the latent space grid, defined by the responsibility vector of item *i*: R_{in} being the level of association

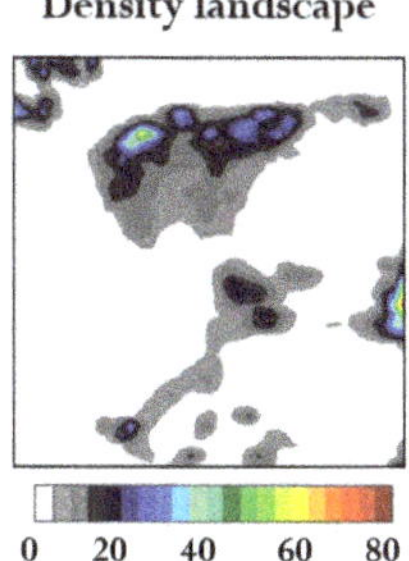

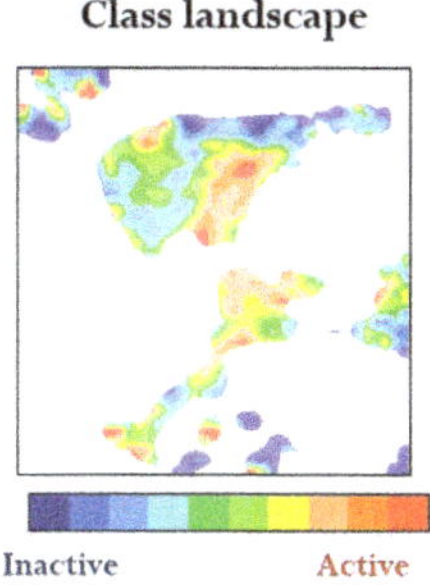

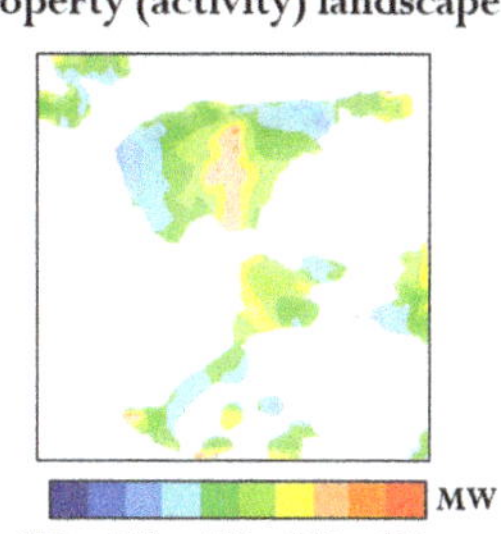

FIGURE 7.3 The three categories of GTM landscapes used to highlight "interesting" chemical space zones. Density landscapes render the cumulated responsibility of all items within a set and highlight densely versus sparsely populated chemical space zones. In class landscapes, the color reflects the relative populations of items in each class ("actives" versus "inactives", for example), whereas property landscapes are colored by the responsibility-weighted mean property of nodes. These two latter landscape types are drawn only for populated nodes – empty zones are white.

between item *i* and node *n*, with $\Sigma_n R_{in} = 1.0$ (item will forcibly reside *somewhere* on the nodes). This is the first key advantage of GTMs over Kohonen[44,45] SOMs, in which every item resides in one and only one node. Residents within the same node are undistinguishable according to the SOM – hence, a SOM with *N* nodes may form at most *N* distinct clusters into which to assign mapped items. By contrast, there is a virtually infinite number of potential density patterns that can be imagined over the *N* nodes – items associated with the same list of nodes with roughly the same responsibilities are said to be members of the same Responsibility Pattern (RP), representing a GTM-based compound cluster (again, please refer to literature.[53] for mathematical details). It is furthermore possible to declare the "center of mass" (nodes with more responsibility bear more "mass") of the responsibility pattern as the (*x*,*y*) "latent position" of the item on the GTM – which amounts to an effective dimensionality reduction of the descriptor space to two dimensions (like in PCA plots, but non-linearly).

Furthermore, compound properties can be "transferred" to the nodes of residence proportionally to R_{in} values. If the compound is active, it will boost the "active" status of resident nodes. The more actives associated with a node, the more solid the working hypothesis that the chemical space neighborhood of that node is bound to harbor active compounds. The responsibility-driven "dispatching" of compound properties over the map results in obtaining various property landscapes (Figure 7.3), which all refer to the same nodes in descriptor space – thus, nodes can be deemed "of interest" for a drug discovery problem based on multiple objectives (activity, selectivity, bioavailability, etc.).

7.3 AUTOENCODER ARCHITECTURES

An autoencoder[54] is a kind of neural network architecture that defines an internal representation (under the form of a "latent" or "code" vector) of an input sample, from which the sample can be reconstructed. The terms "latent" and "code" vector are used, with the former being more popular – please avoid confusion with the two-dimensional GTM "latent space" (*vide supra*). Thus, the latent vector is the output of the first half of the neural network architecture, the encoder, and the input of the second half, the decoder. The decoder reconstructs an instance from the latent vector computed by the encoder from the same instance. The encoder and the decoder are trained jointly, minimizing the differences between the input instances and their reconstructed images. The dimensionality of the latent vector is usually lower than that of the processed data. Therefore, encoding and decoding are often called "compression" and "decompression", respectively. As the autoencoder is trained, it preserves the most relevant information and ignores details and noise from the input dataset. Important information for data reconstruction includes analysis of the data structure, revealing hidden patterns, and performing noise-signal separation. In particular, sequence-to-sequence encoders-decoders, proven very efficient in natural language processing[55,56] may learn to reproduce the input sequences at its output. Such "seq2seq autoencoders" reversibly "compress" character sequences following the syntactic rules of a given language as latent vectors, herewith intrinsically "learning" the syntactic rules and thus gaining the ability to produce only valid "sentences" on output. An input sequence is fed to a recurrent neural network (RNN) representing the encoder, which updates its internal state after reading and processing each input element. The resulting final state of the encoder is then passed to the decoder RNN through a fully connected layer, which serves as an information bottleneck and recombines the state into the latent vector. SMILES strings are "sentences" obeying a specific syntax, thus are eligible as seq2seq autoencoder input after undergoing "one-hot" preprocessing (binarization as a Kronecker bit matrix δ_{ij} marking whether the character at position i of the input string matches or not the jth entry of the list of all possible characters supported by the language).

For each training item, training characters t_i are iteratively fed to the encoder, the signal propagating through the dense layer to the decoder, which is expected to regenerate the same t_i on output. In order to enhance the learning process (the "teacher forcing" trick[57]), the decoder is additionally fed at each step, with the input character seen by the encoder at the previous step (dummy character at step#1). The output of the decoder is compared to what had been fed in the encoder, and internal ANN weights are tuned to minimize the reconstruction loss function. After convergence, the encoder and decoder can be used as stand-alone tools: the former to convert any SMILES to its latent vector, the latter to construct a SMILES from a given latent vector. Sattarov et al.[58] trained such an architecture on ChEMBL[14] compounds, as illustrated in Figure 7.4. With a 128-dimensional latent vector, SMILES reconstruction accuracy over 100K ChEMBL molecules kept out of the training set was 95.8%, rising above 99.7% with 256 code dimensions.

7.4 IS LATENT VECTOR SPACE USEFUL FOR COMPOUND DISCOVERY?

The goal of the above-mentioned article[58] was to explore the usefulness of the latent vector space as a basis for exploring chemical space. In other words, is it possible to use latent vectors instead of "regular" molecular descriptors and single out

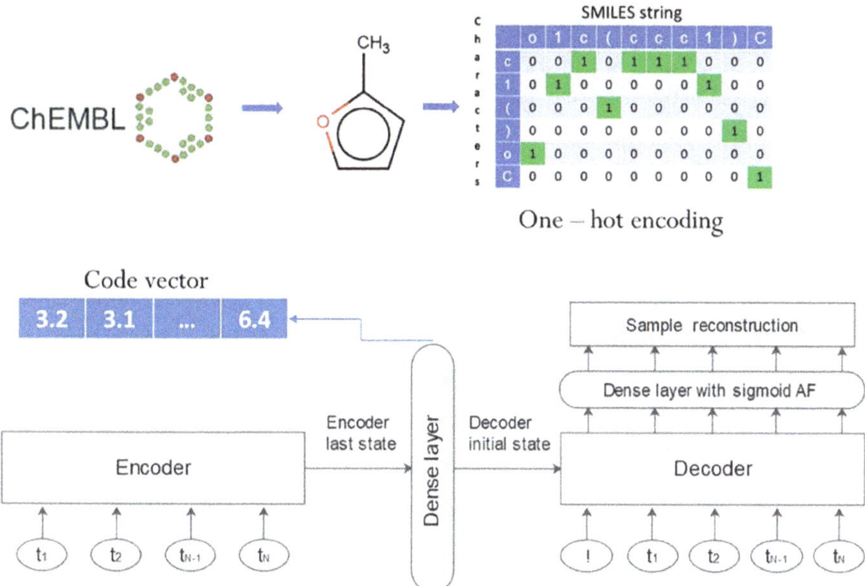

FIGURE 7.4 General scheme of a seq2seq autoencoder architecture processing SMILES strings. The former may be extracted from large compound databases (for example ChEMBL, representing a fully diverse set of medicinal chemistry relevant molecules). Input characters t_i are fed to the Long Short-term Memory (LSTM) Encoder, and further to the Dense Layer containing the "bottleneck" layer of a minimal number of neurons which provides the latent vector. The latter serves as input to the decoder.

"interesting" chemical space zones from which relevant *de novo* structures could be produced by the decoder? Technically, there are no reasons why the latent vector space could not be mapped by GTM onto some 2D "human-readable" map, or used as descriptor space in QSAR model learning. The interest in this scenario is that, herewith, the "hard" part of the inverse QSAR problem (*vide supra*) – finding the structure that corresponds to a given descriptor vector – is implicitly solved by the decoder. The problem with this scenario was that exploiting latent vectors as molecular descriptors is not granted. First, these vectors are intrinsically atom ordering-dependent, whereas molecular descriptors[59] should be absolutely invariant to the brute representation of the molecule. Submitting an alternative SMILES representation of the same molecule will result in a different latent vector. This is intuitively illustrated in Figure 7.5, where three different SMILES representations of the same compound are seen to project into distinct areas of a latent vector-based GTM. The projections seen to significantly diverge – the interest of visual monitoring of the positions in the 2D latent space of the GTM is precisely to convey an intuitive feeling of dissimilarity, unlike the abstract number of a Tanimoto score between latent vectors. Furthermore, version A of the SMILES projects into a latent vector space zone more densely populated by ChEMBL compounds than alternatives B and C (ChEMBL compounds contributing to the density landscape were projected from canonical SMILES, *vide infra*).

A: c1cc(C(NC(C(OC)=O)CCSC)=O)c(-c2ccccc2)cc1NCc1cncn1Cc1ccc(C)cc1

B: N(Cc1cncn1Cc1ccc(C)cc1)c1cc(-c2ccccc2)c(C(=O)NC(C(OC)=O)CCSC)cc1

C: c1cc(C)ccc1Cn1cncc1CNc1ccc(C(=O)NC(CCSC)C(OC)=O)c(-c2ccccc2)c1

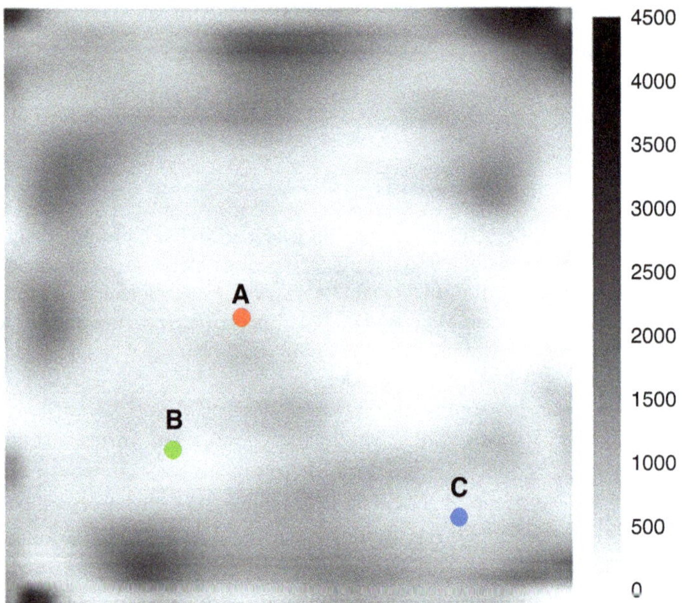

FIGURE 7.5 Latent vectors issued from three different valid SMILES strings denoting the same molecule are significantly different and project into distinct areas of the code-vector-based chemical space rendered by the GTM above (the background landscape represents local density of ChEMBL compounds – from canonical SMILES).

Strict usage of canonical SMILES (as implemented in the cited article) only partially fixes the problem (very similar molecules may have radically different canonical SMILES strings – if, for example, one added methyl group completely redefines the longest linear path in the graph).

Moreover, GTM-based monitoring of the latent vector space revealed that its different zones – herein conveniently defined as neighborhoods of GTM node latent vectors – are not equally well "reversible". The likelihood to have the decoder produce a valid SMILES may strongly depend on the reverted latent vector space zone (Figure 7.6).

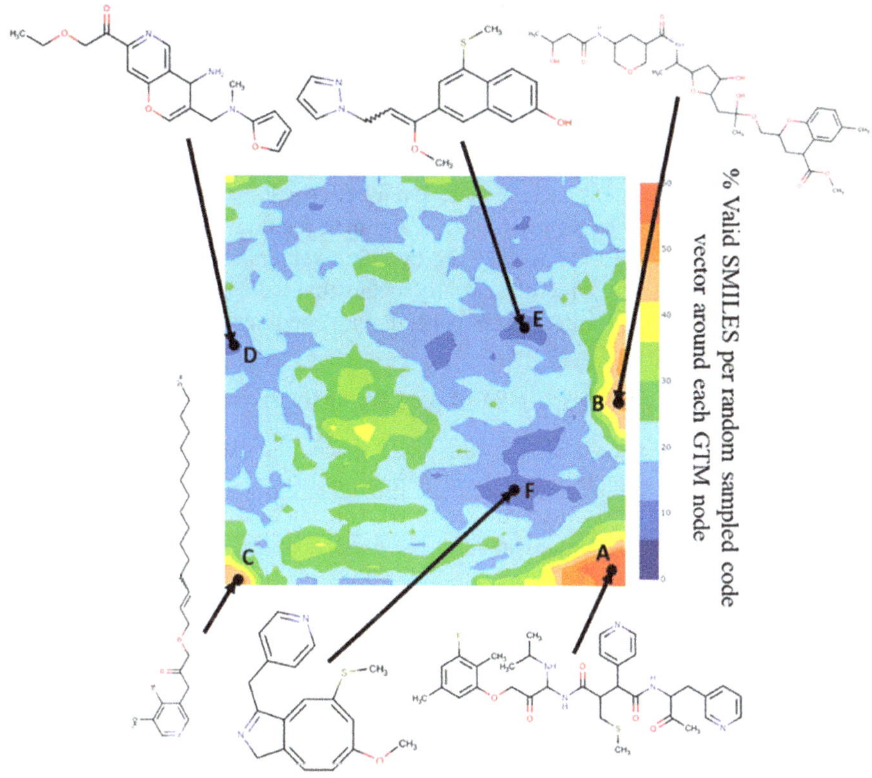

FIGURE 7.6 2D latent space rendering of the latent vector-based chemical space, colored by the likelihood to return a valid SMILES string from randomly drawn latent vectors in the neighborhood of each GTM node latent vector. Examples of valid structures from both the easily revertible (red) and the difficult to revert (blue) latent vector space zones are shown.

Above, "valid" simply means syntactically correct SMILES corresponding to molecular graphs with no valence violations – there is no question of actual synthesizability here. It can be observed that latent vector space zones that are difficult to revert are the ones populated by compounds with condensed rings – the complex syntax of correct ring closure is challenging for the decoder. This makes sense but raises a red flag – it is thus unlikely that chemical space sampling with autoencoders will be unbiased: possible structures are not equally likely to be returned by the decoder.

Furthermore, while high reconstruction rates prove that latent vectors represent a near lossless compression of the molecular structure, it is unclear how this chemical information is compressed in the latent vector so that it can be used to relate latent vectors to measured molecular properties. To this purpose, it was attempted to generate "universal" polypharmacological competent GTMs based on the 128-dimensional latent vector space, following the same protocol[51] as used with ISIDA[60] fragment count descriptors. Not unsurprisingly, the resulting code vector-space-based maps were shown to discriminate between tested actives and tested inactive associated with more than 600 biological targets (out of which only 236 served for training), with balanced accuracy scores matching rather closely the ones obtained with regular descriptors. For example, for the adenosine receptor A2a, separation of the population of about 1,700 "active" *versus* 3,100 "inactive" tested compounds occurred with a balanced accuracy of 0.72, which is in line with performances of various ISIDA descriptor spaces (0.68…0.76). This is one of the most remarkable proofs of NB compliance of the latent vector space, given both the large size of the A2a dataset and the fact that it was not used to train any map (neither with ISIDA, nor with code descriptors). Chemical space defined by latent vectors thus appears to be NB compliant and mappable – which essentially means that the negative impact of atom ordering artifacts can be limited when working with canonical SMILES only.

7.4.1 A Hike in Latent vector Space and Its Trace on the Map

An additional test of the viability of this code space was the staging of a "walk" between two unrelated molecules – here, penicillin (origin) and ibuprofen (target). This exercise (Figure 7.7) is interesting in as far as it can be assimilated to "molecular morphing", the chemical equivalent of the popular process of transforming one

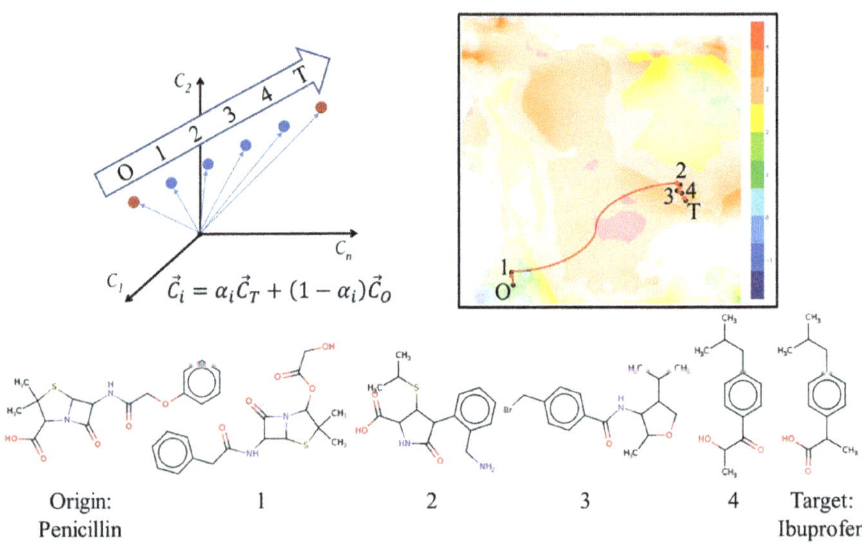

FIGURE 7.7 A walk-in latent vector space (left top), starting at the origin latent vector of penicillin O and targeting the one of ibuprofen, T. At four intermediate steps of equal length taken along the T-O line ($\alpha_i = i/5$) corresponding structures (bottom) were generated by the decoder. The upper right corner of the Figure represents a landscape colored by calculated logP values of ChEMBL compounds (red areas – zones populated by hydrophobic, blue areas – by predominantly polar species) on latent vector space-based "universal" GTM. The species on the explored path are rendered as dots at the center of their responsibility blobs (not shown) in the map latent space. Red arrows render the projection of the linear path in latent vector space on the (non-linearly bent) manifold.

image into another, while watching out for intriguing and unusual effects in the intermediate hybrids.

Here, the penicillin-ibuprofen hybrids are not particularly unusual – on the contrary, they appear to be regular, *a priori* stable, and feasible molecules, which is not granted in any way by autoencoder techniques. NB compliance is clearly observable, as the first step away from penicillin returns a penicillin-like analog, whereas the step before arrival is already within the zone of close ibuprofen analogs. It can be observed how molecular complexity (and the number of rings) decreases from the origin towards the target, while hydrophobicity increases (as measured by LogP). The latter trend can be directly read from the background logP landscape of the latent vector-based GTM, where the trace of linear walk in the high-dimensional latent vector space is rendered as a non-linear path. This is no contradiction, as neither distances in latent vector space nor latent distances on the map are "the absolutely correct" definition of molecular similarity –such a thing does not exist. Nonetheless, relative distances to T in map latent space are still monotonically decreasing in the expected order O≥1>2>3>4. Map rendering suggests that the step between structures 1 and 2 is the most significant – arguably rightly, as this witnesses the sharpest drop in complexity and loss of the condensed ring scaffold. It is however unlikely to observe any smooth transition from antibiotic to anti-inflammatory effect over this path, as witnessed for the estimated logP (NB compliance with respect to activity cliff-prone biological activity is notoriously more difficult to obtain). However, the key point here is that latent vector space can be intuitively "visited" by coupling a seq2seq autoencoder with GTM technology by placing abstract moves in an artificial chemical space back on a property-colored map for which every zone has a clear chemical identity.

7.4.2 Inverse QSAR in Latent vector Space

Encouraged by the successful validation of latent vector space as a meaningful way to render chemical space, the logical continuation of the study was to generate actual *de novo* proposals of molecules likely to bind to some biological receptors shown to have well-separable actives and inactives on the latent vector-based universal GTM. As already mentioned, the chosen target was the adenosine receptor A2a, CHEMBL251. With the decoder mechanism in place to solve the "hard" part of inverse QSAR, it remains to solve the so-called "easy" sampling of latent vectors associated with high A2a activity likelihood. The general solution to this problem which can be applied to any machine-learned QSAR model – black-box mathematical model or GTM landscape-based predictor – is to perform a global search in latent vector space for optima of an objective function $y=f(x_1,x_2,\ldots x_n)$ expressing likelihood to be active in terms of latent vector space coordinates. As soon as such optima $y^*=f(x_1^*,x_2^*,\ldots x_n^*)$ are found, it suffices to feed $(x_1^*,x_2^*,\ldots x_n^*)$ into the seq2seq decoder in order to obtain a (hopefully feasible) novel chemical structure. The flowchart of the whole *de novo* design procedure is illustrated in Figure 7.8.

In the mentioned work, one approach to optimum search involved a genetic algorithm encoding the latent vector as a "chromosome" of 128 real numbers. Coordinates encoded by this "chromosome" are projected on the universal GTM, like any regular

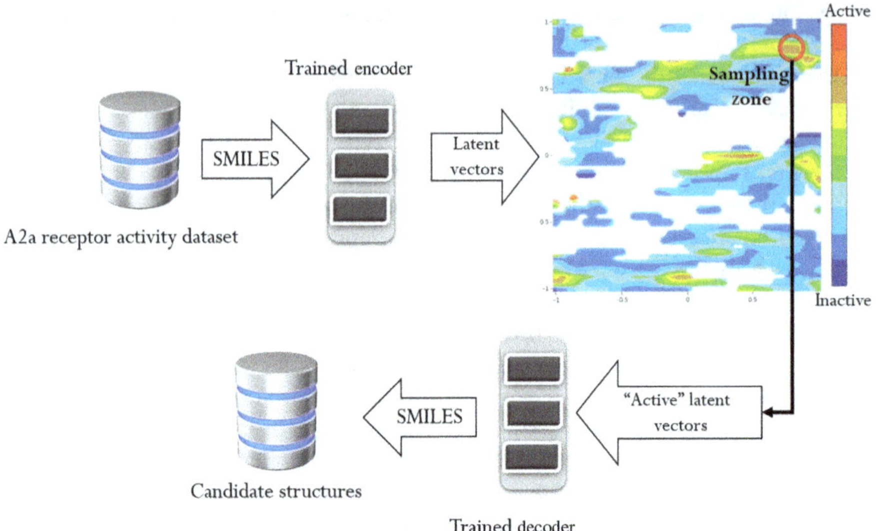

FIGURE 7.8 Flowchart of the *de novo* A2a ligand design procedure exploring the chemical space defined by autoencoder latent vectors, throughout a GTM landscape in which zones predominately populated by already known A2a actives emerge. These can be used to back-track the latent vector coordinates of relevant chemical space zones, to be fed into the decoder in order to obtain the SMILES of candidate structures.

latent vector of an existing molecular structure. GTM nodes of high responsibility to the projected item are selected and analyzed in terms of their (pre-computed) relative occupation by A2a actives and inactives, respectively. If the chromosome projects onto nodes that are all void of any A2a-related molecules, the predictor will assume that the latent vector is irrelevant and set its activity likelihood to zero. In other words, the GTM-based predictor implicitly includes an Applicability Domain[61] check. Otherwise, this likelihood will be the responsibility-weighted average of the (normalized) ratio of active *versus* total A2a residents in the node (the information that makes up the activity landscape). The higher the responsibilities for active-dominated nodes, the higher the returned activity likeness score. Intuitively, the activity likeness is "read out" from the color of the map zone into which the latent vector projects. The sampling heuristics may be allowed to search the latent vector space until it harvests a significant population of latent vectors associated with high activity likeness scores.

The elegance of the GTM-based property predictor lies however in the fact that neither the absolute nor other relevant optima $y^*=f(x_1^*,x_2^*,\ldots x_n^*)$ do *not* need to be searched for in an above-mentioned way: they are known by default. Since, in the above-mentioned example, the likelihood to be active is extrapolated from the relative populations in nodes, it is evident that the absolute maximal y value corresponds to latent vectors mapping with 100% of responsibility onto the node with the largest relative population of A2a training set actives. Or, this node is known and easily recognizable by its "extreme" color according to the spectrum used to plot the landscape. Taking the node coordinates in code space is a direct solution to the "easy" inverse QSAR problem! Also, other nodes that are highly enriched in terms of "active" residents automatically represent other possible starting points to be fed into the decoder. These node coordinates do not correspond to the latent vector of any training set compound – they should be understood as vectors pointing towards active-enriched chemical space zones. They can be used as such or – in order to harvest multiple possible analogues perturbed by some random noise – to be fed into the decoder in order to generate likely active and original structures.

Both these solutions – global search and local exploration around the "best" node – were explored. The former has the advantage to also visit zones that may be rather far from any GTM node yet surrounded by "active" nodes and hence extrapolated to be "active" as well. The latter is much more effective in quickly returning interesting solutions. In both cases, the approach may explore chemical space zones being relatively densely populated by state-of-art A2a inhibitors yet not bound to the immediate neighborhood of either of these known molecules. Therefore, the risk of having the decoder returning chemically impossible structures is much higher than when perturbing the latent vector of a known molecule. Yet, effectivefiltering of the output using SMART-based detection of reactive or chemically unstable groups was used to rapidly select chemically sound potential A2a binders of significant originality. In the work, local exploration around the best node (β-sampling, in the article text) was seen to return species of significantly higher Synthetic Accessibility (SA) score[26] (more difficult to synthesize) than average ChEMBL compounds, by contrast to global sampling. This difference is, however, artificial and stems from the fact that in the latter case, compounds of the SA index above a given threshold were considered "unfit" even though their estimated activity likelihood was high. None of these structures were so far synthetized or tested, but they were further validated by "orthogonal" *in silico* prediction methods – A2a binding pharmacophore matching and docking, which confirmed the high potential interest in these structures. Figure 7.9 illustrates a confirmed A2a

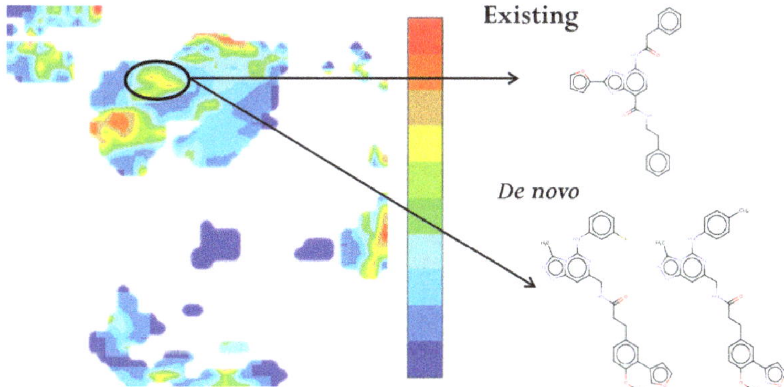

FIGURE 7.9 An example of a confirmed A2a inhibitor ("existing") *versus* some *de novo* generated structures, seen to project into the same "active" node of the A2a activity landscape on a universal GTM based on ISIDA descriptors.

binder next to two *de novo* generated candidates. The latter are clearly "original" in terms of overall molecular topology, although the species share many common substructures (yet reconnected in different ways). These species are neighbors not only on the latent vector-based GTM used in *de novo* design but also on the "regular" ISIDA fragment descriptor-based universal GTM shown below.

7.5 INVERSE QSAR WITH REGULAR MOLECULAR DESCRIPTORS

Even though latent vector spaces may occasionally support robust QSAR modeling, as described previously, this cannot be taken for granted. Atom order dependence remains a serious issue, and working with canonical SMILES comes with specific drawbacks[62] (the autoencoder will "learn" the formal SMILES canonization rules instead of chemistry rules defining valid compounds, thus have the tendency to cover less chemical space on output). Abandoning line formulae in favor of graph convolutional tools[19] implies a significant increase in computational effort without completely eliminating atom order dependence. In spite of the latest attempts to simplify graph neural networks – for example, by using hydrogen-annotated heavy atom nodes and herewith rendering bond orders implicit[63] – some atom order dependence still subsists. Also, the state-of-art, confirmed QSAR models in use worldwide are historically based on expert-designed molecular descriptors. Therefore, the question of how to solve the "hard" problem of finding the chemical structure matching a given molecular descriptor vector is important. One way to achieve this is using a Conditional Variational AutoEncoder (CVAE, Figure 7.10). This approach, advocated[64] by Bort et al. is fed, upon training, with the SMILES and, in parallel, with its calculated molecular descriptor vector. The SMILES is processed by a Gated Recurrent Unit (GRU) into a "target latent vector", generated such as to follow a hyperspherical distribution with zero mean and variance of one. The descriptor

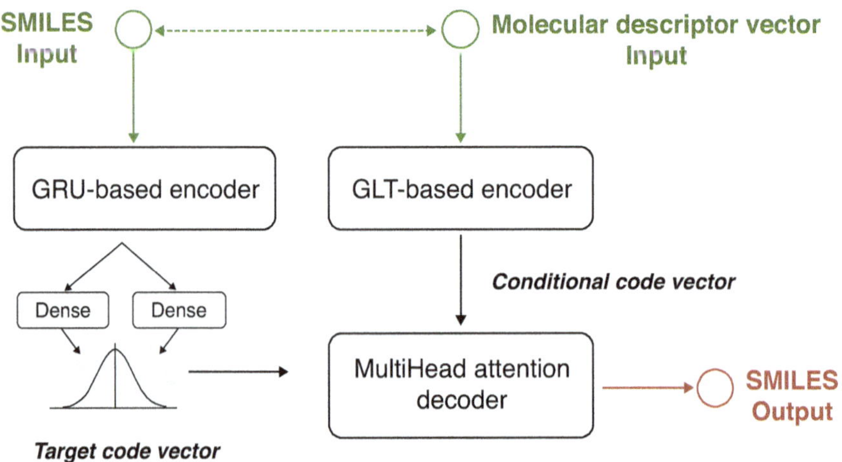

FIGURE 7.10 Schematic representation of an attention-based conditional variational encoder.

vector is fed into a Grouped Linear Transformation (GLT) layer in order to be converted to the "conditional latent vector". Both latent vectors need to be input to the Multihead Attention Decoder able to regenerate the original SMILES. After training, the decoder needs to be provided with the targeted vector from the molecular descriptor space as "conditional" input and will be able to generate sets of SMILES strings from random hyperspherically distributed target latent vectors. Although the input target latent vectors are random, it is expected that under the influence of the conditional input, resulting SMILES will match structures having their actual molecular descriptor vector in the neighborhood of the input descriptor vector (and therefore will have the properties expected for a molecule of that chemical space zone).

An example considered activity landscapes of the ABL tyrosine kinase 1 (CHEMBL1862), for which two classes of predictive models were developed: a Support Vector Regression[12] (SVR) quantitative predictor of the thermodynamic inhibition constant (pK_i) of ligands and a Classification model ("active" *versus* "inactive") ligands using the corresponding activity class landscape on the universal GTM. Both these approaches used ISIDA[65] fragment descriptor vectors (vector elements represent occurrence counts of associated substructures – sequences, atom-centered fragments – in the molecule). The SVR "black box" model operates in the 7,372-dimensional space of counts of atom-centered fragments of radius ≤3. Herein, the "easy" inverse QSAR problem was tackled by a genetic algorithm in search for vectors $x_1^*, x_2^*, \ldots x_n^*$ returning high predicted pK_i "fitness" values. The universal GTM used is based on atom sequence counts with a length of two to three atoms labeled by CVFF force field types and formal charge status. As previously discussed, randomly perturbed coordinates of the GTM node most strongly enriched in "active" ABL-Tk1 inhibitors were the vectors sampled here. In addition, randomly perturbed coordinates of the top active individual training set compounds were also considered as a straightforward and fast approximation for $x_1^*, x_2^*, \ldots x_n^*$.

Irrespective of the actual model and the approach of addressing the "easy" inverse QSAR problem, it is important to point out that the obtained "optimal" vectors are certainly vectors of the molecular descriptor space but *never* actual descriptor vectors associated with a real molecule. For example, any vector in which $x_1=0$ and $x_2=3$ is a well-defined vector of the ISIDA atom sequence count space. It can be submitted to the GLT encoder and converted to a conditional latent vector. But, knowing that x_1 stands for the number of occurrences of the CCO sequence while x_2 counts the occurrences of the CCOC substructure, it is obvious that there is no molecule corresponding to it. The incoherence is not of chemical but of logical nature: as substructure#1 is contained in substructure#2, *no* vector with $x_1 < x_2$ may be the descriptor of any logically coherent graph. Even more blatantly, in "optimal" vectors $x_1^*, x_2^*, \ldots x_n^*$ are real numbers, whereas fragment counts are, by definition, integers. Indeed, the CVAE mechanism is not expected to return a "precise" match upon decoding, but a stochastic set of SMILES representing structures having their descriptor as close as possible to the seed used to generate them. Therefore, it is important to first verify – as already discussed in the other chapters of this book – whether the returned structure is chemically sound, non-reactive and of moderate SA index. If so, the next step required is to check how far the actual molecular descriptors of the structure are located with respect to its seed vector, and to make sure whether it

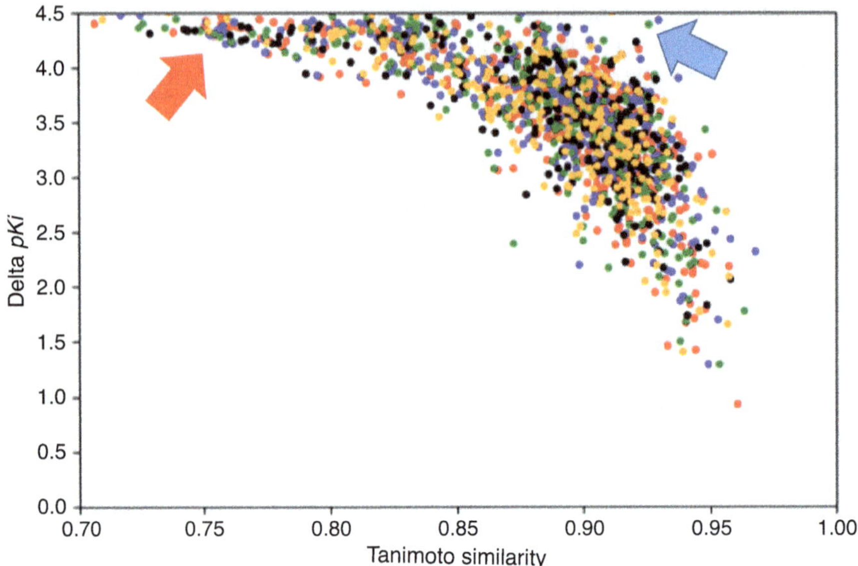

FIGURE 7.11 Monitoring the discrepancies between seed vectors and actual descriptors of CVAE-decoded structures. For various seed vectors, the associated set of decoded structures is plotted with the same color. On X, the Tanimoto similarity between their actual descriptor to the seed vector. On Y, the difference between the SVR-predicted pK_i value for the seed and actual descriptors, respectively. The blue arrow signals cases where the decoder successfully produced a compound with descriptor closely matching the seed, and yet predicted to be much less active by the SVR model (predicted activity cliff). The red arrow shows examples of strong deviation from the original seed upon decoding – systematically accompanied by a predicted activity loss.

remains within a relevant chemical space zone. This can be achieved by comparing the activity predicted for the seed vector $y^*=f(x_1^*,x_2^*,\ldots x_n^*)$ to the one predicted for the actual descriptor vector of the decoded SMILES. The difference can be plotted against the Tanimoto similarity of the vectors – sometimes, predicted activity differences can be large if seed and actual descriptor vector remain similar but find themselves separated by a (predicted) activity cliff (Figure 7.11).

More intuitively, the above question can be visually answered by mapping actual descriptor vectors and seed vectors (or simply highlighting the source node for node-sampled seed vectors) (Figure 7.12). Using the ABL-Tk1 landscape as a background, it is immediately obvious to show how often the decoding procedure failed to find real molecules in the targeted chemical space neighborhood – and, additionally, see whether failures resulted in *de novo* compounds still within the ABL-Tk1 chemical space (but resembling more to tested inactive) or in completely different species, mapping into white zones where no compound related to this target is known so far.

Interestingly, the approach lives up to its expectation to – predominantly – generate structures within the targeted chemical space zones and with desired predicted properties. "Outliers" do occur but are easy to detect and discard by either of the two

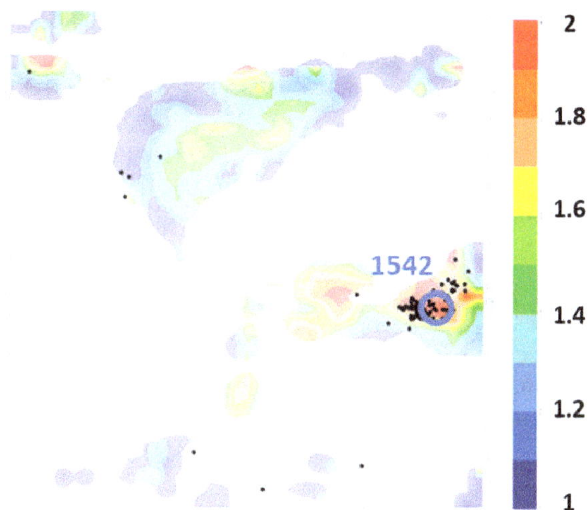

FIGURE 7.12 Positioning of the structures decoded from seed vectors around node 1542 of the universal GTM – one of the nodes harboring the highest relative populations of ABL-Tk1 "actives". The background landscape is the ABL-Tk1 fuzzy activity landscape, with red areas harboring "actives", blue areas "inactives" and yellow-green zones accommodating a mix of both classes. White zones are void of any molecule reportedly tested on ABL-Tk1 (but may accommodate drug-like compounds associated to other targets, not shown here).

approaches highlighted in the two preceding Figures. It can be concluded that CVAEs may serve as generators of *de novo* focused libraries that are heavily biased towards the expected chemical space zone but should be further refined by additional virtual screening steps – applying the actual model at their origin, GTM landscape contextualization, or any other affinity predictor. In the mentioned study, it could thus be shown that the CVAE approach was indeed capable to propose original structures which match ABL-Tk1 3D pharmacophore models, or dock into the kinase active site while satisfying key interactions. The final structures have not yet been synthesized and tested (they were not depicted here – please refer to the original[64] publication). Intriguingly, they are "original" with respect to training ABL-Tk1 binders roughly in the same manner as previously discussed A2a inhibitors generated from optimal latent vectors relate to their training compounds: structures are indeed novel, of differing molecular topology but "reshuffle" many of the functional groups and scaffolds in the original structures. This "reshuffling" per se is not a priori guaranteed to lead to active compounds – however, some of the output structures matched binding pharmacophores and docked well. These needed to be selected – the (valid) output of the encoder/decoder is certainly not 100% ABL-TK1-like, but it is sufficiently enriched in compounds passing "classical" virtual screening tests.

7.6 *DE NOVO* DESIGN OF CHEMICAL REACTIONS

Compound design and synthesis are two deeply complementary problems in (medicinal) chemistry, but the chemoinformatics of chemical reactions is the more difficult topic – unsurprisingly, given that reactions involve several molecules and a sometimes highly empirical synthesis protocol. True, computer-aided synthesis is an important field of chemoinformatics – yet it still is a compound-design oriented problem.[66,67] Forward synthesis protocols, as discussed in the Introduction, are just a means to navigate chemical space in favoring feasibility, whereas retrosynthesis[68,69] is meant to suggest paths leading to a designed compound. Chemical reaction databases[70] were also an important research domain but tightly focused on retrieving reported or similar chemical transformations for the use of the synthetic chemist.

7.6.1 Condensed Graphs of Reaction

However, a key concept – the Condensed Graph of Reaction[71,72] (CGR) – has recently been shown to facilitate the study of chemical reactions per se – for prediction[73] of their thermodynamic or kinetic parameters, clustering[74] and definition of a "chemical reaction" space conceptually equivalent to the chemical space of organic molecules. Simply put, a CGR is nothing but a "hyper-molecule" regrouping both reagents and products within the same graph, assigning particular bond types to the "dynamic" bonds formed, broken, or undergoing a change of bond order during the transformation. The CGR concept is illustrated in Figure 7.13 for a Suzuki reaction. The (imbalanced) Suzuki reaction given above implies a phenyl-pyridyl bond formation,

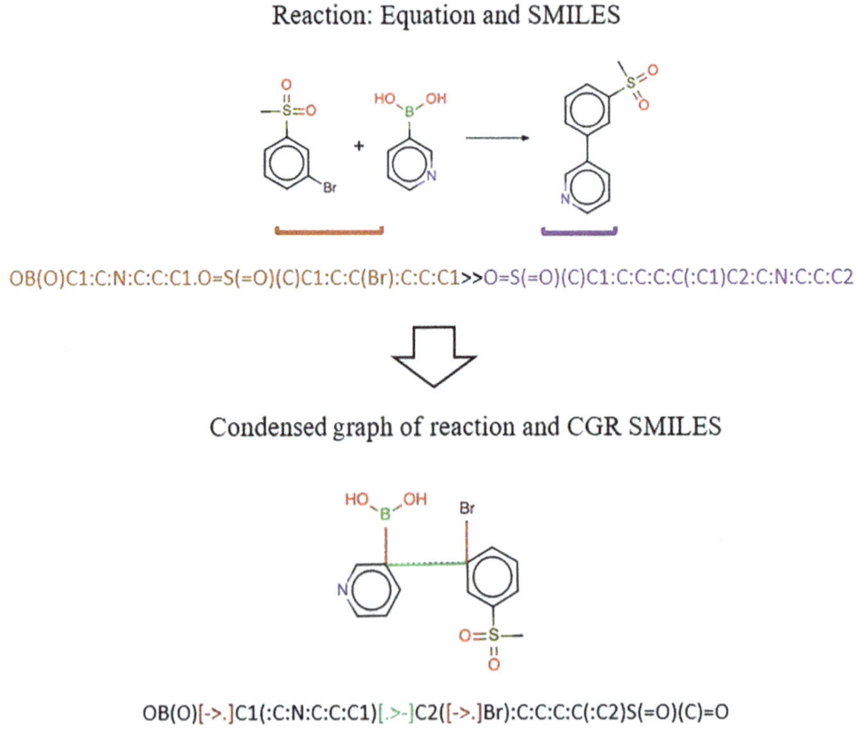

FIGURE 7.13 Illustration of the concept of condensed graph of reaction.

whereas C-B and C-Br will be broken. Formally, this information is fully captured in the CGR below, which can be processed like any "regular" molecule by any software modified to accept the non-standard bond orders for the dynamic bonds. Recently,[72] an extension of the SMILES language to cover dynamic bond types, has been proposed: [->.] stands for "single broken, [.>-] means "single formed" bond. As can be seen, the CGR SMILES is typically only half as long as the standard reaction SMILES, and furthermore, (a) does not suffer from imbalance, and (b) clearly defines the reaction center with all atoms involved in the transformation. Rendering the latter information in a regular reaction SMILES is not possible without atom mapping[75] (in fact, a CGR can be easily translated into an atom-mapped, balanced standard reaction SMILES – but the reciprocal does not apply).

Strictly speaking, the reaction above is not only incomplete because leaving groups were not rendered – it actually misses an important reagent, a nucleophilic species RO^-, leading to the elimination of $ROB(OH)_2$. This will have consequences on the way in which this reaction is being perceived by AI tools, herewith "learning" from the unbalanced process that the chemically meaningless $B(OH)_2$ is a product of the Suzuki reaction. The reality is nonetheless the one depicted above: reaction databases are never rigorous, and the chemoinformatics of reactions is equally linked to limitations in Artificial Intelligence and the excessive sloppiness of chemists (*Homo sapiens*).

7.6.2 An AutoEncoder and a Chemical Reaction Map Based on CGR SMILES

Clearly, CGR SMILES are only slightly more complex than regular molecular SMILES, and were actually proven[76] to be suitable as autoencoder input. This does not apply to regular chemical reaction SMILES – too long, missing key information unless properly balanced and with marked atoms, not only atom- but outright reagent and product order-dependent. Trained on >2M CGRs obtained by curating the USPTO[77] (a public database of patented reactions), the autoencoder displayed reasonable reconstruction rates of ~98% for training and test reactions, respectively, which is remarkable given the additional complexity induced by the multicharacter labels for dynamic bonds. A 100K randomly selected reaction dataset annotated by type (substitution, elimination, cycloaddition, etc.) was used to cartograph the chemical reaction space: a GTM was trained on the 100K latent vectors produced by the autoencoder, in order to maximize the separation between the different reaction classes. The resulting map displays well-separated areas pertaining to each reaction category and is herewith NB-compliant. This GTM-derived map could be used to help chemists acquire a bird's eye view of the pool of reactions reported in the database. In Figure 7.14, the central GTM landscape of the reaction space zones predominantly hosting Suzuki reactions (according to USPTO) are colored in blue, while red areas harbor all other reaction types. There are several "islands" such as those harboring Suzuki reactions, which is expected from such a versatile process allowing aryl, alkenyl, and alkynyl halides to with aryl, alkenyl, or alkynyl boronic acids, which are well separated on the map. This landscape might also serve as a machine-learned classifier of chemical reactions into Suzuki *versus* non-Suzuki types.

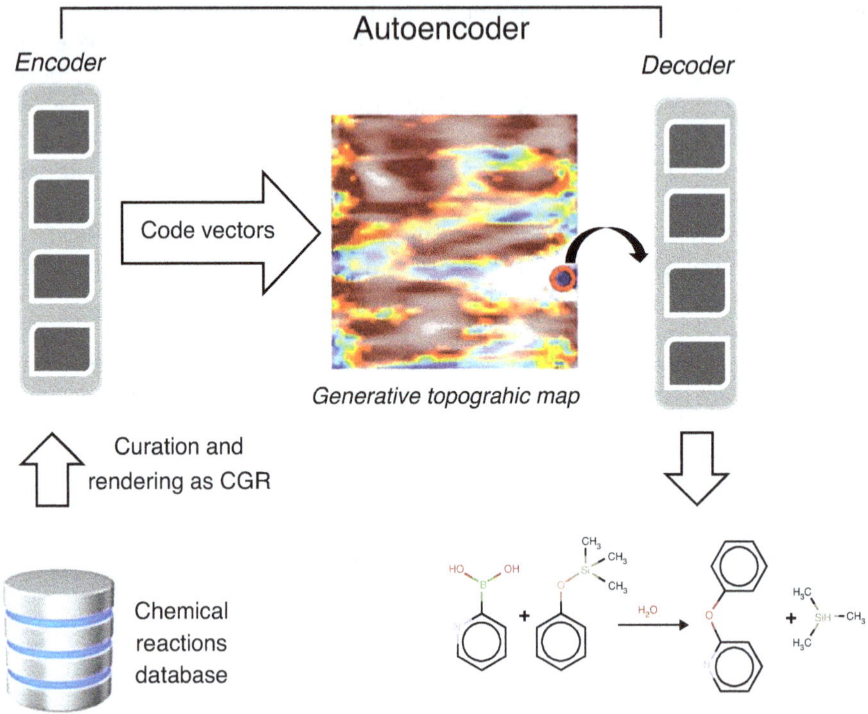

FIGURE 7.14 CGR SMILES-driven autoencoder architecture challenged to suggest "new" Suzuki-like chemical reactions by decoding vectors near the latent vectors of Suzuki-reaction-"inhabited" GTM nodes.

However, the goal of the above-cited work was not Suzuki reaction cartography, but rather to explore what CGRs can be obtained by reverting specific latent vectors of this chemical reaction space. Are those CGR valid depictions of coherent chemical transformations? Could the Artificial Intelligence herewith "imagine" new reactions? The highlighted node harboring only USPTO reactions of Suzuki type was used as the source of latent vectors by randomly perturbing the node coordinates, as already discussed in the A2a inhibitor design study.

These latent vectors were not corresponding to any given reaction but were representatives of a "Suzuki consensus zone" in reaction space. Therefore, only roughly 11% of the output text represented valid CGR SMILES. This is in line with the already mentioned increased difficulty to learn CGR SMILES syntax – but, finally, this is not a liability because the invalid output can be easily discarded algorithmically using the CGRTools package.[72]

The valid CGR strings represent intriguing "reinterpretations" of Suzuki reactions. Two such examples are shown below (Figure 7.15, please refer to the original publication[76] for more)

The first example is, technically, certainly *not* a Suzuki process, and its SciFinder-reported counterpart is not operating under Suzuki conditions. A C–Br

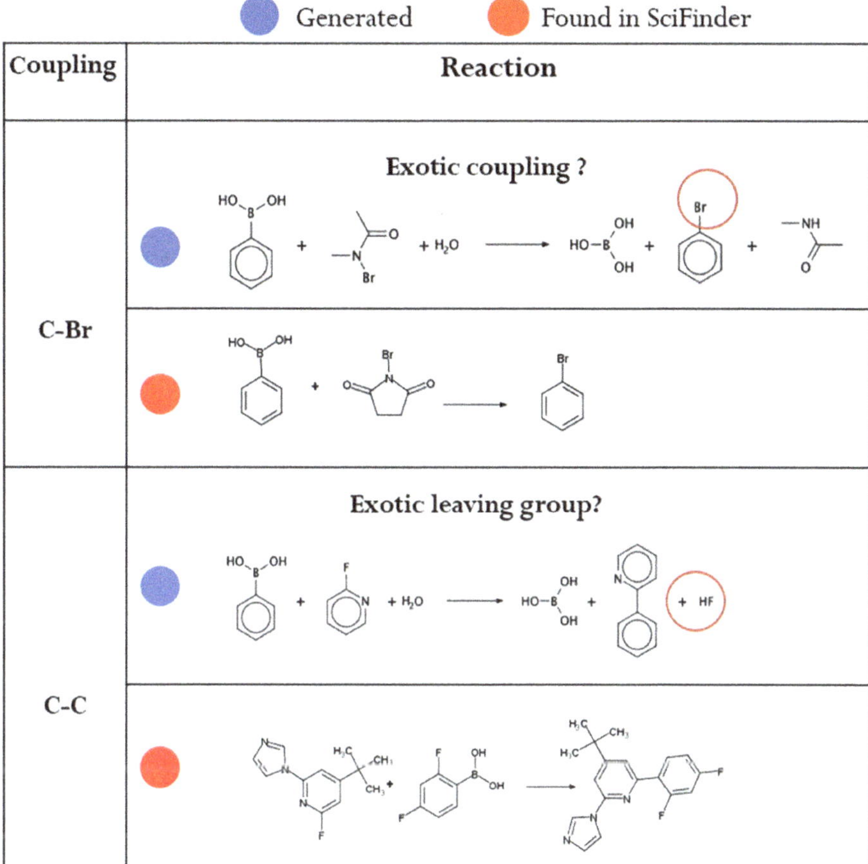

FIGURE 7.15 Suzuki reaction "reinterpreted" by the CGR-driven autoencoder – two unexpected examples next to existing, reported analog processes, showing that eventually, the decoder output is not that far-fetched. Note that the "water" molecule was added manually to properly render the elimination of boric acid – the automated process would have predicted the elimination of the unstable $B(OH)_2$, according to the CGR in Figure 7.14, because of the original imbalanced way to enter chemical reactions in databases.

bond is formed instead of the expected C–C, with the alleged bromination agent being a N-bromoamide (probably less reactive than the standard N-Bromo succinimide). Formally, however, this process does resemble a Suzuki reaction.

The second example features a putative Suzuki process with the unexpected fluoride as the leaving group. This is certainly only possible because of its position is ortho to the activating pyridine nitrogen – and such processes really occur, albeit, again, it is not certain whether they deserve to be called Suzuki reactions on the basis of their mechanism.

As already mentioned, autoencoders are (like many other chemoinformatics approaches) bound to recognize and reproduce specific *patterns* in input data, all while being fully agnostic (or naïve) of the chemistry and mechanism. In this sense, the herein developed method stood up to its challenge – to propose intriguing yet not obviously unfeasible "new" chemical reactions, under GTM "guidance" in chemical reaction space.

7.7 CONCLUSIONS

The unprecedented progress in deep learning has opened new ways to approach chemical structure enumeration. Instead of tedious modifications of a molecular graph by addition, cyclizations, or deletions of fragments – with a largely uncertain outcome in terms of chemical meaningfulness of the result – the autoencoder paradigm enables chemoinformaticians to navigate in a real-number vector "latent" space reversibly associated to chemical structure. True, the chemical feasibility of the proposed structures is still an unresolved issue, although the deep learning process tends to learn chemically stable patterns rather than random atom enchainments. However, radical transformations "walking" between two radically unrelated molecules, hardly envisageable by successive small-step tinkering with the SMILES or the graph, are now as easily accessible as enumerating a set of points by a linear combination of two position vectors. Innovative approaches such as conditional autoencoders may even link structure to classical chemical spaces based on expert-defined descriptors, providing for the first time an elegant solution to the "hard" inverse QSAR problem. In this context, "grasping" this chemical space defined by molecular descriptors (latent vectors or classical expert-defined ones) becomes of paramount importance – now that we have learned to walk, it is even more important to understand where to go. Fortunately, in the shadow of the "deep learning hype", chemical cartography has also steadily progressed – with the notable introduction of Generative Topographic Mapping by Bishop. The latter was eventually adapted for chemical cartography, notably by designing parameterization procedures tuning the degrees of freedom in map construction (including, most importantly, descriptor selection) in order to optimize map quality. Or, a key strength of GTMs, a fuzzy-logics-based "grid" method, similar to Kohonen maps, is their ability to host multiple and diverse predictive landscapes. The predictive propensity of the latter has been successfully used as objective functions to "grow" universal maps, proven to be NB-compliant, simultaneously, with respect to many hundreds of biological properties of small molecules.

Coupling of the two technologies – structure-descriptor-structure autoencoders with descriptor-landscape intuitive and predictive maps – seems to represent a novel and powerful paradigm of exploring the universe of organic molecules (drug-like, or not). This represented the topic of the present chapter, featuring some remarkably positive results, First, encoder-produced latent vectors, albeit not representing ideal molecular descriptors (likely because of their atom ordering dependence) may nonetheless, when based on canonical SMILES, serve as the basis for useful, NB-complaint GTMs. The coordinates of nodes preferentially populated by "actives" become straightforward markers of interesting chemical neighborhoods from which novel structures can be extracted by the decoder module. Many other interesting chemical space features can be explored by following GTM landscapes – notably the "empty" spaces on the map, onto which none of so-far reported compounds of medicinal chemistry interest (ChEMBL) seem to reside. Would reverting coordinates of empty nodes return not yet imagined chemotypes, or rather chemical nonsense? Confirmed universal GTMs based on classical molecular descriptors (ISIDA fragment counts) may be used likewise in conjunction with a CVAE approach operating the translation from descriptor space to structure. Eventually, it was shown that key progress in manipulating chemical reactions under the form of CGR and the specifically developed dynamic bond-sensitive CGR SMILES enables the generalization of autoencoder approaches to chemical reactions. We have also demonstrated that these can be successfully and reversibly translated to latent vectors, and mapped onto a GTM of chemical reaction space, with sharp separations of reactions by type. Suzuki reactions, a hallmark of modern synthetic chemistry, have several "dedicated" nodes that they mainly or even exclusively populate. Decoding of latent vectors sampled in their vicinity indeed returned several examples of unexpected but not unrealistic "Suzuki-like" processes.

Therefore, it can be concluded that GTMs are effective tools to guide autoencoder-driven exploration of chemical space. Is the Artificial Intelligence behind autoencoders able to come up with novel, revolutionary molecules or reactions? Novel, certainly in the commonly accepted terminology (without any blatantly similar neighbors in compound databases). Revolutionary most often not, simply because radical novelty will, in most cases, imply that the compound (or reaction) is chemically meaningless/unstable or at least not achievable within reasonable synthetic effort. This is, of course, not unexpected that the "deep learning" protocols are only deep in terms of pattern recognition but remarkably shallow when it comes to learning about the experimental properties of molecules. The reason for this is not because of the fundamental limitations of the deep learner, but likely due to variable and noisy experimental data. There are potentially billions of SMILES to learn from, but only a few tens to thousands of active compounds of a biological target to define the GTM landscape. Submitting those few data to be directly learned by the ANN would, in most cases, not bring any benefit, on the contrary, it will likely create a black-box model to be trusted blindly. Reaction databases hardly annotate the stored processes by mechanism (which is mostly unknown), but this is the least critical problem in noisy databases with imbalanced reactions and sketchy reaction condition reports. Therefore, autoencoder-generated *de novo* structures may often be considered as a "paraphrasing" of known actives, using the same structural elements, but "reshuffled" in unexpected ways. This is per se not a guarantee of activity – therefore, *de novo* structures must be filtered by standard virtual screening methods (pharmacophore match, docking) in order to select the best candidates. This can, in many cases, return molecules a medicinal chemist would not have envisaged, and if feasible, they may open novel opportunities for drug discovery. Learning, whether deep or shallow, by the machine or the human, cannot ever be better than the knowledge available for training, and GTM-piloted autoencoders are, in our opinion, a good way to make the best with the data at hand at the present time.

REFERENCES

1. So, S.-S.; Karplus, M. Genetic neural networks for quantitative structure-activity relationships: Improvements and application of benzodiazepine affinity for benzodiazepine/GABAA receptors. *J. Med. Chem.* **1996**, *39* (26), 5246–5256.

2. Cherqaoui, D.; Villemin, D. Use of a neural network to determine the boiling point of alkanes. *J. Chem. Soc., Faraday Trans.* **1994**, *90*, 97–102.
3. Gakh, A. A.; Gakh, E. G.; Sumpter, B. G.; Noid, D. W. Neural network-graph theory approach to the prediction of the physical properties of organic compounds. *J. Chem. Inf. Comput. Sci.* **1994**, *34* (4), 832–839.
4. Rogers, G. W.; Szu, H. H.; Priebe, C. E.; Solka, J. L. Nonparametric density estimation by a self-consistent neural network. In *Proceedings of the International Joint Conference on Neural Networks*, 1993; Vol. 2, pp. 2001–2004.
5. Specht, D. A general regression neural network. *IEEE T. Neural Networks* **1991**, *2*, 568–576.
6. Todeschini, R.; Consonni, V.; Mannhold, R.; Kubinyi, H.; Timmerman, H. *Handbook of Molecular Descriptors*, John Wiley & Sons, 2008.
7. Hansch, C.; Leo, A. *Exploring QSAR: Fundamentals and Applications in Chemistry and Biology*, American Chemical Society, 1995.
8. Hansch, C.; Maloney, P. P.; Fujita, T.; Muir, R. M. Correlation of biological activity of phenoxyacetic acids with Hammett substituent constants and partition coefficients. *Nature* **1962**, *194*, 178–180.
9. Butkiewicz, M.; Lowe, E. W.; Mueller, R.; Mendenhall, J. L.; Teixeira, P. L.; Weaver, C. D.; Meiler, J. Benchmarking ligand-based virtual high-throughput screening with the PubChem database. *Molecules* **2013**, *18*, 735–756.
10. Hastie, T.; Tibshirani, R.; Friedman, J. H. *The Elements of Statistical Learning: Data Mining, Inference, and Prediction*, Springer, 2001.
11. Zhou, X.; Liu, H.; Shi, C.; Liu, J. Chapter 2 - The basics of deep learning. In *Deep Learning on Edge Computing Devices*, Zhou, X., Liu, H., Shi, C., Liu, J., Eds., Elsevier, 2022, pp. 19–36.
12. Ivanciuc, O. Applications of support vector machines in chemistry. In *Reviews in Computational Chemistry*, Lipkowitz, K. B., Cundary, T. R., Eds., Wiley-VCH: Weinheim, 2007, Vol. 23, pp. 291–400.
13. Breiman, L. Random forests. *Mach. Learn.* **2001**, *45* (1), 5–32.
14. Gaulton, A.; Bellis, L. J.; Bento, A. P.; Chambers, J.; Davies, M.; Hersey, A.; Light, Y.; McGlinchey, S.; Michalovich, D.; Al-Lazikani, B.; et al. ChEMBL: A large-scale bioactivity database for drug discovery. *Nucleic Acids Res.* **2011**, *40* (D1), D1100–D1107. DOI:10.1093/nar/gkr777.
15. NIH. *The PubChem Project.* https://pubchem.ncbi.nlm.nih.gov/ (accessed 2010).
16. Heyndrickx, W.; Mervin, L.; Morawietz, T.; Sturm, N.; Friedrich, L.; Zalewski, A.; Pentina, A.; Humbeck, L.; Oldenhof, M.; Niwayama, R.; et al. MELLODDY: Cross-pharma Federated Learning at Unprecedented Scale Unlocks Benefits in QSAR without Compromising Proprietary Information. *Journal of Chemical Information and Modeling* **2024**, *64* (7), 2331–2344. DOI: 10.1021/acs.jcim.3c00799
17. Goodfellow, I.; Pouget-Abadie, J.; Mirza, M.; Xu, B.; Warde-Farley, D.; Ozair, S.; Courville, A.; Bengio, Y. Generative adversarial networks. *Commun. ACM* **2020**, *63* (11), 139–144. DOI:10.1145/3422622.
18. Brown, T. B.; Mann, B.; Ryder, N.; Subbiah, M.; Kaplan, J.; Dhariwal, P.; Neelakantan, A.; Shyam, P.; Sastry, G.; Askell, A.; et al. Language models are few-shot learners. In *Proceedings of the 34th International Conference on Neural Information Processing Systems*, Vancouver, BC, Canada, 2020.
19. Zhou, J.; Cui, G.; Hu, S.; Zhang, Z.; Yang, C.; Liu, Z.; Wang, L.; Li, C.; Sun, M. Graph neural networks: A review of methods and applications. *AI Open* **2020**, *1*, 57–81. DOI:10.1016/j.aiopen.2021.01.001.
20. Weininger, D. SMILES, A chemical language and information system. 1. Introduction to methodology and encoding rules. *J. Chem. Inf. Comput. Sci.* **1988**, *28* (1), 31–36.

21. Krenn, M.; Ai, Q.; Barthel, S.; Carson, N.; Frei, A.; Frey, N. C.; Friederich, P.; Gaudin, T.; Gayle, A. A.; Jablonka, K. M.; et al. SELFIES and the future of molecular string representations. *Patterns* **2022**, *3* (10), 100588. DOI:10.1016/j.patter.2022.100588.
22. Badrinarayanan, V.; Kendall, A.; Cipolla, R. Segnet: A deep convolutional encoder-decoder architecture for image segmentation. *IEEE Trans. Pattern Anal. Mach. Intell.* **2017**, *39* (12), 2481–2495.
23. DayLight. *SMARTS*. Daylight Chemical Information Systems, 2007. https://www.daylight.com/dayhtml/doc/theory.smarts.html (accessed October 2014).
24. Hartenfeller, M.; Zettl, H.; Walter, M.; Rupp, M.; Reisen, F.; Proschak, E.; Weggen, S.; Stark, H.; Schneider, G. DOGS: Reaction-driven de novo design of bioactive compounds. *PLoS Comput Biol* **2012**, *8* (2), e1002380.
25. Brown, N.; Fiscato, M.; Segler, M. H. S.; Vaucher, A. C. GuacaMol: Benchmarking models for de novo molecular design. *J. Chem. Inform. Model.* **2019**, *59* (3), 1096–1108. DOI:10.1021/acs.jcim.8b00839.
26. Ertl, P.; Schuffenhauer, A. Estimation of synthetic accessibility score of drug-like molecules based on molecular complexity and fragment contributions. *J. Cheminform.* **2009**, *1* (1), 8. DOI:10.1186/1758-2946-1-8.
27. Polishchuk, P. Control of synthetic feasibility of compounds generated with CReM. *J. Chem. Inform. Model.* **2020**, *60* (12), 6074–6080. DOI:10.1021/acs.jcim.0c00792.
28. Eshel, I. L.; Milo, A. Predicting synthetic viability. *Nat. Synth.* **2023**, *2* (6), 473–474. DOI:10.1038/s44160-023-00297-4.
29. Kaneko, H. Data visualization, regression, applicability domains and inverse analysis based on generative topographic mapping. *Mol. Inform.* **2019**, *38* (3), e1800088. DOI:10.1002/minf.201800088.
30. Miyao, T.; Kaneko, H.; Funatsu, K. Inverse QSPR/QSAR analysis for chemical structure generation (from y to x). *J. Chem. Inform. Model.* **2016**, *56* (2), 286–299. DOI:10.1021/acs.jcim.5b00628.
31. Skvortsova, M. I.; Baskin, I. I., Palyulin, V. A.; Slovokhotova, O. L.; Zefirov, N. S. Structural design. Inverse problems for topological indices in QSAR/QSPR studies. In *AIP Conference Proceedings 330. E.C.C.C.1 Computational Chemistry F.E.C.S. Conference*, Nancy, France, Bernardi, F., Rivail, J.-L., Eds., AIP Press, 1995, pp. 486–499.
32. Karlov, D. S.; Sosnin, S.; Tetko, I. V.; Fedorov, M. V. Chemical space exploration guided by deep neural networks. *RSC Adv.* **2019**, *9* (9), 5151–5157. DOI:10.1039/C8RA10182E.
33. Kireeva, N.; Baskin, I.; Gaspar, H. A.; Horvath, D.; Marcou, G.; Varnek, A. Generative topographic mapping (GTM): Universal tool for data visualization, structure-activity modeling and dataset comparison. *Mol. Inf.* **2012**, *31* (3–4), 301–312. DOI:10.1002/minf.201100163.
34. Agrafiotis, D. K. Stochastic proximity embedding. *J. Comput. Chem.* **2003**, *24* (10), 1215–1221. DOI:10.1002/jcc.10234.
35. Agrafiotis, D. K.; Rassokhin, D. N.; Lobanov, V. S. Multidimensional scaling and visualization of large molecular similarity tables. *J. Comput. Chem.* **2001**, *22* (5), 488–500. DOI: 10.1002/1096-987x(20010415)22:5<488::aid-jcc1020>3.0.co;2-4.
36. Zabolotna, Y.; Bonachera, F.; Horvath, D.; Lin, A.; Marcou, G.; Klimchuk, O.; Varnek, A. Chemspace atlas: Multiscale chemography of ultralarge libraries for drug discovery. *J. Chem. Inf. Model.* **2022**, *62* (18), 4537–4548. DOI:10.1021/acs.jcim.2c00509.
37. Papadatos, G.; Cooper, A. W. J.; Kadirkamanathan, V.; Macdonald, S. J. F.; McLay, I. M.; Pickett, S. D.; Pritchard, J. M.; Willett, P.; Gillet, V. J. Analysis of neighborhood behavior in lead optimization and array design. *J. Chem. Inf. Model.* **2009**, *49* (2), 195–208, Proceedings Paper. DOI:10.1021/ci800302g.

38. Patterson, D. E.; Cramer, R. D.; Ferguson, A. M.; Clark, R. D.; Weinberger, L. E. Neighborhood behavior: A useful concept for validation of "molecular diversity" descriptors. *J. Med. Chem.* **1996**, *39* (16), 3049–3059.
39. Johnson, M. A.; Maggiora, G. M. *Concepts and Applications of Molecular Similarity*, Wiley Interscience: New York, 1990.
40. Gaspar, H. A.; Baskin, I. I.; Marcou, G.; Horvath, D.; Varnek, A. GTM-based QSAR models and their applicability domains. *Mol. Inform.* **2015**, *34* (6–7), 348–356. DOI:10.1002/minf.201400153.
41. Oprea, T. I.; Gottfries, J. Chemography: The art of navigating in chemical space. *J. Combin. Chem.* **2001**, *3* (2), 157–166.
42. Jolliffe, I. T. *Principal Component Analysis*, Springer Verlag, 2002.
43. van der Maaten, L.; Hinton, G. Visualizing data using t-SNE. *J. Mach. Learn. Res.* **2008**, *9*, 2579–2605.
44. de Sousa, J. M. A. Data visualization and analysis using Kohonen self-organizing maps. *Tut. Chemoinform.* **2017**, 119–126. DOI:10.1002/9781119161110.ch7 (acccessed 2020/02/06).
45. Kohonen, T. *Self-Organizing Maps*, Springer, 2001.
46. Gaspar, H. A.; Baskin, I. I.; Marcou, G.; Horvath, D.; Varnek, A. Chemical data visualization and analysis with incremental generative topographic mapping: Big data challenge. *J. Chem. Inf. Model.* **2014**, *55* (1), 84–94. DOI:10.1021/ci500575y.
47. Gaspar, H. A.; Marcou, G.; Horvath, D.; Arault, A.; Lozano, S.; Vayer, P.; Varnek, A. Generative topographic mapping-based classification models and their applicability domain: Application to the biopharmaceutics drug disposition classification system (BDDCS). *J. Chem. Inform. Model.* **2013**, *53* (12), 3318–3325. DOI:10.1021/ci400423c.
48. Bishop, C. M.; Svensén, M.; Williams, C. K. GTM: The generative topographic mapping. *Neural Comput.* **1998**, *10* (1), 215–234.
49. Bishop, C. M.; Svensén, M.; Williams, C. K. I. Developments of the generative topographic mapping. *Neurocomputing* **1998**, *21* (1–3), 203–224. DOI:10.1016/S0925-2312(98)00043-5.
50. Casciuc, I.; Zabolotna, Y.; Horvath, D.; Marcou, G.; Bajorath, J.; Varnek, A. Virtual Screening with generative topographic maps: How many maps are required? *J. Chem. Inf. Model.* **2019**, *59* (1), 564–572. DOI:10.1021/acs.jcim.8b00650.
51. Sidorov, P.; Gaspar, H.; Marcou, G.; Varnek, A.; Horvath, D. Mappability of drug-like space: Towards a polypharmacologically competent map of drug-relevant compounds. *J. Comp.-Aided Mol. Des.* **2015**, *29* (12), 1087–1108. DOI:10.1007/s10822-015-9882-z.
52. Zabolotna, Y.; Ertl, P.; Horvath, D.; Bonachera, F.; Marcou, G.; Varnek, A. NP navigator: A new look at the natural product chemical space. *Mol. Inform.* **2021**, *40*, e2100068. DOI:10.1002/minf.202100068.
53. Klimenko, K.; Marcou, G.; Horvath, D.; Varnek, A. Chemical space mapping and structure-activity analysis of the ChEMBL antiviral compound set. *J. Chem. Inf. Model.* **2016**, *56* (8), 1438–1454. DOI:10.1021/acs.jcim.6b00192.
54. Bengio, Y.; Courville, A.; Vincent, P. Representation learning: A review and new perspectives. *IEEE Trans. Pattern Anal. Mach. Intell.* **2013**, *35*, 1798–1828. DOI:10.1109/TPAMI.2013.50.
55. Sutskever, I.; Vinyals, O.; Le, Q. V. Sequence to sequence learning with neural networks. In *Proceedings of the 27th International Conference on Neural Information Processing Systems - Volume 2*, Montreal, Canada, 2014.
56. Amiriparian, S.; Freitag, M.; Cummins, N.; Schuller, B. Sequence to Sequence Autoencoders for Unsupervised Representation Learning from Audio. In *Detection and Classification of Acoustic Scenes and Events*, München, Germany, 2017.
57. Williams, R. J.; Zipser, D. A learning algorithm for continually running fully recurrent neural networks. *Neural Comput.* **1989**, *1*, 270–280.

58. Sattarov, B.; Baskin, II; Horvath, D.; Marcou, G.; Bjerrum, E. J.; Varnek, A. De novo molecular design by combining deep autoencoder recurrent neural networks with generative topographic mapping. *J. Chem. Inf. Model.* **2019**, *59* (3), 1182–1196. DOI:10.1021/acs.jcim.8b00751.
59. Todeschini, R.; Consonni, V. *Handbook of Molecular Descriptors*, Wiley-VCH Publishers, 2000.
60. Ruggiu, F.; Marcou, G.; Varnek, A.; Horvath, D. Isida property-labelled fragment descriptors. *Mol. Inform.* **2010**, *29* (12), 855–868.
61. Horvath, D.; Marcou, G.; Varnek, A. Trustworthiness, the key to grid-based map-driven predictive model enhancement and applicability domain control. *J. Chem. Inf. Model.* **2020**, *60* (12), 6020–6032. DOI:10.1021/acs.jcim.0c00998.
62. Arús-Pous, J.; Johansson, S.; Prykhodko, O.; Bjerrum, E. J.; Tyrchan, C.; Reymond, J.-L.; Chen, H.; Engkvist, O. Improving deep generative models with randomized SMILES. In *Artificial Neural Networks and Machine Learning – ICANN 2019: Workshop and Special Sessions*, Cham, Tetko, I. V., Kůrková, V., Karpov, P., Theis, F., Eds., Springer International Publishing, 2019, pp. 747–751.
63. Akhmetshin, T.; Lin, A.; Mazitov, D.; Zabolotna, Y.; Ziaikin, E.; Madzhidov, T.; Varnek, A. HyFactor: A novel open-source, graph-based architecture for chemical structure generation. *J. Chem. Inf. Model.* **2022**, *62* (15), 3524–3534. DOI:10.1021/acs.jcim.2c00744.
64. Bort, W.; Mazitov, D.; Horvath, D.; Bonachera, F.; Lin, A.; Marcou, G.; Baskin, I.; Madzhidov, T.; Varnek, A. Inverse QSAR: Reversing descriptor-driven prediction pipeline using attention-based conditional variational autoencoder. *J. Chem. Inf. Model.* **2022**, *62* (22), 5471–5484. DOI:10.1021/acs.jcim.2c01086.
65. Varnek, A.; Fourches, D.; Horvath, D.; Klimchuk, O.; Gaudin, C.; Vayer, P.; Solov'ev, V.; Hoonakker, F.; Tetko, I. V.; Marcou, G. ISIDA - Platform for virtual screening based on fragment and pharmacophoric descriptors. *Curr. Comp.-Aided Drug Des.* **2008**, *4* (3), 191–198. DOI:10.2174/157340908785747465.
66. Hartenfeller, M.; Proschak, E.; Schueller, A.; Schneider, G. Concept of combinatorial de novo design of drug-like molecules by particle swarm optimization. *Chem. Biol. Drug Des.* **2008**, *72* (1), 16–26. DOI:10.1111/j.1747-0285.2008.00672.x.
67. Coley, C. W.; Barzilay, R.; Jaakkola, T. S.; Green, W. H.; Jensen, K. F. Prediction of organic reaction outcomes using machine learning. *ACS Cent. Sci.* **2017**, *3*, 434.
68. Coley, C. W.; Rogers, L.; Green, W. H.; Jensen, K. F. Computer-assisted retrosynthesis based on molecular similarity. *ACS Cent. Sci.* **2017**, *3* (12), 1237–1245. DOI:10.1021/acscentsci.7b00355.
69. Satoh, K.; Funatsu, K. A novel approach to retrosynthetic analysis using knowledge bases derived from reaction databases. *J. Chem. Inf. Comput. Sci.* **1999**, *39*, 316.
70. Kearnes, S. M.; Maser, M. R.; Wleklinski, M.; Kast, A.; Doyle, A. G.; Dreher, S. D.; Hawkins, J. M.; Jensen, K. F.; Coley, C. W. The open reaction database. *J. Am. Chem. Soc.* **2021**, *143* (45), 18820–18826. DOI:10.1021/jacs.1c09820.
71. Hoonakker, F.; Lachiche, N.; Varnek, A.; Wagner, A. Condensed Graph of Reaction: Considering a Chemical Reaction as One Single Pseudo Molecule, *Int. J. Artif. Intel. T.* **2011** *20* (2), 253–270.
72. Nugmanov, R. I.; Mukhametgaleev, R.; Akhmetshin, T.; Gimadiev, T.; Afonina, V.; Madzhidov, T.; Varnek, A. CGRtools: Python library for molecule, reaction, and condensed graph of reaction processing. *J. Chem. Inf. Model.* **2019**, *59*, 2516.
73. Glavatskikh, M.; Madzhidov, T.; Horvath, D.; Nugmanov, R.; Gimadiev, T.; Malakhova, D.; Marcou, G.; Varnek, A. Predictive models for kinetic parameters of cycloaddition reactions. *Mol. Inf.* **2019**, *38* (1–2), e1800077. DOI:10.1002/minf.201800077.
74. de Luca, A.; Horvath, D.; Marcou, G.; Solovev, V.; Varnek, A. Mining chemical reactions using neighborhood behavior and condensed graphs of reactions approaches. *J. Chem. Inf. Model.* **2012**, *52* (9), 2325–2338. DOI:10.1021/ci300149n.

75. Muller, C.; Marcou, G.; Horvath, D.; Aires-de-Sousa, J. O.; Varnek, A. Models for identification of erroneous atom-to-atom mapping of reactions performed by automated algorithms. *J. Chem. Inf. Model.* **2012**, *52* (12), 3116–3122. DOI:10.1021/ci300418q.
76. Bort, W.; Baskin, II; Gimadiev, T.; Mukanov, A.; Nugmanov, R.; Sidorov, P.; Marcou, G.; Horvath, D.; Klimchuk, O.; Madzhidov, T.; et al. Discovery of novel chemical reactions by deep generative recurrent neural network. *Sci. Rep.* **2021**, *11* (1), 3178. DOI:10.1038/s41598-021-81889-y.
77. Lowe, D. M. *Extraction of Chemical Structures and Reactions from the Literature.* University of Cambridge, 2012.

8 In Silico ADME/Tox in the Generative AI Paradigm

Sean Ekins, Thomas R. Lane, Joshua S. Harris, and Fabio Urbina

8.1 INTRODUCTION

As we enter the era of generative drug discovery, we should be developing molecules with not only the desired bioactivity but also ideal physicochemical and other properties. It is worth briefly reflecting on how we reached this point before we describe where we might go in the future as well as some of the limitations.

As the available datasets and computational software have improved over time, these approaches for drug discovery have evolved considerably since the 1980s. *In vitro,* methods for absorption, distribution, metabolism, excretion, and toxicity (ADME/Tox) started to be adopted in the industry in the late 1980s to early 1990s, which, when combined with the nascent combinatorial chemistry and high throughput screening used at the time, provided the increasing quantities of complex data which then necessitated more sophisticated computational approaches[1] (Figure 8.1). The dramatically increasing costs of drug development and failure rates associated with ADME/Tox attrition were starting to be recognized at the same time,[2] suggesting that these properties could be addressed to filter out poor-performing compounds[3,4] as well as predict drug-drug interactions[5] with an array of approaches.[6–8] It was also proposed that predicting ADME/Tox properties alone or alongside additional experimental data could lead to fewer design-make-test cycles.[9] From the outset, it was felt no single method would lead to success, and the need for multiple approaches was apparent.[10,11] In the late 1990s, the throughput of the ADME assays was in the hundreds of compounds per week in big pharma.[12] It was also appreciated that human biology was more complex. this then necessitated systems biology approaches.[13] Some pharmaceutical companies were early in describing their use of computational ADME/Tox, including Roche, who used computational methods to assess metabolic stability, phospholipidosis, and hERG models based on physiological parameters and structural fragments.[14] While the results of such early approaches were promising, they were not ideal for predicting rare toxicity events at this point.[15]

It was also noted at the same time that data in the public domain was a limiting factor, and by around 2010, pre-competitive initiatives were proposed for ADME/Tox[16] such that publicly available data could enable predictive models. It was found at the same time that open-source software was also on a par with commercial tools for generating these ADME/Tox models.[17] Within a few years, such datasets were

DOI: 10.1201/9781003399346-12

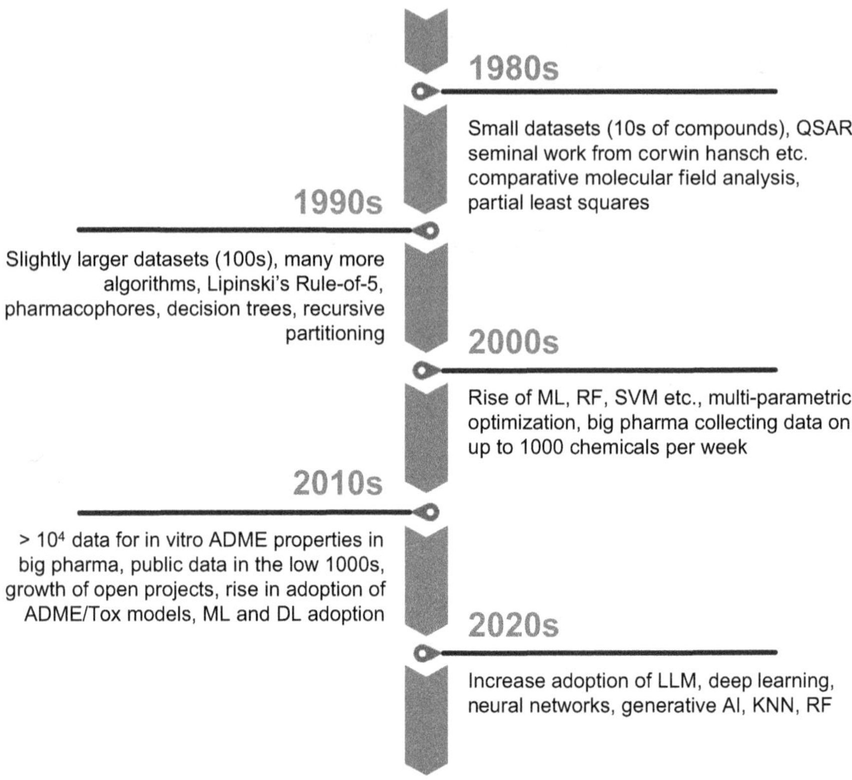

FIGURE 8.1 The evolution of machine learning models over the past decades.

enabling reliable classification models,[18] leading to websites and open software toolkits[19,20] which have subsequently expanded their use further over the years.

Within the last decade, consortia of several large pharmaceutical companies have described their use of ADME models trained on hundreds to thousands of compounds that were available to them.[21] In some cases, these datasets exceeded 100,000 compounds: Pfizer had metabolic stability data for over 200,000 compounds, which resulted in predictive models with open-source software (in 2010).[17] AstraZeneca were able to show that a solubility model could increase this property sevenfold, while a microsomal stability model at Genentech improved compound stability twofold and a CYP3A4 time-dependent inhibition model at Eli Lilly showed a threefold improvement. Other models such as human protein binding, MDCK-MDR1, metabolic stability, and P-glycoprotein efflux were also described.[21] One of the companies with approximately 20 years of experience of computational ADME/Tox is Bayer, who have recently reviewed these efforts, enabling an in-house informatics platform, data warehouse and data visualization tools, combined with other tools where the model quality, relevance, ease of access and interpretability of the results were stressed.[22] Sanofi also recently reviewed their research in this domain as well as the use of newer algorithms such as generative pre-training.[23]

In recent years, there has also been increased focus on the reproducibility of computational models in drug discovery, including ADME/Tox models.[24] Several public-private partnerships have been initiated (iD3-INST) with a focus on modeling pharmacokinetics and cardiac toxicity.[25] In the USA, the National Institutes of Health (NIH) has generated datasets for ADME properties (e.g. PAMPA, rat liver microsome stability, and solubility) which have been used with random forest models and graph-based neural networks.[26] Findable, accessible, interoperable, and reusable (FAIR) principles have been suggested to be applied to toxicology models, and this may influence regulatory acceptance.[27] The importance of computational *in vivo* models of toxicity[28] for regulatory agencies suggest the ultimate goal of replacement of *in vivo* studies in animals[29] which may reduce the use of animals.[30]

8.2 WHAT'S NEW IS OLD AGAIN

In the 1990s, the biggest challenge was likely the lack of data to build ADME/Tox models; and in some ways, this is still true even now. As the industry embraces new chemical modalities, such as the focus on larger molecules (beyond the rule of 5), again we are facing limited data on molecules outside the typical chemistry space of what was previously accepted. In particular, there is limited *in vitro* ADME/Tox data for proteolysis targeting chimeras (PROTACS) outside of the companies that are focused on them exclusively.[31] Even such data on macrocycles, peptides, and natural products is limited. Such, extensive molecule data in public databases is quite limited, which restricts their use for model building. Properties such as the permeability of PROTACS have been predicted computationally,[32] although again, there has been heavy use of proprietary data. There needs to be more data published before we can have confidence in such models for PROTACS, and there also needs to be complete datasets, including solubility, metabolic stability, HERG, transporters and other properties of interest that incorporate these moelcules.

Over 20 years ago, we thought ADME/Tox models would have an important role in the industry[9]; and while it has taken some time to get there, it is now apparent that there is considerable data in the public domain to allow anyone outside of big pharma to build such models. While the amount of public ADME/Tox data is still relatively small compared to what each big pharma has,[17,22] it is a foundation for machine learning model development. As an illustration of what can be achieved with public data, we have recently curated data from ChEMBL[33] and the literature for human intestinal absorption (HIA)[34] and human oral bioavailability (HOB)[35] (Figure 8.2); Blood Brain Barrier (BBB)[36–39] and Plasma Protein Binding (PPB)[40,41] (Figure 8.3); human microsomal stability[33] (Figure 8.4); human clearance $t_{1/2}$ and clearance[33] (Figure 8.5); hERG[42] (Figure 8.6); and P-gp substrate and inhibitors[43–45] (Figure 8.7). This data was rigorously curated using our in-house automated curation pipeline e-Clean.[46–49] The following steps were performed to standardize SMILES: standardize isotopes, remove stereoisomer information, disconnect metals, remove common salts and solvents, identify parent molecules, discard molecules with undesirable elements (inorganic elements), neutralize charges, and canonicalize SMILES. After standardizing SMILES,

Target	Total	Thresholds
Human intestinal absorption (HIA)	578	>80%, >90%
Human oral bioavailability (HOB)	1252	>70%, >50%

Human intestinal absorption (HIA); >80% 578 430/148

Method	AUC	F1	Precision	Recall	Accuracy	Specificity	Cohen's κ	MCC
ada	0.77	0.87	0.79	0.97	0.78	0.24	0.27	0.33
bnb	0.77	0.87	0.79	0.96	0.79	0.27	0.29	0.35
knn	0.76	0.88	0.86	0.9	0.81	0.57	0.49	0.49
lreg	0.8	0.87	0.83	0.92	0.79	0.43	0.39	0.4
DL	0.76	0.88	0.79	0.98	0.8	0.26	0.31	0.4
rf	0.78	0.87	0.83	0.92	0.8	0.45	0.42	0.43
svc	0.77	0.86	0.84	0.87	0.78	0.52	0.4	0.41
xgb	0.8	0.88	0.85	0.92	0.81	0.51	0.47	0.48

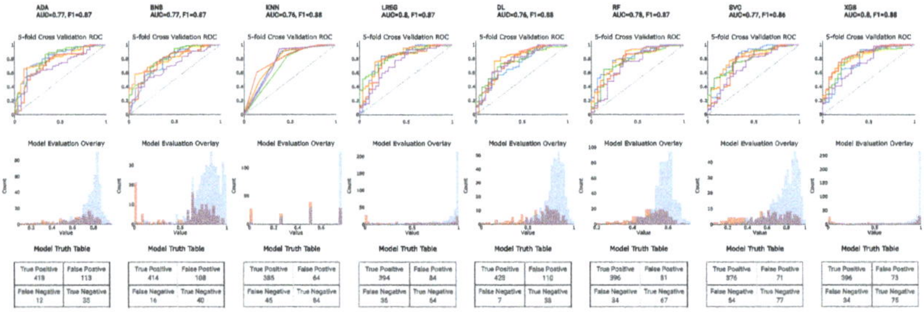

Human oral bio-availability (HOB); >70% 649 316/333

Method	AUC	F1	Precision	Recall	Accuracy	Specificity	Cohen's κ	MCC
ada	0.76	0.68	0.71	0.66	0.7	0.73	0.39	0.4
bnb	0.78	0.69	0.7	0.68	0.7	0.73	0.41	0.41
knn	0.77	0.69	0.71	0.67	0.7	0.73	0.41	0.41
lreg	0.78	0.71	0.70	0.71	0.72	0.74	0.43	0.43
DL	0.77	0.66	0.77	0.59	0.71	0.83	0.42	0.43
rf	0.81	0.72	0.74	0.71	0.73	0.76	0.47	0.47
svc	0.82	0.73	0.73	0.72	0.74	0.75	0.47	0.47
xgb	0.77	0.7	0.69	0.72	0.71	0.69	0.41	0.41

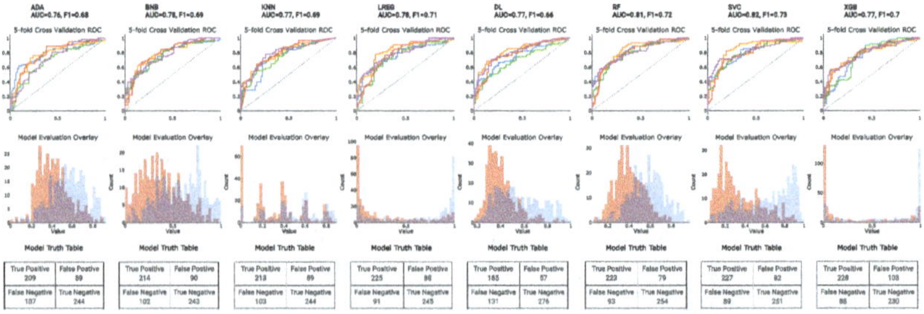

FIGURE 8.2 Human intestinal absorption and human oral bioavailability machine learning models.

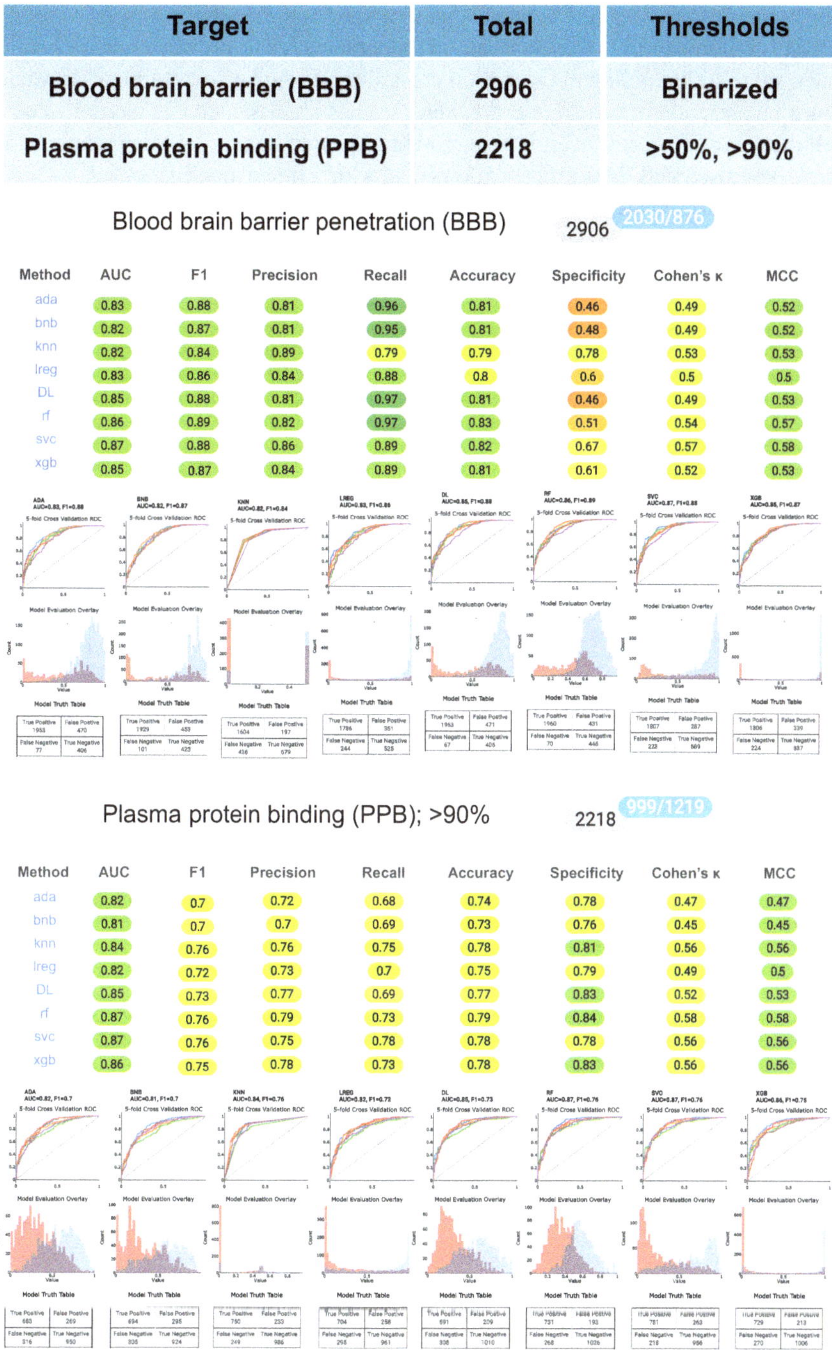

Target	Total	Thresholds
Blood brain barrier (BBB)	2906	Binarized
Plasma protein binding (PPB)	2218	>50%, >90%

Method	AUC	F1	Precision	Recall	Accuracy	Specificity	Cohen's κ	MCC
ada	0.83	0.88	0.81	0.96	0.81	0.46	0.49	0.52
bnb	0.82	0.87	0.81	0.95	0.81	0.48	0.49	0.52
knn	0.82	0.84	0.89	0.79	0.79	0.78	0.53	0.53
lreg	0.83	0.86	0.84	0.88	0.8	0.6	0.5	0.5
DL	0.85	0.88	0.81	0.97	0.81	0.46	0.49	0.53
rf	0.86	0.89	0.82	0.97	0.83	0.51	0.54	0.57
svc	0.87	0.88	0.86	0.89	0.82	0.67	0.57	0.58
xgb	0.85	0.87	0.84	0.89	0.81	0.61	0.52	0.53

Method	AUC	F1	Precision	Recall	Accuracy	Specificity	Cohen's κ	MCC
ada	0.82	0.7	0.72	0.68	0.74	0.78	0.47	0.47
bnb	0.81	0.7	0.7	0.69	0.73	0.76	0.45	0.45
knn	0.84	0.76	0.76	0.75	0.78	0.81	0.56	0.56
lreg	0.82	0.72	0.73	0.7	0.75	0.79	0.49	0.5
DL	0.85	0.73	0.77	0.69	0.77	0.83	0.52	0.53
rf	0.87	0.76	0.79	0.73	0.79	0.84	0.58	0.58
svc	0.87	0.76	0.75	0.78	0.78	0.78	0.56	0.56
xgb	0.86	0.75	0.78	0.73	0.78	0.83	0.56	0.56

FIGURE 8.3 Blood-brain barrier and plasma protein binding machine learning models.

samples are grouped together by molecular structure, and measurement values are converted to common units. Measurements on the same molecule are combined to a single binary value by the following steps: (a) discard exact duplicates, (b) binarize values using a binarization threshold (e.g. all values <1 μM are assigned a binarized value of 1, all others are assigned 0). (c) If binarization was ambiguous (≤60% agreement), the sample was discarded. This process allows data with different qualifiers ("<", ">", "=") to be utilized and condensed to a single classification for each molecule. Our software Assay Central was used to generate multiple additional classification models that have been described in detail previously.[50] The algorithms used included Bernoulli naïve Bayes, Linear Logistic Regression, AdaBoost Decision Tree, Random Forest, Support Vector Machine, Deep Neural Networks, and XGBoost. Machine learning model validation was performed using nested fivefold cross-validation.

Most of these datasets are on the order of thousands of molecules, and yet these represent a small sample of the large number of potential ADME/Tox models that could be generated with public data, as we have excluded models for drug induced liver injury,[51] nephrotoxicity, ecotoxicity[49] and others which may be of utility depending on the context and needs of a project.

Species	Model(s)	Threshold	*Actives/total
Human	Microsomal stability	≥ 70% remaining after 30 min	612/1610
		≥ 70% remaining after 60 min	400/865
	Hepatocyte stability	≥ 9.5 μL/min/mg	196/404
		Clint ≥ 20 ml/min/kg	78/173
	Plasma stability	$t_{1/2}$ ≥ 50 min	231/515
	Whole blood stability	$t_{1/2}$ ≥ 30 min	68/130
	CYP substrate (CYP1A2, 2B6, 2C9, 2C19, 2D6, 3A4)	Variable	Size: 1768–2402 (mean=1959)
	CYP inhibition (CYP1A2, 2B6, 2C9, 2C19, 2D6, 3A4)	Variable	Size: 465-9940 (mean=5131)

FIGURE 8.4 Microsomal stability at 30 (a) and 60 minutes (b) and other related machine learning model datasets.

(Continued)

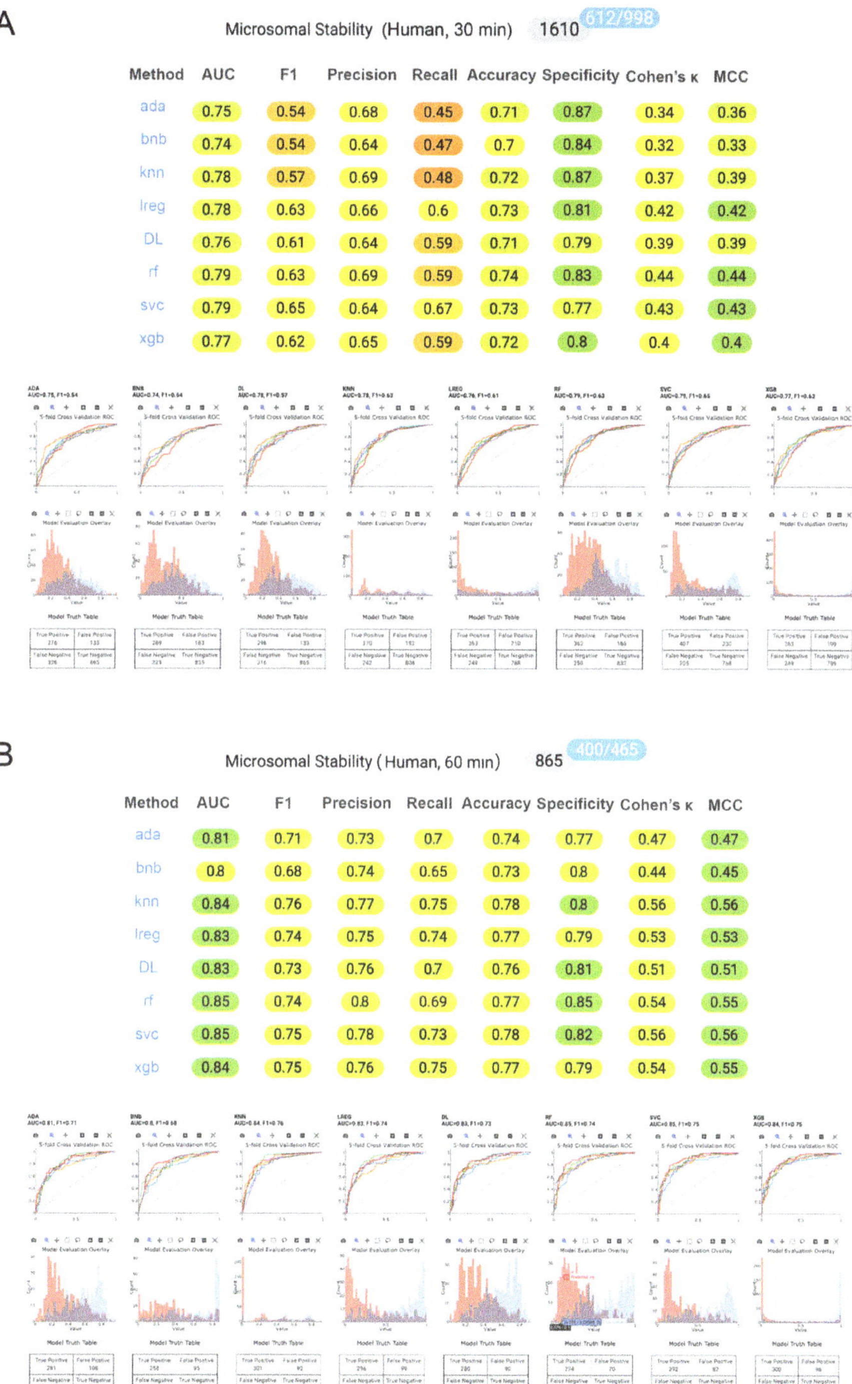

Method	AUC	F1	Precision	Recall	Accuracy	Specificity	Cohen's κ	MCC
ada	0.75	0.54	0.68	0.45	0.71	0.87	0.34	0.36
bnb	0.74	0.54	0.64	0.47	0.7	0.84	0.32	0.33
knn	0.78	0.57	0.69	0.48	0.72	0.87	0.37	0.39
lreg	0.78	0.63	0.66	0.6	0.73	0.81	0.42	0.42
DL	0.76	0.61	0.64	0.59	0.71	0.79	0.39	0.39
rf	0.79	0.63	0.69	0.59	0.74	0.83	0.44	0.44
svc	0.79	0.65	0.64	0.67	0.73	0.77	0.43	0.43
xgb	0.77	0.62	0.65	0.59	0.72	0.8	0.4	0.4

Method	AUC	F1	Precision	Recall	Accuracy	Specificity	Cohen's κ	MCC
ada	0.81	0.71	0.73	0.7	0.74	0.77	0.47	0.47
bnb	0.8	0.68	0.74	0.65	0.73	0.8	0.44	0.45
knn	0.84	0.76	0.77	0.75	0.78	0.8	0.56	0.56
lreg	0.83	0.74	0.75	0.74	0.77	0.79	0.53	0.53
DL	0.83	0.73	0.76	0.7	0.76	0.81	0.51	0.51
rf	0.85	0.74	0.8	0.69	0.77	0.85	0.54	0.55
svc	0.85	0.75	0.78	0.73	0.78	0.82	0.56	0.56
xgb	0.84	0.75	0.76	0.75	0.77	0.79	0.54	0.55

FIGURE 8.4 (*Continued*) Microsomal stability at 30 (a) and 60 minutes (b) and other related machine learning model datasets.

Target	Total	Thresholds
Human clearance ($t_{1/2}$)	688	>2 hr, >4 hr
Human clearance (Cl)	718	>4 mg/min*kg

Human clearance ($t_{1/2}$); >2 hr 688 493/195

Method	AUC	F1	Precision	Recall	Accuracy	Specificity	Cohen's κ	MCC
ada	0.71	0.84	0.75	0.96	0.74	0.2	0.2	0.25
bnb	0.75	0.86	0.77	0.96	0.77	0.3	0.31	0.36
knn	0.76	0.84	0.83	0.84	0.76	0.56	0.41	0.41
lreg	0.76	0.84	0.81	0.87	0.76	0.47	0.36	0.37
DL	0.76	0.85	0.76	0.95	0.75	0.26	0.25	0.3
rf	0.76	0.85	0.8	0.91	0.77	0.43	0.37	0.38
svc	0.78	0.83	0.82	0.85	0.76	0.52	0.38	0.38
xgb	0.76	0.85	0.81	0.89	0.77	0.48	0.4	0.41

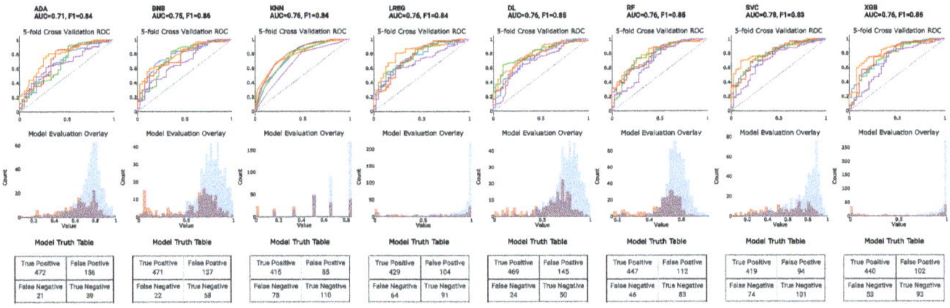

Human clearance (Cl); >4 mg/min*kg 718 360/358

Method	AUC	F1	Precision	Recall	Accuracy	Specificity	Cohen's κ	MCC
ada	0.69	0.62	0.61	0.64	0.62	0.59	0.23	0.24
bnb	0.73	0.65	0.66	0.63	0.65	0.67	0.3	0.3
knn	0.76	0.7	0.71	0.7	0.71	0.72	0.42	0.42
lreg	0.72	0.66	0.66	0.66	0.66	0.65	0.31	0.31
DL	0.73	0.65	0.66	0.66	0.65	0.65	0.31	0.31
rf	0.76	0.69	0.71	0.68	0.7	0.71	0.4	0.4
svc	0.77	0.68	0.7	0.67	0.69	0.72	0.39	0.39
xgb	0.73	0.69	0.68	0.7	0.69	0.68	0.37	0.38

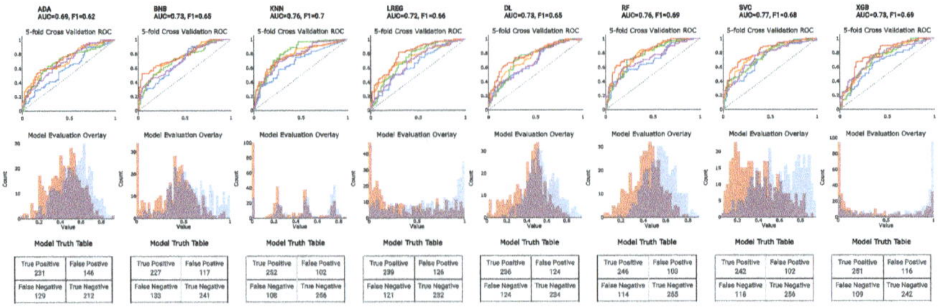

FIGURE 8.5 Human clearance t1/2 and human clearance Cl machine learning models.

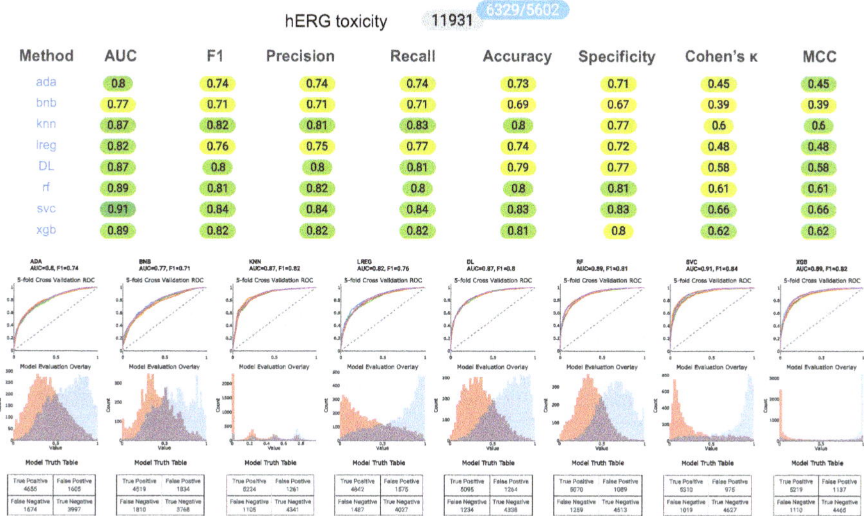

Method	AUC	F1	Precision	Recall	Accuracy	Specificity	Cohen's κ	MCC
ada	0.8	0.74	0.74	0.74	0.73	0.71	0.45	0.45
bnb	0.77	0.71	0.71	0.71	0.69	0.67	0.39	0.39
knn	0.87	0.82	0.81	0.83	0.8	0.77	0.6	0.6
lreg	0.82	0.76	0.75	0.77	0.74	0.72	0.48	0.48
DL	0.87	0.8	0.8	0.81	0.79	0.77	0.58	0.58
rf	0.89	0.81	0.82	0.8	0.8	0.81	0.61	0.61
svc	0.91	0.84	0.84	0.84	0.83	0.83	0.66	0.66
xgb	0.89	0.82	0.82	0.82	0.81	0.8	0.62	0.62

FIGURE 8.6 hERG toxicity machine learning models.

8.3 THE GENERATIVE DRUG DISCOVERY AGE NEEDS ADME/TOX MODELS

In recent years, as our ADME/Tox modeling has been reaching a peak, there have been advances in machine learning in other areas, including image generation[52] and transformer-based large language models (LLMs)[53], which have the potential to accelerate research by scaling models and data.[54–56] The result has led to dramatically improved model capabilities such as question-and-answering, text-to-image translation, language conversion, and emergent properties.[57,58] These advances can be translated to applications in drug discovery with molecules that can be represented as a language (text) using the Simplified Molecular-Input Line-Entry System (SMILES).[59] SMILES captures information about atoms and bonds, aromaticity, and stereochemistry; LLMs trained on SMILES representations of molecules have yielded impressive results for molecular property endpoints and ADME.[60–62] As a new approach to ADME/Tox, the use of such models has been limited to training relatively small datasets. Hoffmann *et al.* revealed transformer-based LLMs scale roughly linearly with dataset size for a fixed compute.[63] The scaling law for SMILES-encoded molecules has not been reported. ADME/Tox data sparsity is likely to limit the predictive power of LLMs for this application.

As big pharma companies have merged, they have been able to combine their ADME/Tox datasets to enable even bigger models. An example of this is Bayer and Schering, with their merger representing an increase in the diversity of the molecules in their combined pipelines[22]; however, this also presents challenges for harmonization. Bringing datasets together from other companies may be possible using approaches like federated learning to create a machine learning model trained on distinct private datasets and not requiring the sharing molecular structures.[64,65]

Enzyme name	Enyzyme ChEMBL ID	Actives/total
P-glycoprotein 1 (substrate)	CHEMBL4302	595/1309
P-glycoprotein 1 (inhibition)	CHEMBL4302	153/877

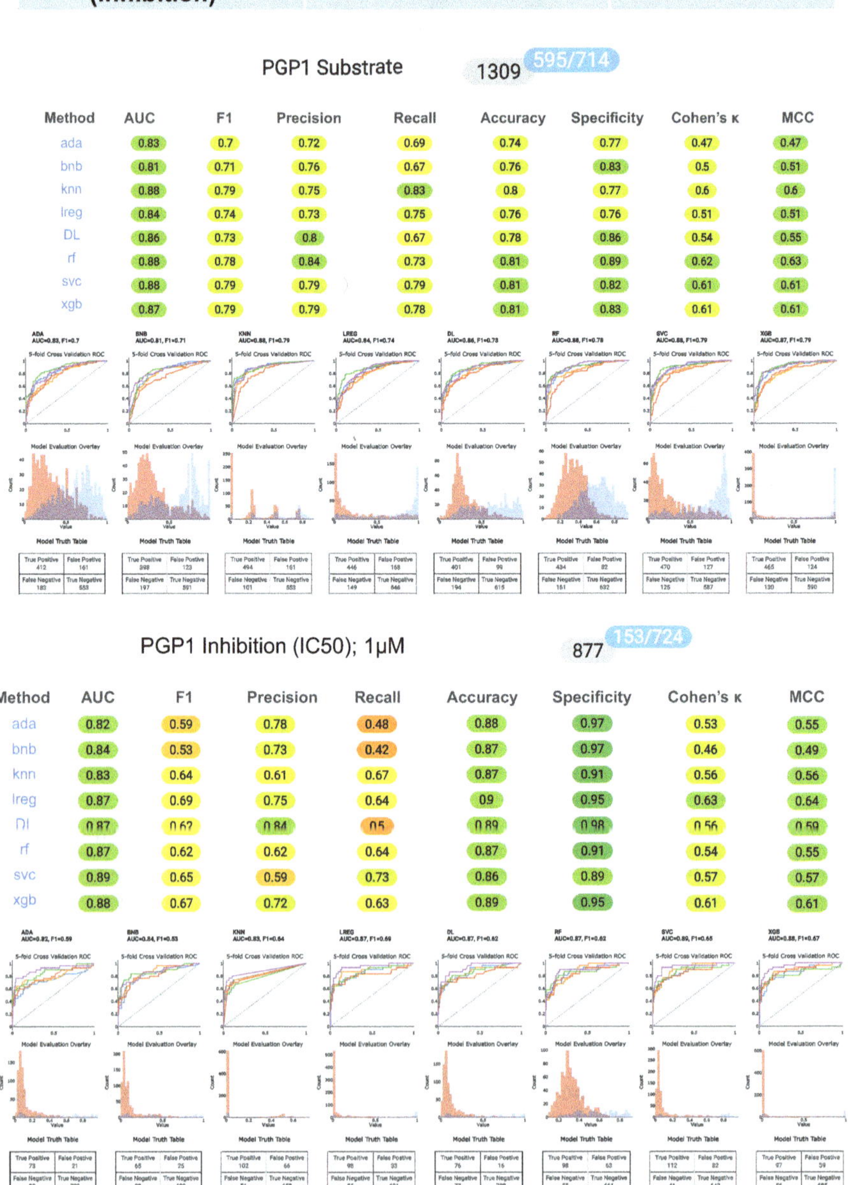

Method	AUC	F1	Precision	Recall	Accuracy	Specificity	Cohen's κ	MCC
ada	0.83	0.7	0.72	0.69	0.74	0.77	0.47	0.47
bnb	0.81	0.71	0.76	0.67	0.76	0.83	0.5	0.51
knn	0.88	0.79	0.75	0.83	0.8	0.77	0.6	0.6
lreg	0.84	0.74	0.73	0.75	0.76	0.76	0.51	0.51
DL	0.86	0.73	0.8	0.67	0.78	0.86	0.54	0.55
rf	0.88	0.78	0.84	0.73	0.81	0.89	0.62	0.63
svc	0.88	0.79	0.79	0.79	0.81	0.82	0.61	0.61
xgb	0.87	0.79	0.79	0.78	0.81	0.83	0.61	0.61

Method	AUC	F1	Precision	Recall	Accuracy	Specificity	Cohen's κ	MCC
ada	0.82	0.59	0.78	0.48	0.88	0.97	0.53	0.55
bnb	0.84	0.53	0.73	0.42	0.87	0.97	0.46	0.49
knn	0.83	0.64	0.61	0.67	0.87	0.91	0.56	0.56
lreg	0.87	0.69	0.75	0.64	09	0.95	0.63	0.64
Dl	0.87	0.62	0.84	0.5	0.89	0.98	0.56	0.59
rf	0.87	0.62	0.62	0.64	0.87	0.91	0.54	0.55
svc	0.89	0.65	0.59	0.73	0.86	0.89	0.57	0.57
xgb	0.88	0.67	0.72	0.63	0.89	0.95	0.61	0.61

FIGURE 8.7 P-glycoprotein substrate and inhibitor machine learning models.

This approach shares encrypted model weights for each host and ultimately aggregates updates from each into a single model. One example is MELLODDY[66], a now-closed cross pharma consortia of 10 companies that collected a data set of over 2.6 billion confidential experimental activity data points, that, in turn, documented over 21 million small molecules and over 40,000 assays.[67] In this case models for ADME showed predictive performance that was improved by combining data across companies using federated learning. While our use of public data is limited and less diverse, we can still create models that cover a large applicability domain. Such models may enable reduced testing of these *in vitro* properties and save valuable resources for other uses.

In our experience, computational ADME/Tox models using different algorithms have multiple applications, with additional data becoming available over time. Certainly, this is likely to continue, but there may also be a point where the model

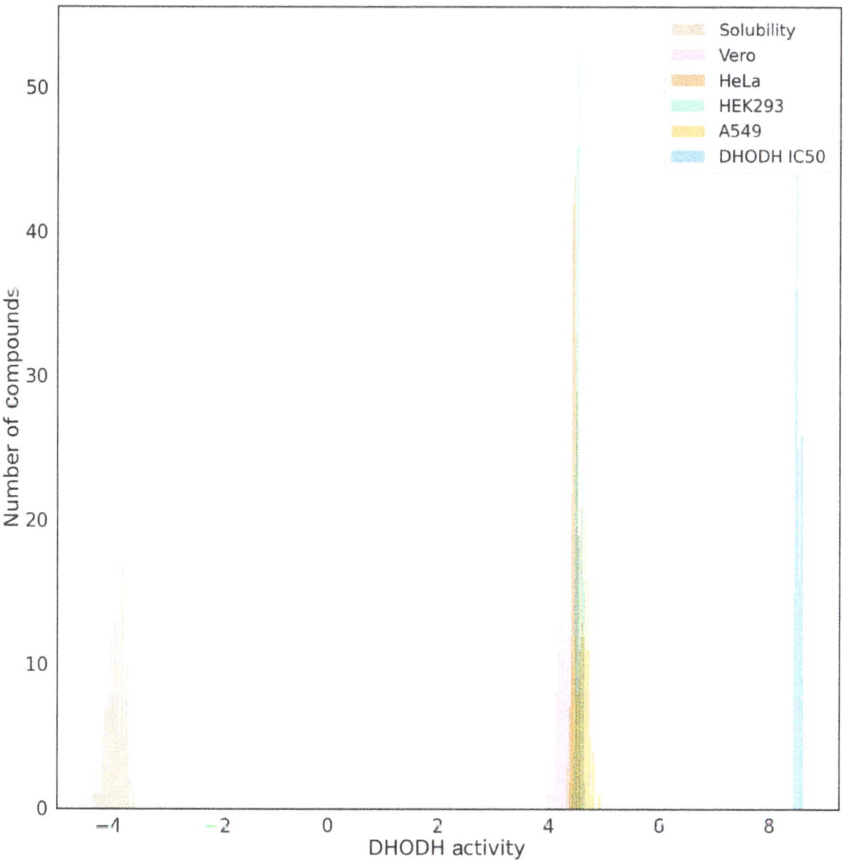

FIGURE 8.8 Generative design: Bioactivity and ADME/Tox model combination showing the distribution of the molecules and their predicted activities.

improvements plateau or even potentially degrade without the addition of some radically different structural classes. We are already seeing the more recent advances in new machine learning algorithms, as well as different software for *de novo* design, combined with the exploration of much larger molecules like PROTACS. This will undoubtedly impact the applicability domain of such machine learning models that are developed. Alternatively, we may need to focus on more local models around these newer classes of molecules as the availability of *in vitro* ADME/Tox increases. Integrating such models into generative models, which are increasingly being used in molecule design, will enable multiparameter optimization. This will likely be seamless for those using the software to design molecules with optimal bioactivity and ADME/Tox properties simultaneously. As an example, we trained our generative software MegaSyn to learn to generate soluble, nontoxic inhibitors of dihydroorotate

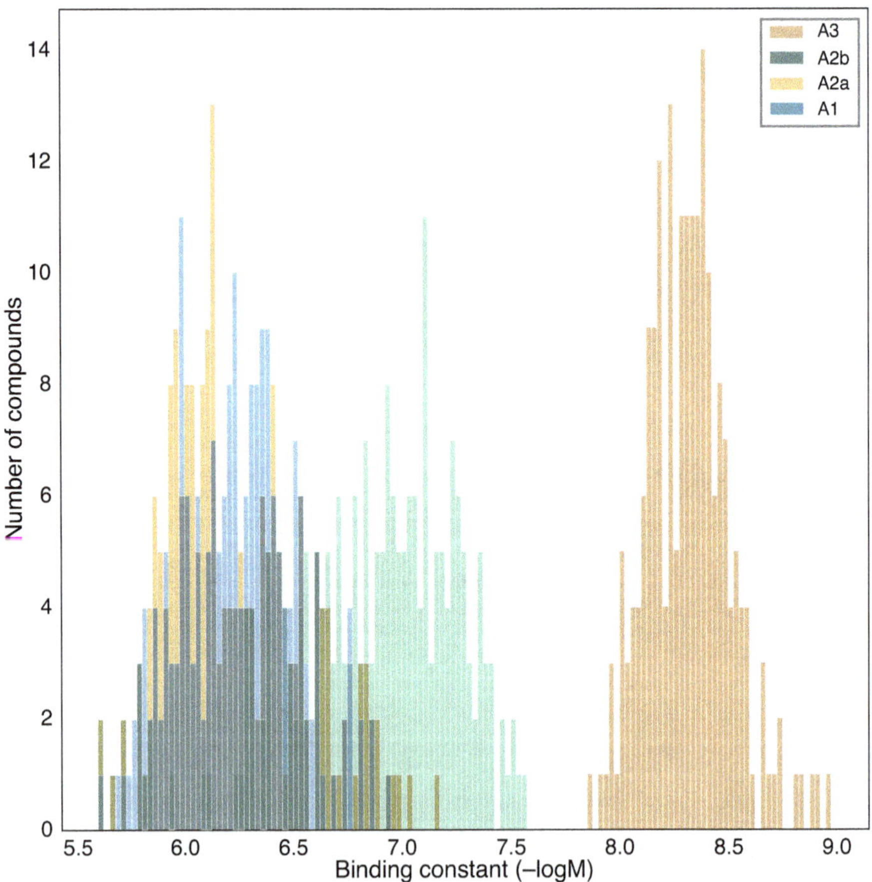

FIGURE 8.9 Selective adenosine receptor A3 selective agonists produced using generative design showing the distribution of the molecules and their predicted activities.

dehydrogenase (DHODH), where we have models for DHODH IC_{50} (> −8 log(M)) as well as ADME/Tox targets such as Cytotoxicity (A549, HEK293, HeLa, Vero) (< −5 log(M)) and Solubility (> −4 logS). In this case, we used MegaSyn to optimize each goal simultaneously; then we used the trained generative model to generate a sample of 200 compounds, for which we plotted a histogram of DHODH, cytotoxicity, and solubility predictions (Figure 8.8). The histogram demonstrates that the molecules in the sample are potent DHODH inhibitors while maintaining high solubility and low cytotoxicity.

Another example deals with the challenge of developing a selective adenosine A3 agonist that circumvents patents that cover virtually every potent structure in the training set for the model. We trained MegaSyn to optimize A3 binding and agonism as well as adenosine A3 selectivity (A1/A2a/A2b), while filtering out patented substructures during training. Again, a sample of 200 molecules was drawn from the trained model, and a histogram of adenosine receptor binding constants was plotted for the sample (Figure 8.9). The histogram shows that the molecules in the sample are predicted as potent and selective towards adenosine A3 agonists; moreover, every generated molecule circumvents existing patents (based on comparison to SureChEMBL) and is predicted to be an adenosine A3 agonist. In this case, we did not incorporate ADME/Tox models as part of the process due to the challenges of finding novel structures with selectivity towards adenosine A3 agonists. However, even when ADME/Tox models are not used directly in training a generative model, they can be readily used after the fact to screen molecules in a generated sample, which would be the case here.

8.4 CONCLUSION

As we are seeing elsewhere in other fields, the barriers to using generative AI have been dramatically lowered in drug discovery, enabling large language models to have increased accessibility, which in turn allows for the development of tools with diverse capabilities to be more cost-effective. These new tools may provide computational chemists and drug designers with the ability to request the prediction of ideal molecules with certain predetermined required properties or the improvement of known molecules with certain toxicity liabilities or non-ideal physiochemical properties. This may also increase our scientific creativity rather than make us redundant. Reaching this point will require such models to be trained on increasing quantities of ADME/Tox or physicochemical property data with sufficient structural diversity. We can learn much from the earlier days of building ADME/Tox models, where we were constrained in all dimensions (dataset size, molecule diversity, compute power, understanding of biology, etc.). In contrast, the algorithms being developed today with the data currently available in many public databases are likely themselves capable of learning so much more than we could visualize due to the complexity of the relationships between different molecular properties. Ultimately, these generative models are just another more advanced "tool" to help the drug designers of the future, whether that is a chemist, biologist, or computer (with or without the interference of a human).

FUNDING

We kindly acknowledge NIH funding from R44GM122196-02A1 from NIGMS and 1R44ES031038-01 from NIEHS for our machine learning software development and applications. "Research reported in this publication was supported by the National Institute of Environmental Health Sciences of the National Institutes of Health under Award Number R44ES031038.

REFERENCES

1. Ekins S, Ring BJ, Grace J, McRobie-Belle DJ, Wrighton SA. Present and future in vitro approaches for drug metabolism. *J Pharmacol Toxicol Methods.* 2000;44(1):313–24. Epub 2001/03/29. doi:S1056-8719(00)00110-6 [pii]. PubMed PMID: 11274898.
2. Kennedy T. Managing the drug discovery/development interface. *Drug Discovery Today.* 1997;2(10):436–44. doi:10.1016/S1359-6446(97)01099-4.
3. Lipinski CA, Lombardo F, Dominy BW, Feeney PJ. Experimental and computational approaches to estimate solubility and permeability in drug discovery and development settings. *Adv Drug Deliv Rev.* 1997;23(1):3–25. doi:10.1016/S0169-409X(96)00423-1.
4. Ekins S, Waller CL, Swaan PW, Cruciani G, Wrighton SA, Wikel JH. Progress in predicting human ADME parameters in silico. *J Pharmacol Toxicol Methods.* 2000;44(1):251–72. Epub 2001/03/29. doi:10.1016/s1056-8719(00)00109-x. PubMed PMID: 11274894.
5. Ekins S, Wrighton SA. Application of in silico approaches to predicting drug–drug interactions. *J Pharmacol Toxicol Methods.* 2001;45(1):65–9. Epub 2001/08/08. doi:S1056-8719(01)00119-8 [pii]. PubMed PMID: 11489666.
6. Ekins S, de Groot MJ, Jones JP. Pharmacophore and three-dimensional quantitative structure activity relationship methods for modeling cytochrome p450 active sites. *Drug Metab Dispos.* 2001;29(7):936–44. Epub 2001/06/16. PubMed PMID: 11408357.
7. Selick HE, Beresford AP, Tarbit MH. The emerging importance of predictive ADME simulation in drug discovery. *Drug Discov Today.* 2002;7(2):109–16. Epub 2002/01/16. doi:10.1016/s1359-6446(01)02100-6. PubMed PMID: 11790621.
8. Dickins M, Modi S. The importance of predictive ADME simulation. *Drug Discov Today.* 2002;7(14):755–6. Epub 2003/01/28. doi:10.1016/s1359-6446(02)02357-7. PubMed PMID: 12547029.
9. Ekins S, Boulanger B, Swaan PW, Hupcey MA. Towards a new age of virtual ADME/TOX and multidimensional drug discovery. *J Comput Aided Mol Des.* 2002;16(5–6):381–401. PubMed PMID: 12489686.
10. Butina D, Segall MD, Frankcombe K. Predicting ADME properties in silico: methods and models. *Drug Discov Today.* 2002;7(11):S83–8. Epub 2002/06/06. doi:10.1016/s1359-6446(02)02288-2. PubMed PMID: 12047885.
11. van de Waterbeemd H, Gifford E. ADMET in silico modelling: towards prediction paradise? *Nat Rev Drug Discov.* 2003;2(3):192–204. Epub 2003/03/04. doi:10.1038/nrd1032. PubMed PMID: 12612645.
12. Yu H, Adedoyin A. ADME-Tox in drug discovery: integration of experimental and computational technologies. *Drug Discov Today.* 2003;8(18):852–61. Epub 2003/09/10. doi:10.1016/s1359-6446(03)02828-9. PubMed PMID: 12963322.
13. Ekins S, Nikolsky Y, Nikolskaya T. Techniques: application of systems biology to absorption, distribution, metabolism, excretion and toxicity. *Trends Pharmacol Sci.* 2005;26(4):202–9. Epub 2005/04/06. doi:10.1016/j.tips.2005.02.006. PubMed PMID: 15808345.

14. Stahl M, Guba W, Kansy M. Integrating molecular design resources within modern drug discovery research: The Roche experience. *Drug Discov Today*. 2006;11(7–8):326–33. Epub 2006/04/04. doi:10.1016/j.drudis.2006.02.008. PubMed PMID: 16580974.
15. Muster W, Breidenbach A, Fischer H, Kirchner S, Muller L, Pahler A. Computational toxicology in drug development. *Drug Discov Today*. 2008;13(7–8):303–10. PubMed PMID: 18405842.
16. Ekins S, Williams AJ. Precompetitive preclinical ADME/Tox data: set it free on the web to facilitate computational model building and assist drug development. *Lab Chip*. 2010;10(1):13–22. Epub 2009/12/22. doi:10.1039/b917760b. PubMed PMID: 20024044.
17. Gupta RR, Gifford EM, Liston T, Waller CL, Hohman M, Bunin BA, Ekins S. Using open source computational tools for predicting human metabolic stability and additional absorption, distribution, metabolism, excretion, and toxicity properties. *Drug Metab Dispos*. 2010;38(11):2083–90. Epub 2010/08/10. doi:10.1124/dmd.110.034918. PubMed PMID: 20693417.
18. Ekins S. Progress in computational toxicology. *J Pharmacol Toxicol Methods*. 2014;69(2):115–40. doi:10.1016/j.vascn.2013.12.003. PubMed PMID: 24361690.
19. Landrum G. RDkit 2020. Available from: https://www.rdkit.org.
20. Willighagen EL, Mayfield JW, Alvarsson J, Berg A, Carlsson L, Jeliazkova N, Kuhn S, Pluskal T, Rojas-Cherto M, Spjuth O, Torrance G, Evelo CT, Guha R, Steinbeck C. The Chemistry Development Kit (CDK) v2.0: Atom typing, depiction, molecular formulas, and substructure searching. *J Cheminform*. 2017;9(1):33. Epub 2017/11/01. doi:10.1186/s13321-017-0220-4. PubMed PMID: 29086040; PMCID: PMC5461230.
21. Lombardo F, Desai PV, Arimoto R, Desino KE, Fischer H, Keefer CE, Petersson C, Winiwarter S, Broccatelli F. In silico absorption, distribution, metabolism, excretion, and pharmacokinetics (ADME-PK): Utility and best practices. An industry perspective from the international consortium for innovation through quality in pharmaceutical development. *J Med Chem*. 2017;60(22):9097–113. Epub 2017/06/14. doi:10.1021/acs.jmedchem.7b00487. PubMed PMID: 28609624.
22. Goller AH, Kuhnke L, Montanari F, Bonin A, Schneckener S, Ter Laak A, Wichard J, Lobell M, Hillisch A. Bayer's in silico ADMET platform: A journey of machine learning over the past two decades. *Drug Discov Today*. 2020;25(9):1702–9. Epub 2020/07/12. doi:10.1016/j.drudis.2020.07.001. PubMed PMID: 32652309.
23. Pillai N, Dasgupta A, Sudsakorn S, Fretland J, Mavroudis PD. Machine learning guided early drug discovery of small molecules. *Drug Discov Today*. 2022;27(8):2209–15. Epub 2022/04/02. doi:10.1016/j.drudis.2022.03.017. PubMed PMID: 35364270.
24. Schaduangrat N, Lampa S, Simeon S, Gleeson MP, Spjuth O, Nantasenamat C. Towards reproducible computational drug discovery. *J Cheminform*. 2020;12(1):9. Epub 2021/01/13. doi: 10.1186/s13321-020-0408-x. PubMed PMID: 33430992; PMCID: PMC6988305.
25. Komura H, Watanabe R, Kawashima H, Ohashi R, Kuroda M, Sato T, Honma T, Mizuguchi K. A public-private partnership to enrich the development of in silico predictive models for pharmacokinetic and cardiotoxic properties. *Drug Discov Today*. 2021;26(5):1275–83. Epub 2021/02/01. doi:10.1016/j.drudis.2021.01.024. PubMed PMID: 33516857.
26. Siramshetty V, Williams J, Nguyen Eth T, Neyra J, Southall N, Mathe E, Xu X, Shah P. Validating ADME QSAR models using marketed drugs. *SLAS Discov*. 2021;26(10):1326–36. Epub 2021/06/29. doi:10.1177/24725552211017520. PubMed PMID: 34176369.

27. Cronin MTD, Belfield SJ, Briggs KA, Enoch SJ, Firman JW, Frericks M, Garrard C, Maccallum PH, Madden JC, Pastor M, Sanz F, Soininen I, Sousoni D. Making in silico predictive models for toxicology FAIR. *Regul Toxicol Pharmacol.* 2023;140:105385. Epub 2023/04/11. doi:10.1016/j.yrtph.2023.105385. PubMed PMID: 37037390.
28. Mansouri K, Karmaus A, Fitzpatrick J, Patlewicz G, Pradeep P, Alberga D, Alepee N, Allen TEH, Allen D, Alves VM, Andrade CH, Auernhammer TR, Ballabio D, Bell S, Benfenati E, Bhattacharya S, Bastos JV, Boyd S, Brown JB, Capuzzi SJ, Chushak Y, Ciallella H, Clark AM, Consonni V, Daga PR, Ekins S, Farag S, Fedorov M, Fourches D, Gadaleta D, Gao F, Gearhart JM, Goh G, Goodman JM, Grisoni F, Grulke CM, Hartung T, Hirn M, Karpov P, Korotcov A, Lavado GJ, Lawless M, Li X, Luechtefeld T, Lunghini F, Mangiatordi GF, Marcou G, Marsh D, Martin T, Mauri A, Muratov EN, Myatt GJ, Nguyen DT, Nicolotti O, Note R, Pande P, Parks AK, Peryea T, Polash A, Rallo R, Roncaglioni A, Rowlands C, Ruiz P, Russo D, Sayed A, Sayre R, Sheils T, Siegel C, Silva AC, Simeonov A, Sosnin S, Southall N, Strickland J, Tang Y, Teppen B, Tetko IV, Thomas D, Tkachenko V, Todeschini R, Toma C, Tripodi I, Trisciuzzi D, Tropsha A, Varnek A, Vukovic K, Wang Z, Wang L, Waters KM, Wedlake AJ, Wijeyesakere SJ, Wilson D, Xiao Z, Yang H, Zahoranszky-Kohalmi G, Zakharov AV, Zhang FF, Zhang Z, Zhao T, Zhu H, Zorn KM, Casey W, Kleinstreuer NC. Erratum: CATMoS: Collaborative acute toxicity modeling suite. *Environ Health Perspect.* 2021;129(7):79001. Epub 2021/07/10. doi:10.1289/EHP9883. PubMed PMID: 34242083; PMCID: PMC8270350.
29. Minerali E, Foil DH, Zorn KM, Ekins S. Evaluation of assay Central® machine learning models for rat acute oral toxicity prediction. *ACS Sustain Chem Eng.* 2020;8:16020–7.
30. Lane TR, Harris J, Urbina F, Ekins S. Comparing LD50/LC50 machine learning models for multiple species. *ACS Chem Health Saf.* 2023;30(2):83–97. doi:10.1021/acs.chas.2c00088.
31. Volak LP, Duevel HM, Humphreys S, Nettleton D, Phipps C, Pike A, Rynn C, Scott-Stevens P, Zhang D, Zientek M. Industry perspective on the pharmacokinetic and ADME characterization of heterobifunctional protein degraders. *Drug Metab Dispos.* 2023. Epub 2023/04/12. doi:10.1124/dmd.122.001154. PubMed PMID: 37041086.
32. Poongavanam V, Kolling F, Giese A, Goller AH, Lehmann L, Meibom D, Kihlberg J. Predictive modeling of PROTAC cell permeability with machine learning. *ACS Omega.* 2023;8(6):5901–16. Epub 2023/02/24. doi:10.1021/acsomega.2c07717. PubMed PMID: 36816707; PMCID: PMC9933238.
33. Zdrazil B, Felix E, Hunter F, Manners EJ, Blackshaw J, Corbett S, de Veij M, Ioannidis H, Lopez DM, Mosquera JF, Magarinos MP, Bosc N, Arcila R, Kiziloren T, Gaulton A, Bento AP, Adasme MF, Monecke P, Landrum GA, Leach AR. The ChEMBL database in 2023: A drug discovery platform spanning multiple bioactivity data types and time periods. *Nucleic Acids Res.* 2024;52(D1):D1180–92. doi:10.1093/nar/gkad1004. PubMed PMID: 37933841; PMCID: PMC10767899.
34. Shen J, Cheng F, Xu Y, Li W, Tang Y. Estimation of ADME properties with substructure pattern recognition. *J Chem Inf Model.* 2010;50(6):1034–41. doi:10.1021/ci100104j. PubMed PMID: 20578727.
35. Wei M, Zhang X, Pan X, Wang B, Ji C, Qi Y, Zhang JZH. HobPre: Accurate prediction of human oral bioavailability for small molecules. *J Cheminform.* 2022;14(1):1. Epub 20220106. doi:10.1186/s13321-021-00580-6. PubMed PMID: 34991690; PMCID: PMC8740492.
36. Wang Z, Yang H, Wu Z, Wang T, Li W, Tang Y, Liu G. In silico prediction of blood-brain barrier permeability of compounds by machine learning and resampling methods. *ChemMedChem.* 2018;13(20):2189–201. Epub 20180921. doi:10.1002/cmdc.201800533. PubMed PMID: 30110511.

37. Martins IF, Teixeira AL, Pinheiro L, Falcao AO. A Bayesian approach to in silico blood-brain barrier penetration modeling. *J Chem Inf Model.* 2012;52(6):1686–97. PubMed PMID: 22612593.
38. Kumar R, Sharma A, Alexiou A, Bilgrami AL, Kamal MA, Ashraf GM. DeePred-BBB: A blood brain barrier permeability prediction model with improved accuracy. *Front Neurosci.* 2022;16:858126. Epub 20220503. doi:10.3389/fnins.2022.858126. PubMed PMID: 35592264; PMCID: PMC9112838.
39. Shaker B, Yu MS, Song JS, Ahn S, Ryu JY, Oh KS, Na D. LightBBB: Computational prediction model of blood-brain-barrier penetration based on LightGBM. *Bioinformatics.* 2021;37(8):1135–9. doi:10.1093/bioinformatics/btaa918. PubMed PMID: 33112379.
40. Sun L, Yang H, Li J, Wang T, Li W, Liu G, Tang Y. In silico prediction of compounds binding to human plasma proteins by QSAR models. *ChemMedChem.* 2018;13(6):572–81. Epub 20171110. doi:10.1002/cmdc.201700582. PubMed PMID: 29057587.
41. Votano JR, Parham M, Hall LM, Hall LH, Kier LB, Oloff S, Tropsha A. QSAR modeling of human serum protein binding with several modeling techniques utilizing structure-information representation. *J Med Chem.* 2006;49(24):7169–81. doi:10.1021/jm051245v. PubMed PMID: 17125269.
42. Iftkhar S, de Sa AGC, Velloso JPL, Aljarf R, Pires DEV, Ascher DB. cardioToxCSM: A web server for predicting cardiotoxicity of small molecules. *J Chem Inf Model.* 2022;62(20):4827–36. Epub 20221011. doi:10.1021/acs.jcim.2c00822. PubMed PMID: 36219164.
43. Poongavanam V, Haider N, Ecker GF. Fingerprint-based in silico models for the prediction of P-glycoprotein substrates and inhibitors. *Bioorg Med Chem.* 2012;20(18):5388–95. Epub 20120329. doi:10.1016/j.bmc.2012.03.045. PubMed PMID: 22595422; PMCID: PMC3445814.
44. Wang Z, Chen Y, Liang H, Bender A, Glen RC, Yan A. P-glycoprotein substrate models using support vector machines based on a comprehensive data set. *J Chem Inf Model.* 2011;51(6):1447–56. Epub 20110603. doi:10.1021/ci2001583. PubMed PMID: 21604677.
45. Levatic J, Curak J, Kralj M, Smuc T, Osmak M, Supek F. Accurate models for P-gp drug recognition induced from a cancer cell line cytotoxicity screen. *J Med Chem.* 2013;56(14):5691–708. Epub 20130708. doi:10.1021/jm400328s. PubMed PMID: 23772653.
46. Vignaux PA, Lane TR, Urbina F, Gerlach J, Puhl AC, Snyder SH, Ekins S. Validation of acetylcholinesterase inhibition machine learning models for multiple species. *Chem Res Toxicol.* 2023;36(2):188–201. Epub 20230203. doi:10.1021/acs.chemrestox.2c00283. PubMed PMID: 36737043; PMCID: PMC9945174.
47. Kazakova E, Lane TR, Jones T, Puhl AC, Riabova O, Makarov V, Ekins S. 1-Sulfonyl-3-amino-1H-1,2,4-triazoles as yellow fever virus inhibitors: Synthesis and structure-activity relationship. *ACS Omega.* 2023;8(45):42951-65. Epub 2023/11/29. doi:10.1021/acsomega.3c06106. PubMed PMID: 38024733; PMCID: PMC10653066.
48. Jones T, Tavis JE, Li Q, Riabova O, Monakhova N, Bradley DP, Lane TR, Makarov V, Ekins S. Antiviral evaluation of dispirotripiperazines against hepatitis B virus. *J Med Chem.* 2023;66(17):12459–67. Epub 2023/08/23. doi:10.1021/acs.jmedchem.3c00974. PubMed PMID: 37611244.
49. Lane TR, Harris J, Urbina F, Ekins S. Comparing LD(50)/LC(50) machine learning models for multiple species. *J Chem Health Saf.* 2023;30(2):83–97. Epub 2023/07/17. doi:10.1021/acs.chas.2c00088. PubMed PMID: 37457397; PMCID: PMC10348353.
50. Lane T, Russo DP, Zorn KM, Clark AM, Korotcov A, Tkachenko V, Reynolds RC, Perryman AL, Freundlich JS, Ekins S. Comparing and validating machine learning models for mycobacterium tuberculosis drug discovery. *Mol Pharm.* 2018;15(10):4346–60. Epub 2018/04/20. doi:10.1021/acs.molpharmaceut.8b00083. PubMed PMID: 29672063; PMCID: PMC6167198.

51. Minerali E, Foil DH, Zorn KM, Lane TR, Ekins S. Comparing machine learning algorithms for predicting drug-induced liver injury (DILI). *Mol Pharm.* 2020;17(7):2628–37. Epub 20200608. doi:10.1021/acs.molpharmaceut.0c00326. PubMed PMID: 32422053; PMCID: PMC7702310.
52. Ramesh A, Dhariwal P, Nichol A, Chu C, Chen M. Hierarchical Text-Conditional Image Generation with CLIP Latents. 2022. Available from: https://arxiv.org/abs/2204.06125.
53. Vaswani A, Shazeer N, Parmar N, Uszkoreit J, Jones L, HGomez AN, Kaiser L, Plusukhin I. Attention is all you need. *ArXiv*, 2017;1706.03762.
54. Brown TB, Mann B, Ryder N, Subbiah M, Kaplan J, Dhariwal P, Neelakantan A, Shyam P, Sastry G, Askell A, Agarwal SR, Herbert-Voss A, Kreueger G, Henighan T, Child R, Ramesh A, Ziegler DM, Wiu J, Winter C, Hesse C, Chen M, Sigler E, Litwin M, Gray S, Chess B, Clark J, Berner C, McCandlish S, Radford A, Sutkever I, Amodei D. Language Models are Few-Shot Learners. 2020. Available from: https://arxiv.org/abs/2005.14165.
55. Bubeck S, Chandrasekaran V, Eldan R, Gehrke J, Horvitz E, Kamar E, Lee P, Lee YT, Li Y, Lundberg SM, Nori H, Palangi H, Ribeiro MT, Zhang Y. Sparks of Artificial General Intelligence: Early Experiments with GPT-4. 2023. https://arxivorg/abs/230312712.
56. Lewis M, Liu Y, Goyal N, Gazvininejad M, Levy O, Stoyanov V, Zettlemoyer L. BART: Denoising Sequence-to-Sequence Pre-training for Natural Language Generation, Translation, and Comprehension. 2019. https://arxivorg/abs/191013461.
57. Chowdhery A, Narang S, Devlin J, Bosma M, Mishra G, Roberts A, Barham P, Chung HW, Sutton C, Gehrmann S, Schuh P, Shi K, Tsvyashchenko S, Maynez J, Rao A, Barnes P, Tay Y, Shazeer N, Prabhakaran V, Reif E, Du N, Hutchinson B, Pope R, Bradbury J, Austin J, Isard M, Gur-Ari G, Yin P, Duke T, Levskaya A, Ghemawat S, Dev S, Michalewski H, Garcia X, Misra V, Robinson K, Fedus L, Zhou D, Ippolito D, Luan D, Lim H, Zoph B, Spiridonov A, Sepassi R, Dohan D, Agrawal S, Omernick M, Dai AM, Sankaranarayana Pillai T, Pellat M, Lewkowycz A, Moreira E, Child R, Polozov O, Lee K, Zhou Z, Wang X, Saeta B, Diaz M, Firat O, Catasta M, Wei J, Meier-Hellstern K, Eck D, Dean J, Petrov S, Fiedel N. PaLM: Scaling Language Modeling with Pathways. 2022, 2022:[arXiv:2204.02311 p.]. Available from: https://ui.adsabs.harvard.edu/abs/2022arXiv220402311C.
58. Srivastava A, Rastogi A, Rao A, Shoeb AAM, Abid A, Fisch A, Brown AR, Santoro A, Gupta A, Garriga-Alonso A, Kluska A, Lewkowycz A, Agarwal A, Power A, Ray A, Warstadt A, Kocurek AW, Safaya A, Tazarv A, Xiang A, Parrish A, Nie A, Hussain A, Askell A, Dsouza A, Slone A, Rahane A, Iyer AS, Andreassen A, Madotto A, Santilli A, Stuhlmüller A, Dai A, La A, Lampinen A, Zou A, Jiang A, Chen A, Vuong A, Gupta A, Gottardi A, Norelli A, Venkatesh A, Gholamidavoodi A, Tabassum A, Menezes A, Kirubarajan A, Mullokandov A, Sabharwal A, Herrick A, Efrat A, Erdem A, Karakaş A, Roberts BR, Loe BS, Zoph B, Bojanowski B, Özyurt B, Hedayatnia B, Neyshabur B, Inden B, Stein B, Ekmekci B, Yuchen Lin B, Howald B, Orinion B, Diao C, Dour C, Stinson C, Argueta C, Ferri Ramírez C, Singh C, Rathkopf C, Meng C, Baral C, Wu C, Callison-Burch C, Waites C, Voigt C, Manning CD, Potts C, Ramirez C, Rivera CE, Siro C, Raffel C, Ashcraft C, Garbacea C, Sileo D, Garrette D, Hendrycks D, Kilman D, Roth D, Freeman D, Khashabi D, Levy D, Moseguí González D, Perszyk D, Hernandez D, Chen D, Ippolito D, Gilboa D, Dohan D, Drakard D, Jurgens D, Datta D, Ganguli D, Emelin D, Kleyko D, Yuret D, Chen D, Tam D, Hupkes D, Misra D, Buzan D, Coelho Mollo D, Yang D, Lee D-H, Schrader D, Shutova E, Dogus Cubuk E, Segal E, Hagerman E, Barnes E, Donoway E, Pavlick E, Rodola E, Lam E, Chu E, Tang E, Erdem E, Chang E, Chi EA, Dyer E, Jerzak E, Kim E, Engefu Manyasi E, Zheltonozhskii E, Xia F, Siar F, Martínez-Plumed F, Happé F, Chollet F, Rong F, Mishra G, Indra Winata G, de Melo G, Kruszewski G, Parascandolo G, Mariani G, Wang G, Jaimovitch-López G, Betz G, Gur-Ari G, Galijasevic H, Kim H, Rashkin H, Hajishirzi H, Mehta H, Bogar

H, Shevlin H, Schütze H, Yakura H, Zhang H, Wong HM, Ng I, Noble I, Jumelet J, Geissinger J, Kernion J, Hilton J, Lee J, Fernández Fisac J, Simon JB, Koppel J, Zheng J, Zou J, Kocoń J, Thompson J, Wingfield J, Kaplan J, Radom J, Sohl-Dickstein J, Phang J, Wei J, Yosinski J, Novikova J, Bosscher J, Marsh J, Kim J, Taal J, Engel J, Alabi J, Xu J, Song J, Tang J, Waweru J, Burden J, Miller J, Balis JU, Batchelder J, Berant J, Frohberg J, Rozen J, Hernandez-Orallo J, Boudeman J, Guerr J, Jones J, Tenenbaum JB, Rule JS, Chua J, Kanclerz K, Livescu K, Krauth K, Gopalakrishnan K, Ignatyeva K, Markert K, Dhole KD, Gimpel K, Omondi K, Mathewson K, Chiafullo K, Shkaruta K, Shridhar K, McDonell K, Richardson K, Reynolds L, Gao L, Zhang L, Dugan L, Qin L, Contreras-Ochando L, Morency L-P, Moschella L, Lam L, Noble L, Schmidt L, He L, Oliveros Colón L, Metz L, Kerem Şenel L, Bosma M, Sap M, ter Hoeve M, Farooqi M, Faruqui M, Mazeika M, Baturan M, Marelli M, Maru M, Ramírez Quintana MJ, Tolkiehn M, Giulianelli M, Lewis M, Potthast M, Leavitt ML, Hagen M, Schubert M, Orduna Baitemirova M, Arnaud M, McElrath M, Yee MA, Cohen M, Gu M, Ivanitskiy M, Starritt M, Strube M, Swędrowski M, Bevilacqua M, Yasunaga M, Kale M, Cain M, Xu M, Suzgun M, Walker M, Tiwari M, Bansal M, Aminnaseri M, Geva M, Gheini M, Varma T M, Peng N, Chi NA, Lee N, Gur-Ari Krakover N, Cameron N, Roberts N, Doiron N, Martinez N, Nangia N, Deckers N, Muennighoff N, Shirish Keskar N, Iyer NS, Constant N, Fiedel N, Wen N, Zhang O, Agha O, Elbaghdadi O, Levy O, Evans O, Moreno Casares PA, Doshi P, Fung P, Liang PP, Vicol P, Alipoormolabashi P, Liao P, Liang P, Chang P, Eckersley P, Mon Htut P, Hwang P, Miłkowski P, Patil P, Pezeshkpour P, Oli P, Mei Q, Lyu Q, Chen Q, Banjade R, Etta Rudolph R, Gabriel R, Habacker R, Risco R, Millière R, Garg R, Barnes R, Saurous RA, Arakawa R, Raymaekers R, Frank R, Sikand R, Novak R, Sitelew R, LeBras R, Liu R, Jacobs R, Zhang R, Salakhutdinov R, Chi R, Lee R, Stovall R, Teehan R, Yang R, Singh S, Mohammad SM, Anand S, Dillavou S, Shleifer S, Wiseman S, Gruetter S, Bowman SR, Schoenholz SS, Han S, Kwatra S, Rous SA, Ghazarian S, Ghosh S, Casey S, Bischoff S, Gehrmann S, Schuster S, Sadeghi S, Hamdan S, Zhou S, Srivastava S, Shi S, Singh S, Asaadi S, Gu SS, Pachchigar S, Toshniwal S, Upadhyay S, Shyamolima, Debnath, Shakeri S, Thormeyer S, Melzi S, Reddy S, Priscilla Makini S, Lee S-H, Torene S, Hatwar S, Dehaene S, Divic S, Ermon S, Biderman S, Lin S, Prasad S, Piantadosi ST, Shieber SM, Misherghi S, Kiritchenko S, Mishra S, Linzen T, Schuster T, Li T, Yu T, Ali T, Hashimoto T, Wu T-L, Desbordes T, Rothschild T, Phan T, Wang T, Nkinyili T, Schick T, Kornev T, Tunduny T, Gerstenberg T, Chang T, Neeraj T, Khot T, Shultz T, Shaham U, Misra V, Demberg V, Nyamai V, Raunak V, Ramasesh V, Uday Prabhu V, Padmakumar V, Srikumar V, Fedus W, Saunders W, Zhang W, Vossen W, Ren X, Tong X, Zhao X, Wu X, Shen X, Yaghoobzadeh Y, Lakretz Y, Song Y, Bahri Y, Choi Y, Yang Y, Hao Y, Chen Y, Belinkov Y, Hou Y, Hou Y, Bai Y, Seid Z, Zhao Z, Wang Z, Wang ZJ, Wang Z, Wu Z. Beyond the Imitation Game: Quantifying and Extrapolating the Capabilities of Language Models. 2022 June 01, 2022:[arXiv:2206.04615 p.]. Available from: https://ui.adsabs.harvard.edu/abs/2022arXiv220604615S.

59. Weininger D. SMILES, a chemical language and information system. 1. Introduction to methodology and encoding rules. *J Chem Inf Comp Sci.* 1988;28(1):31–6. doi:10.1021/ci00057a005.

60. Irwin R, Dimitriadis S, He J, Bjerrum EJ. Chemformer: A pre-trained transformer for computational chemistry. *Mach Learn: Sci Technol.* 2022;3(1):015022. doi:10.1088/2632-2153/ac3ffb.

61. Lu J, Zhang Y. Unified deep learning model for multitask reaction predictions with explanation. *J Chem Inf Model.* 2022;62(6):1376–87. doi:10.1021/acs.jcim.1c01467.

62. He J, Nittinger E, Tyrchan C, Czechtizky W, Patronov A, Bjerrum EJ, Engkvist O. Transformer-based molecular optimization beyond matched molecular pairs. *J Cheminformatics.* 2022;14(1):18. doi:10.1186/s13321-022-00599-3.

63. Hoffmann J, Borgeaud S, Mensch A, Buchatskaya E, Cai T, Rutherford E, de Las Casas D, Hendricks LA, Welbl J, Clark A, Hennigan T, Noland E, Millican K, van den Driessche G, Damoc B, Guy A, Osindero S, Simonyan K, Elsen E, Rae JW, Vinyals O, Sifre L. Training Compute-Optimal Large Language Models. 2022, March 01, 2022:[arXiv:2203.15556 p.]. Available from: https://ui.adsabs.harvard.edu/abs/2022arXiv220315556H.
64. Mittone G, Svoboda F, Aldinucci M, Lane ND, Lio P. A Federated Learning Benchmark for Drug-Target Interaction. 2023, February 01, 2023:[arXiv:2302.07684 p.]. Available from: https://ui.adsabs.harvard.edu/abs/2023arXiv230207684M.
65. Konečný J, McMahan B, Ramage D. Federated Optimization:Distributed Optimization Beyond the Datacenter. 2015, November 01, 2015:[arXiv:1511.03575 p.]. Available from: https://ui.adsabs.harvard.edu/abs/2015arXiv151103575K.
66. Oldenhof M, Ács G, Pejó B, Schuffenhauer A, Holway N, Sturm N, Dieckmann A, Fortmeier O, Boniface E, Mayer C, Gohier A, Schmidtke P, Niwayama R, Kopecky D, Mervin L, Rathi PC, Friedrich L, Formanek A, Antal P, Rahaman J, Zalewski A, Heyndrickx W, Oluoch E, Stößel M, Vančo M, Endico D, Gelus F, de Boisfossé T, Darbier A, Nicollet A, Blottière M, Telenczuk M, Tien Nguyen V, Martinez T, Boillet C, Moutet K, Picosson A, Gasser A, Djafar I, Simon A, Arany Á, Simm J, Moreau Y, Engkvist O, Ceulemans H, Marini C, Galtier M. Industry-Scale Orchestrated Federated Learning for Drug Discovery. 2022 October 01, 2022:[arXiv:2210.08871 p.]. Available from: https://ui.adsabs.harvard.edu/abs/2022arXiv221008871O.
67. Heyndrickx W, Mervin L, Morawietz T, Sturm N, Friedrich L, Zalewski A, Pentina A, Humbeck L, Oldenhof M, Niwayama R, Schmidtke P, Fechner N, Simm J, Arany A, Drizard N, Jabal R, Afanasyeva A, Loeb R, Verma S, Harnqvist S, Holmes M, Pejo B, Telenczuk M, Holway N, Dieckmann A, Rieke N, Zumsande F, Clevert DA, Krug M, Luscombe C, Green D, Ertl P, Antal P, Marcus D, Do Huu N, Fuji H, Pickett S, Acs G, Boniface E, Beck B, Sun Y, Gohier A, Rippmann F, Engkvist O, Goller AH, Moreau Y, Galtier MN, Schuffenhauer A, Ceulemans H. MELLODDY: Cross-pharma federated learning at unprecedented scale unlocks benefits in QSAR without compromising proprietary information. *J Chem Inf Model*. 2024;64(7):2331–44. Epub 20230829. doi:10.1021/acs.jcim.3c00799. PubMed PMID: 37642660; PMCID: PMC11005050.

9 The Dark Side
Dual Use Implications of Generative Drug Discovery

Sean Ekins

9.1 INTRODUCTION

You may be fresh out of graduate school with a PhD and embarking on a postdoc or alternatively have started that dream job in the pharmaceutical industry, or biotech and you think you know everything about artificial intelligence (AI). On the other hand, you might be a mid-career scientist/entrepreneur who has used computational approaches for decades and is far down the pathway of understanding the importance of AI for drug discovery. Then, out of the blue comes the opportunity to do something neither of you had considered "in the interests of science," and overnight everything changes. You are suddenly thrust into the world of dual-use, which can be any research or technology with the potential to either help or harm us.[1,2] Dual-use research of concern (DURC) can be defined as research, predominantly in the life sciences, that has the potential to be misused for harmful purposes.[1] Principal examples of this are the synthesis of poliovirus,[3] the synthesis of mousepox,[2] gain-of-function studies with H5N1 in ferrets,[5] the generation of the 1918 influenza virus[4] and the synthesis of horsepox, the viral cousin of smallpox.[6] These seminal events all involved the physical synthesis of a biological agent but what if other technologies could have dual use potential but were not physical?

When we think of science, we virtually always associate the positive uses it can be put towards, but clearly, if history has taught us anything there are also negative impacts as well, some of which might not have been considered or understood at the time of discovery or implementation. For example, leaded gasoline and chlorofluorocarbons, which have had a clear detrimental impact on life and the environment, were initially thought of as important technological developments. In the space of healthcare, developing new treatments for human diseases is a rapidly evolving field. The lag between the discovery of new technologies and their commercialization is highly variable and can be adopted rapidly as in the case of mRNA vaccines for COVID, for example, or it can take up to a decade or more, as in the case of clustered regularly interspaced short palindromic repeats (CRISPR).[3] The field of drug discovery is no exception, and new technological adoption "hype cycles" are common. If you have been in the field of drug discovery for long enough, you may ultimately see one or more hype cycles for a technology applied either in your domain of expertise or elsewhere. The current revolution is "generative AI in drug discovery", which covers a wide array of applications from drug discovery through development. For example,

DOI: 10.1201/9781003399346-13

there have been considerable efforts in both academia and industry to develop and apply generative AI approaches that can be used to design new molecules[4–12] using algorithms such as Variational Autoencoder,[13] Generative Adversarial Networks[14] and Recurrent Neural Networks[5,11,15–18] as examples (see Chapter one). There have been several recent reviews that summarize the numerous publications in this area, which is rapidly developing[19–21] such that we have recently described this as part of what we termed the commoditization of AI for molecule design.[22]

9.2 SPIEZ INVITATION

In 2021, we were invited to present at the Swiss Federal Institute for NBC-Protection—Spiez Laboratory, part of the 'Convergence' conference series[23] set up by the Swiss government to identify developments in chemistry, biology, and enabling technologies, which may have implications for the Chemical and Biological Weapons Conventions.[24,25] This conference meets every two years and brings together an international group of scientific and disarmament experts to explore the current state of the art in the chemical and biological fields and their trajectories. This enables them to think through any potential security implications there might be and to consider how these can most effectively be managed internationally. At the time of the invitation we were particularly interested in the efforts of both academia and industry to develop and apply generative AI approaches used to design new molecules.[19] My company—Collaborations Pharmaceuticals, Inc—had recently published several machine learning models for toxicity prediction (and these likely got the attention of Spiez), and, in developing the presentation to the Spiez meeting, I opted to explore how AI could be used to design more toxic molecules. The running of a small company left limited time to put together an example that could suggest how the technology might be misused. Ultimately, I proposed three examples that could be used as a demonstration, and implemented the first suggestion because it seemed the most readily accessible.

At that time, it was evident there was an acceleration in interest in both academia and industry to develop and apply generative AI approaches to design new molecules.[22] We had previously designed a *de novo* molecule generator called MegaSyn[26], which integrates machine learning models for individual properties, namely bioactivity and toxicity, while also allowing a focus on specific molecule properties, such as drug-likeness, hydrophobicity, etc (see chapter 6). This generative model normally penalizes predicted toxicity and rewards predicted target activity. We simply proposed to invert this logic using the same approach to design *de novo* molecules, but now guiding the model to reward both toxicity and bioactivity instead. Such techniques are very fast and require relatively modest computer resources. We trained the AI with ~2M molecules from the public ChEMBL database, a collection of primarily drug-like molecules (drug-like meaning synthesizable and likely to be absorbed) and their bioactivities (Figure 9.1). We opted to score the designed molecules with a rat oral LD_{50} model originally developed as part of CATMoS,[27] an NIEHS online resource, and an acetylcholinesterase (AChE) inhibition model using data from ChEMBL and published recently to help derive compounds for treatment of Alzheimer's disease.[28] The underlying generative software has similar

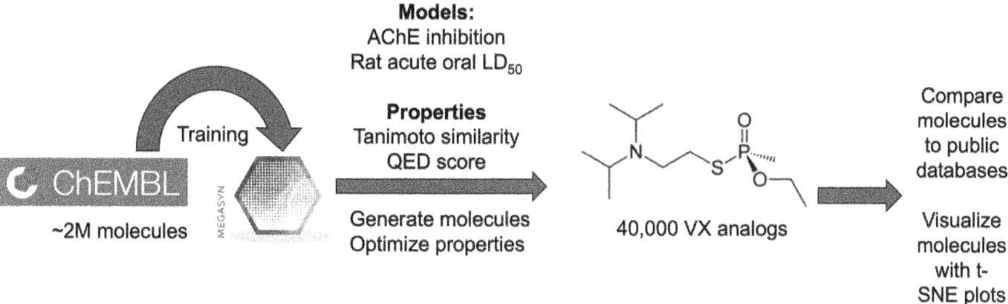

FIGURE 9.1 *De novo* design of VX and analogs using a generative AI (MegaSyn).

open-source software easily available.[29] To narrow the universe of molecules, we chose to drive the generative model towards those with high similarity to the nerve agent VX, one of the most toxic chemical warfare agents developed during the 20th century, were 6–10 mg[30] is sufficient to kill a person. Absorbed through the skin, VX inhibits AChE, an enzyme that breaks down the neurotransmitter acetylcholine (ACh). The subsequent build-up of ACh throughout the nervous system causes nerves to continually 'fire', leading to paralysis and death within a matter of minutes. Nerve agents using this mechanism have been in the headlines recently.[31] We also had an interest in the metabolism of pesticides and chemical weapons as we were funded by DTRA to work on computational and in vitro approaches to predict metabolism.

We literally pressed 'GO', and in less than 6 hours, our generative model finished training and generated forty thousand molecules that scored within our desired threshold. In the process, not only the AI designed VX, but also many other known chemical warfare agents that we identified through simple visual confirmation with structures in PubChem (Figure 9.1). Many new VX analog molecules were also designed to look equally plausible. These new molecules were predicted to be more potent AChE inhibitors and more toxic based on the predicted LD_{50} in comparison to publicly known chemical warfare agents. This was unexpected as the datasets we used for training the AI did not include these nerve agents. The virtual molecules even occupied a region of molecular property space that was entirely separate from the many thousands of molecules in the rat LD_{50} model, which is mainly made up of pesticides, environmental toxins, and drugs. The experiment was presented at the Convergence conference (by Zoom) and drew considerable immediate interest and was subsequently written up with significant input and guidance from Dr. Filippa Lentzos and Dr. Cedric Invernizzi, who are experts on arms control and dual-use. Our brief commentary called for the need for more discussion around the repurposing potential of AI in drug discovery.[32] While we did not explore that the approach could also be applied elsewhere, it was implied that it could certainly be used to design other illicit molecules that could also be considered chemical threats (e.g. synthetic opioids – fentanyl analogs, amphetamines readily came to mind when we were putting the thought experiment together) and then lead to the development of novel molecules that are not listed by the Chemical Weapons Convention. While we did not identify or disclose any synthetic routes or, indeed, the synthesizability for the over 40 thousand molecules designed, the rediscovery of known molecules like

VX and precursors pointed to the actual feasibility of the designs. As we did not make or test any of the new analogs, there is no experimental data on the toxicity of the molecules. The thought experiment also demonstrated the speed and relative ease with which such software that was based on open-source tools and datasets from the public domain could be misused to then create existing and novel potential biochemical threats. Our thought experiment was not one we had considered before, in fact we had not used any machine learning approaches previously to do anything other than predict activities that would be beneficial for human health.

9.3 THE BIGGER PICTURE

That we were able to generate a known chemical weapon VX and precursors of this and other agents (using the computer) relatively easily came as a surprise,[32] although in hindsight, the task is no different than using these same technologies to generate potential therapeutics which opens up a bigger picture to discuss. Our toxicity models were obviously originally created to avoid any toxicity, enabling us to better virtually screen molecules before ultimately confirming their toxicity through *in vitro* testing (e.g. whether cytotoxicity models or specific toxicities like hERG, drug-induced liver injury, etc.). The inverse, however, has always been true though: the better we can predict any toxicity, the better we can steer our generative model to design new molecules in a region of chemical space 'populated by predominantly lethal' molecules. We had just frankly not thought of this before. We did not assess the molecules for synthesizability or explore how to make them with retrosynthesis software, if we had more time, we probably would have done so. Both steps have many examples of available commercial and open-source software, which can be easily integrated into the *de novo* design process for making new molecules.[33] We also did not physically synthesize any of the molecules but with the massive number of global CROs offering chemical synthesis, it would not have been a difficult step to undertake. Importantly, we had a human-in-the-loop on the software side (and a supervisor) who could ultimately intervene and stop the process. But we also thought about if the human was removed from the loop, or replaced with someone (or a machine) who behaved unethically? We were concerned that with current breakthroughs and research into autonomous chemical synthesis,[34] a complete design-make-test cycle applicable to making not only drugs, but toxins, was entirely within reach of current technology and had not been considered before. We had also given some thought to the potential of a rogue AI to go beyond where we had stopped. Our thought experiment provided a literal wake-up call for the 'AI in drug discovery' community[35] pointing to how some expertise in chemistry or biology is still required to generate toxic substances or biological agents that can cause significant harm, but when these fields collide with generative machine learning models, all that is needed is the ability to use programs and to understand the output of the models themselves, they dramatically lower technical thresholds enabling relatively inexperienced people to participate. Open-source machine learning software is the primary route for learning and creating new models like ours, and the public toxicity datasets such as ToxCast[36] and ChEMBL[37] and others that enable providing a baseline model for toxicity predictions for a range of targets are readily available to anyone. While this proof of concept was only tested on VX we could have applied the approach to any other small molecule, peptide, polymer etc. We have also seen how the retrosynthesis tools are improving in parallel (see chapter 4 and 5), which allows new synthesis routes to be investigated for any known molecules or chemical warfare agents, hence potentially circumventing national and international lists of watched or controlled precursors for known synthesis routes. This was a major issue for us.

We were also concerned about the bigger picture as a very small company in an ecosystem of thousands of pharmaceutical companies globally that are using AI software for drug discovery. We wondered how many other companies had even considered how these generative AI approaches could be repurposed or misused in this way. We think it was probably likely that there had not been much forethought in this area. Bigger companies will have access to more funding, but as we showed, you do not need an abundance of funding to misuse generative AI,; you do not even need access to powerful computers, as most of what we demonstrated was done on a 2015 Apple desktop. What we did was demonstrate how the generative AI could find pockets of chemical space that can be filled with molecules that were predicted to be orders of magnitude more toxic than VX ($LD_{50}=0.022$ mg/kg in mice).[38] How many people possess the know-how to do that because it is certainly not something that could be done manually.

Much of the earlier discussion of the societal impact of AI had quite rightly focused on aspects like safety, privacy, discrimination, and potential criminal misuse,[39] but not discussion if any had been around AI and chemical weapons and their impact on national and international security. Previously, when we thought about drug discovery, we had not considered technology misuse potential and generative AI was just the latest incarnation of machine learning being undertaken by us. As scientists, specifically in the writer's case, a 'clinical pharmacologist' we had not been trained to think about the misuse potential. So, as this project developed, we felt it would be likely important to share this experience with other companies and individuals. We definitely saw denial, actual public relations people at a certain VC group that went out to suggest what we published was not important or relevant. Now of course, the VC in question had funded several companies working on generative AI to the tune of several billion dollars so there was really no conflict there! We had focused some of our concern around the use of AI generative machine learning tools for drug discovery, but we also imagine that other industries, such as consumer products and agrochemicals also have a major interest in designing and making new molecules with specific physicochemical properties.

We shone a light on this topic and are left to ponder the implications? The open-source software tools and datasets populate public databases with no oversight. If the threat of harm, or actual harm, occurs with ties back to machine learning, what impact will this have on how this technology is perceived? Our concern was, will the hype in the press on AI-designed drugs suddenly flip to AI-designed toxins, leading to potential for public shaming and decreased investment in these technologies? As a field, we felt that it would be prudent to open a conversation on this topic because the reputational risk is there, and it only takes one bad apple who takes what we have described to the next logical step, or a state looking for a technological edge. Generative AI could be that edge so how can we prevent this from happening?

We would have a hard time locking away all the software and data. Even monitoring who has access to these software and data would be difficult let alone restricting access. We had seen how some of the developing generative AI models, like GPT-3[40] had been restricting access. Even considering our work on toxicology machine learning models, we were not aware of any discussions around concerns of abuse or dual use, let alone ensuring that misuse was prevented and the models were only used for good. There was clearly a bigger picture to consider, and we had embarked on uncovering part of it.

9.4 ETHICS

Once we had generated the molecules in our thought experiment, we knew that we had gone as far as we dared, ethically without crossing a line. We now understood how to do it and have not tried anything remotely similar since. The molecules created were saved and encrypted and have only been analyzed further as we produced additional articles. We immediately felt there was a need to share our work at scientific conferences to foster a dialogue between industry and academia about the implications of our computational tools and the policies needed for safety. We did not imagine that we would enable even higher levels of visibility for potential dual use.[41] Our initial thoughts leaned heavily on ethics and guidelines, such as The Hague Ethical Guidelines.[42] We also considered that AI-focused drug discovery, pharmaceutical, and possibly other companies might want to agree to a code of conduct to train their employees, while at the same time securing their technology and prevent access and potential misuse. On a larger scale, we imagined the need for a connection to alert the authorities, which might have seemed alarmist. We felt that, in particular, universities should be at the forefront in applying ethical training to their science and computing students so that they become aware of the potential misuse of AI as early as possible.

9.5 MISSING FROM THE PAPER

Our initial commentary was in review for about five months before it finally saw the light of day when it was published in March 2022,[32] and when it surfaced, it was accidentally released by the journal as they did not alert any of the authors. It went viral and was the first we knew that it had been published when it appeared on the "in the pipeline" blog.[43] Many elements were either toned down by reviewers or removed by the journal to provide less information that could be misused. We also did not point out that only minimal computing resources were used, and we did not describe the several VX precursor molecules produced. Afterward, we went back to show that the AI explored other areas of chemistry space where other different known nerve agents were located, but these themselves were not rediscovered.[35] We also did not describe that the rat acute oral toxicity LD_{50} dataset[44] included VX and several analogs, providing us with some confidence that the predictions were likely more realistic as we had some coverage with molecules and were likely, not extrapolating. While we focused on chemical weapons, we could and perhaps should have also drawn attention to how the work may have also been used to propose new countermeasures for nerve agent or pesticide exposure, using datasets for AChE reactivators as an example. We raised awareness of the dual-use of AI in the drug discovery community[45,46], but others quickly followed up to add more detail and context.[47]

9.6 THE AFTERMATH

We have been asked to talk about many aspects of the paper, such as our motivations for the experiment, the molecules that were designed, and the ethical implications to groups from the White House Office of Science and Technology Policy and National Security Council (who advise the president), the Organization for the Prohibition of Chemical Weapons (OPCW), the Australia Group on export controls, the U.S. Defense Threat Reduction Agency, U.S. Department of State, U.S. Army and other U.S. National Laboratories. The work was also highlighted in a 2023 documentary on Netflix (Unknown: Killer Robots), which in itself was an adventure of its own. More recently the author was invited to present at the National Academies of Science, Engineering and Medicine as the concern over generative AI and biosecurity has increased.

The follow on from this has led us to consider how we manage such technologies as a company. We have described our example as a teachable moment for the field of dual-use on a par with earlier physical examples which had generated viruses, for example.

On the one hand, the misuse of any technology is possible; it does not have to be just generative AI. As a scientific community, we have focused for so long on sharing and openness of both data and algorithms that we have not considered the negative implications. It is long overdue for a correction. Our mission as drug discovery scientists is clear: we can develop technologies and generate data that have valuable applications in isolation, but we also need to think about the potential other side of the coin. Generative AI clearly needs quality data to generate predictive models, and they in turn, can be just as easily flipped to design drugs or toxins. We need to be ahead of the technology development curve. Today it is generative AI for drug discovery; tomorrow, it will be something else that is perhaps already in development or being used. We must remain vigilant and consider dual-use potential as early as possible in the development of technologies. Denial of the potential for dual use is not an option.

9.7 RECOMMENDATIONS

Rather than wait for organizations to respond, our experiences led us to question what we should do as scientists to deal with the dual-use risk of AI being used to develop new molecules that may be toxic to humans. We came up with 10 recommendations for regulatory agencies and other scientists to consider before others apply the technology to their own ends.[48] These efforts themselves could also be considered as steps on the way to some form of self-regulation and this may lead to the creation of an organization that could do this (e.g. the American Bar Association and others)

1. Use existing ethical guidelines from the OPCW[42] as an example, which include the key elements, sustainability, education, awareness and engagement, ethics, safety and security, accountability, oversight, and exchange of information.
2. Partner with AI ethics groups that may also have their own guidelines, such as the Montreal AI Ethics Institute,[49]; the Future of Life Institute,[50]; the institute for Ethics in AI,[51]; and the Institute for Ethical AI and Machine Learning.[52] There may be limited experience around AI in warfare.[53]
3. Increase the ethical training of computing and drug discovery students at universities.
4. Provide training for scientists in pharmaceutical companies on the potential dual-use potential of generative AI.
5. Keeping humans in the loop at all times provides another level of control.
6. Use waitlists to limit and control access to such technologies.
7. Create a public-facing API generative AI software to control access
8. Use approaches like federated learning that allow continued dataset use for model training while restricting sensitive structure-activity relationships.[54]
9. Limiting access through other methods such as confidentiality, and trade secrets and requiring security clearance to access it.
10. Disclose consideration of dual-use potential when publishing, which is already addressed in some other areas where 'risk' and 'misuse' is commented on.[55]

9.8 DISCUSSION

The initial publication has been noted by the World Health Organization[56] and the European Commission[57] in recent policy documents and has also provided justification for politicians in the US to call for legislation to control generative AI. Why stop at small molecules when AI is also being used to design proteins (the developers of these tools were even recently awarded Nobel prizes) which has led us to consider how some of these (predominantly consisting of large language model approaches like those used in ChatGPT) may also be misused[58] and how some of our earlier recommendations may have applicability to this domain as well.[59] What could we do in the future to ensure that the release of new technologies are not misused? One approach uses "red teaming" (i.e. willfully misusing a technology to access their vulnerabilities). Research papers from Anthropic.com explore red teaming in which they use temporary workers to act as red teamers who perform 'attacks' on their AI language models to test resistance against misuse and ultimately harmful content.[60] When used in this context to support chemical and biological security, such red teaming might replicate how an actor would breach Chemical and Biological Weapons Conventions [24,25] These efforts can also help strengthen how we respond to misuse, but there is also a risk that comes from training thousands of people to do this, so it is important that they understand the ethical and legal consequences of their role which in turn should be well controlled and monitored.

In conclusion, my company uses AI to help identify drugs to treat disease and *not* create weapons. The company is therefore very careful with whom we work and has close control over our software. By exploring the dual use potential of such generative AI in our industry we have alerted the world to this potential hopefully in time for us to take sufficient actions before someone puts what we have shown into practice. In that respect I feel we can clearly justify what we have undertaken as a public service, even though at the time we were perhaps unaware of where it would lead us.

ACKNOWLEDGMENTS

Dr. Fabio Urbina, Dr. Cédric Invernizzi, Dr. Filippa Lentzos and Dr. Max Brackmann are thanked for their collaborations on this project which resulted in several of the papers cited herein.

FUNDING

We kindly acknowledge NIH funding from R44GM122196-02A1 from NIGMS and 1R43ES031038-01 and 1R43ES033855-01 from NIEHS for our machine learning software development and applications. "Research reported in this publication was supported by the National Institute of Environmental Health Sciences of the National Institutes of Health under Award Number R43ES031038 and 1R43ES033855-01. The content is solely the responsibility of the authors and does not necessarily represent the official views of the National Institutes of Health."

STATEMENT ON DUAL-USE

The generative AI software described in this work has potential dual-use capabilities. We therefore propose to implement restrictions such as API's and waitlists to control who can access the software and what applications it is used for. We believe these precautions are necessary and will likely evolve over time as we integrate software features to address and limit repurposing potential.

REFERENCES

1. National Research Council. *Biotechnology Research in an Age of Terrorism*, The National Academies Press, Washington, DC, **2004**.
2. Rath, J.; Ischi, M.; Perkins, D. Evolution of different dual-use concepts in international and national law and its implications on research ethics and governance. *Sci Eng Ethics* **2014**, *20*, 769–790.
3. DiEuliis, D.; Giordano, J. Gene editing using CRISPR/Cas9: implications for dual-use and biosecurity. *Protein Cell* **2018**, *9* (3), 239–240. DOI:10.1007/s13238-017-0493-4.
4. Olivecrona, M.; Blaschke, T.; Engkvist, O.; Chen, H. Molecular de-novo design through deep reinforcement learning. *J Cheminf* **2017**, *9* (1), 48. DOI:10.1186/s13321-017-0235-x.
5. Segler, M. H. S.; Kogej, T.; Tyrchan, C.; Waller, M. P. Generating focused molecule libraries for drug discovery with recurrent neural networks. *ACS Cent Sci* **2018**, *4* (1), 120–131. DOI:10.1021/acscentsci.7b00512.
6. Krenn, M.; Häse, F.; Nigam, A.; Friederich, P.; Aspuru-Guzik, A. Self-referencing embedded strings (SELFIES): a 100% robust molecular string representation. *Mach Learn Sci Technol* **2020**, *1* (4), 045024. DOI:10.1088/2632-2153/aba947.

7. Jin, W.; Barzilay, R.; Jaakola, T. *Junction Tree Variational Autoencoder for Molecular Graph Generation*, **2019**. https://arxiv.org/pdf/1802.04364.pdf.
8. Hochreiter, S.; Schmidhuber, J. Long short-term memory. *Neural Comput* **1997**, *9*, 1735–1780.
9. Blaschke, T.; Olivecrona, M.; Engkvist, O.; Bajorath, J.; Chen, H. Application of generative autoencoder in de novo molecular design. *Mol Inform* **2018**, *37* (1–2), 1700123. DOI:10.1002/minf.201700123.
10. Sanchez-Lengeling, B.; Outeiral, C.; Guimaraes, G. L.; Aspuru-Guzik, A. *Optimizing Distributions Over Molecular Space. An Objective-Reinforced Generative Adversarial Network for Inverse-Design Chemistry (ORGANIC)*, **2017**. https://chemrxiv.org/engage/chemrxiv/article-details/60c73d91702a9beea7189bc2.
11. Winter, R.; Montanari, F.; Steffen, A.; Briem, H.; Noé, F.; Clevert, D.-A. Efficient multi-objective molecular optimization in a continuous latent space. *Chem Sci* **2019**, *10* (34), 8016–8024. DOI:10.1039/C9SC01928F.
12. Gao, K.; Nguyen, D. D.; Tu, M.; Wei, G.-W. Generative network complex for the automated generation of drug-like molecules. *J Chem Inform Model* **2020**, *60* (12), 5682–5698. DOI:10.1021/acs.jcim.0c00599.
13. Gomez-Bombarelli, R.; Wei, J. N.; Duvenaud, D.; Hernandez-Lobato, J. M.; Sanchez-Lengeling, B.; Sheberla, D.; Aguilera-Iparraguirre, J.; Hirzel, T. D.; Adams, R. P.; Aspuru-Guzik, A. Automatic chemical design using a data-driven continuous representation of molecules. *ACS Cent Sci* **2018**, *4* (2), 268–276. DOI:10.1021/acscentsci.7b00572.
14. Prykhodko, O.; Johansson, S. V.; Kotsias, P. C.; Arus-Pous, J.; Bjerrum, E. J.; Engkvist, O.; Chen, H. A de novo molecular generation method using latent vector based generative adversarial network. *J Cheminform* **2019**, *11* (1), 74. DOI:10.1186/s13321-019-0397-9.
15. Gupta, A.; Muller, A. T.; Huisman, B. J. H.; Fuchs, J. A.; Schneider, P.; Schneider, G. Erratum: Generative recurrent networks for de novo drug design. *Mol Inform* **2018**, *37* (1–2), 1880141. DOI:10.1002/minf.201880141.
16. Bjerrum, E. J.; Threlfall, R. Molecular generation with recurrent neural networks (RNNs). *arXiv* **2017**, *1705.04612*.
17. Domenico, A.; Nicola, G.; Daniela, T.; Fulvio, C.; Nicola, A.; Orazio, N. De novo drug design of targeted chemical libraries based on artificial intelligence and pair-based multiobjective optimization. *J Chem Inf Model* **2020**, *60* (10), 4582–4593. DOI:10.1021/acs.jcim.0c00517.
18. Maziarka, L.; Pocha, A.; Kaczmarczyk, J.; Rataj, K.; Danel, T.; Warchol, M. Mol-CycleGAN: a generative model for molecular optimization. *J Cheminform* **2020**, *12*, 2.
19. Meyers, J.; Fabian, B.; Brown, N. De novo molecular design and generative models. *Drug Discov Today* **2021**, *26* (11), 2707–2715. DOI:10.1016/j.drudis.2021.05.019.
20. Bhisetti, G.; Fang, C. Artificial intelligence-enabled de novo design of novel compounds that are synthesizable. *Methods Mol Biol* **2022**, *2390*, 409–419. DOI:10.1007/978-1-0716-1787-8_17.
21. Palazzesi, F.; Pozzan, A. Deep learning applied to ligand-based de novo drug design. *Methods Mol Biol* **2022**, *2390*, 273–299. DOI:10.1007/978-1-0716-1787-8_12.
22. Urbina, F.; Ekins, S. The commoditization of AI for molecule design. *Artif Intell Life Sci* **2022**, *2*, 100031.
23. Anon. *Spiez Convergence*, **2021**. https://www.spiezlab.admin.ch/en/home/meta/refconvergence.html.
24. Anon. *Chemical Weapons Convention*, **2024**. https://www.opcw.org/chemical-weapons-convention.

25. Anon. *Biological Weapons Convention.* https://www.nti.org/education-center/treaties-and-regimes/convention-prohibition-development-production-and-stockpiling-bacteriological-biological-and-toxin-weapons-btwc/
26. Urbina, F.; Lowden, C. T.; Culberson, J. C.; Ekins, S. *MegaSyn: Integrating Generative Molecule Design, Automated Analog Designer and Synthetic Viability Prediction,* **2021**. https://doi.org/10.33774/chemrxiv-2021-nlwvs.
27. Mansouri, K.; Karmaus, A.; Fitzpatrick, J.; Patlewicz, G.; Pradeep, P.; Alberga, D.; Alepee, N.; Allen, T. E. H.; Allen, D.; Alves, V. M.; et al. Erratum: CATMoS: collaborative acute toxicity modeling suite. *Environ Health Perspect* **2021**, *129* (7), 79001. DOI:10.1289/EHP9883.
28. Vignaux, P. A.; Minerali, E.; Lane, T. R.; Foil, D. H.; Madrid, P. B.; Puhl, A. C.; Ekins, S. The antiviral drug tilorone is a potent and selective inhibitor of acetylcholinesterase. *Chem Res Toxicol* **2021**, *34* (5), 1296–1307. DOI:10.1021/acs.chemrestox.0c00466.
29. Blaschke, T.; Arus-Pous, J.; Chen, H.; Margreitter, C.; Tyrchan, C.; Engkvist, O.; Papadopoulos, K.; Patronov, A. REINVENT 2.0: an AI tool for de novo drug design. *J Chem Inf Model* **2020**, *60* (12), 5918–5922. DOI:10.1021/acs.jcim.0c00915.
30. National Research Council (US) Committee on Toxicology. *Review of Acute Human-Toxicity Estimates for VX.* National Academies Press (US), Washington, DC, **1997**. https://www.ncbi.nlm.nih.gov/books/NBK233724/.
31. Aroniadou-Anderjaska, V.; Apland, J. P.; Figueiredo, T. H.; De Araujo Furtado, M.; Braga, M. F. Acetylcholinesterase inhibitors (nerve agents) as weapons of mass destruction: history, mechanisms of action, and medical countermeasures. *Neuropharmacology* **2020**, *181*, 108298. DOI:10.1016/j.neuropharm.2020.108298.
32. Urbina, F.; Lentzos, F.; Invernizzi, C.; Ekins, S. Dual use of artificial-intelligence-powered drug discovery. *Nat Mach Intell* **2022**, *4* (3), 189–191. DOI:10.1038/s42256-022-00465-9.
33. Genheden, S.; Thakkar, A.; Chadimova, V.; Reymond, J. L.; Engkvist, O.; Bjerrum, E. AiZynthFinder: a fast, robust and flexible open-source software for retrosynthetic planning. *J Cheminform* **2020**, *12* (1), 70. DOI:10.1186/s13321-020-00472-1.
34. Coley, C. W.; Thomas, D. A., 3rd; Lummiss, J. A. M.; Jaworski, J. N.; Breen, C. P.; Schultz, V.; Hart, T.; Fishman, J. S.; Rogers, L.; Gao, H.; et al. A robotic platform for flow synthesis of organic compounds informed by AI planning. *Science* **2019**, *365* (6453), eaax1566. DOI:10.1126/science.aax1566.
35. Urbina, F.; Lentzos, F.; Invernizzi, C.; Ekins, S. AI in drug discovery: a wake-up call. *Drug Discov Today* **2023**, *28* (1), 103410. DOI:10.1016/j.drudis.2022.103410.
36. Dix, D. J.; Houck, K. A.; Martin, M. T.; Richard, A. M.; Setzer, R. W.; Kavlock, R. J. The ToxCast program for prioritizing toxicity testing of environmental chemicals. *Toxicol Sci* **2007**, *95* (1), 5–12.
37. Gaulton, A.; Hersey, A.; Nowotka, M.; Bento, A. P.; Chambers, J.; Mendez, D.; Mutowo, P.; Atkinson, F.; Bellis, L. J.; Cibrian-Uhalte, E.; et al. The ChEMBL database in 2017. *Nucleic Acids Res* **2017**, *45* (D1), D945–D954. DOI:10.1093/nar/gkw1074.
38. Pike, D. W. Physical protection against acetylcholinesterases. In *Clinincal and Experimental Toxicology of Organophosphates and Carbamates*, Ballantyne, B., Marrs, T. C., Eds., Butterworth-Heinemann Ltd., Oxford, **1992**, pp. 414–420.
39. Hutson, M. *Who Should Stop Unethical A.I.?* **2021**. https://www.newyorker.com/tech/annals-of-technology/who-should-stop-unethical-ai.
40. Brown, T. B.; Mann, B.; Ryder, N.; Subbiah, M.; Kaplan, J.; Dhariwal, P.; Neelakantan, A.; Shyam, P.; Sastry, G.; Askell, A.; et al. *Language Models are Few-Shot Learners*, **2020**. https://arxiv.org/abs/2005.14165.
41. EPA. *Policy and Procedures for Managing Dual Use Research of Concern*, **2021**. https://www.epa.gov/research/policy-and-procedures-managing-dual-use-research-concern.
42. Anon. *The Hague Ethical Guidelines*, **2021**. https://www.opcw.org/hague-ethical-guidelines.

43. Lowe, D. *Deliberately Optimizing for Harm*, **2022**. https://www.science.org/content/blog-post/deliberately-optimizing-harm.
44. Mansouri, K.; Karmaus, A. L.; Fitzpatrick, J.; Patlewicz, G.; Pradeep, P.; Alberga, D.; Alepee, N.; Allen, T. E. H.; Allen, D.; Alves, V. M.; et al. CATMoS: collaborative acute toxicity modeling suite. *Environ Health Perspect* **2021**, *129* (4), 47013. DOI:10.1289/EHP8495.
45. Tackling the perils of dual use in AI. *Nat Mach Intell* **2022**, *4* (4), 313–313. DOI:10.1038/s42256-022-00484-6.
46. Urbina, F.; Lentzos, F.; Invernizzi, C.; Ekins, S. A teachable moment for dual use. *Nat Mach Intell* **2022**, *4*, 607. DOI:10.1038/s42256-022-00465-9.
47. Blum, M.-M. No chemical killer AI (yet). *Nat Mach Intell* **2022**, *4*, 506–507.
48. Urbina, F.; Lentzos, F.; Invernizzi, C.; Ekins, S. Preventing AI from creating biochemical threats. *J Chem Inf Model* **2023**, *63* (3), 691–694. DOI:10.1021/acs.jcim.2c01616.
49. Anon. *Montreal AI Ethics Institute*, **2022**. https://montrealethics.ai.
50. Anon. *The Future of Life Institute*, **2022**. https://futureoflife.org.
51. Anon. *Institute for Ethics in AI*, **2022**. https://www.schwarzmancentre.ox.ac.uk/ethicsinai.
52. Anon. *The Institute for Ethical AI & Machine Learning*, **2022**. https://ethical.institute.
53. Lentzos, F. AI and biological weapons. In *Armament, Arms Control and Artificial Intelligence: The Janus-faced Nature of Machine Learning in the Military Realm*, Reinhold, T., Schöring, N., Eds., Springer, Cham, **2022**.
54. Chen, S.; Xue, D.; Chuai, G.; Yang, Q.; Liu, Q. FL-QSAR: a federated learning-based QSAR prototype for collaborative drug discovery. *Bioinformatics* **2020**, *36* (22–23), 5492–5498. DOI:10.1093/bioinformatics/btaa1006 (acccessed 4/10/2022).
55. Ramesh, A.; Dhariwal, P.; Nichol, A.; Chu, C.; Chen, M. *Hierarchical Text-Conditional Image Generation with CLIP Latents*, **2022**. https://arxiv.org/abs/2204.06125.
56. World Health Organization. *Global Guidance Framework for the Responsible Use of the Life Sciences*, **2022**. https://www.interacademies.org/publication/global-guidance-framework-responsible-use-life-sciences.
57. European Commission. *Towards a Green & Digital Future*, European Commission, **2022**. https://op.europa.eu/en/publication-detail/-/publication/58c3af16-f692-11ec-b976-01aa75ed71a1/language-en/format-PDF/source-260501988.
58. Ekins, S.; Lentzos, F.; Brackmann, M.; Invernizzi, C. There's a ChatGPT' for biology. What could go wrong? *Bull Atom Sci* **2023**. https://thebulletin.org/2023/03/chat-gpt-for-biology/
59. Ekins, S.; Brackmann, M.; Invernizzi, C.; Lentzos, F. Generative artificial intelligence-assisted protein design must consider repurposing potential. *GEN Biotechnol* **2023**, *2* (4), 296–300. DOI:10.1089/genbio.2023.0025.
60. Ganguli, D.; Lovitt, L.; Kernion, J.; Askell, A.; Bai, Y.; Kadavath, S.; Mann, B.; Perez, E.; Schiefer, N.; Ndousse, K.; et al. Red teaming language models to reduce harms: methods, scaling behaviors, and lessons learned. *arXiv* **2022**, *2209.07858*.

Part V

The Future

10 Future Labs – Generative Approaches in Self-Driving Labs

Sean Ekins

10.1 INTRODUCTION

Future labs was a workshop held on January 11–12th, 2024, that was chaired by Dr. Milad Abolhasani at NC State University, which brought together a diverse mix of researchers in academia and industry from around the world.[1] The meeting was focused on self-driving labs (SDLs). These are at the intersection of laboratory automation, robotics, and artificial intelligence (AI). In addition to these fields, you could add an area of interest such as biotechnology, chemistry, materials science. My interest in this area stemmed from work several years earlier as part of a DARPA-funded project with Stanford Research International that was focused on developing their automated chemistry synthesis platform called SynFini[2] and some work towards the prediction of UV-VIS spectra for these efforts.[3] In addition, I have over 28 years experience of using computational approaches to assist in the design-make-test-analyze cycle which is increasingly becoming an area with a heavy AI component. I, therefore attended with a limited background to understanding SDL but came away wondering how this might impact drug discovery and the bigger picture of science and innovation in general. What follows is a brief overview of some of the workshop presentations that I attended.

An SDL can be simply defined as a lab without a human in the loop. The human is replaced by robots that can move plates, pipette liquids and perform the experiments under the guidance of an AI. The decline in research productivity[4] and disruptiveness over the last 60 years of patent literature and papers[5] certainly suggests we need to be embracing new approaches to modernize research and development that uses data and is guided by machine learning (ML), which points to SDL.[6]

10.2 EXAMPLES OF SDL

As an example, in the space of making materials like quantum dots, this has led to the development of an Artificial Chemist SDL approach by the Abolhasani group, which uses flow chemistry, *in situ* characterization, real-time processing, and machine learning experiment selection.[7] The approach was able to make new quantum dots without prior knowledge and showed it could reach favorable synthesis conditions to make molecules with ideal properties. SDLs have been applied elsewhere and have been used in synthetic biology with many opportunities and also risks.[8]

DOI: 10.1201/9781003399346-15

SDLs could be considered centralized facilities or decentralized labs that could also be made available to open up access to facilities and capabilities to those from anywhere in the country (or world), akin to how supercomputers were accessible back in the 1980s and 1990s, when a researcher would book time at a facility to do their experiment. One might imagine the same happening with SDLs.

The workshop was primarily heavily focused on materials discovery. Klavs Jensen described his group's recent paper, which used an SDL to both explore and exploit the chemical space to optimize dye-like molecules, an approach with clear parallels in drug discovery.[9] This work led to 303 dye-like molecules and highlighted how commonly used metrics for synthesizability did not improve the reaction planning quality suggesting the need for more efficient methods. Human input was still needed for recovery from errors and restocking of materials in this study, so there will still be jobs for humans! As expected, there were also model applicability domain issues in terms of how far you could extrapolate beyond the molecular properties measured.[9]

As highlighted by Jeff Carbeck (Eastman) companies could use SDL to anticipate and prepare for the end of lifecycle of materials, thereby changing the way companies have developed products historically, which is likely also just as relevant for other industries such as pharmaceutical, agrochemical companies and beyond.

The application of SDL by Martin Burke highlighted the development of automated synthesis for small molecules[10] using specific reactions such as the heteroaryl Suzuki-Miyaura coupling.[10] This SDL approach was able to double the average yield compared with a benchmark and resulted in a 95% success rate.[10] The Burke group and others have also used building block-based synthesis approaches to prepare many derivatives of a compound.[11] The generalized small-molecule synthesizers as automated approaches move us away from traditional methods[12] and have already been integrated into SDL.

SDL uses computational algorithms to decide what to make and then controls the hardware to perform the synthesis, purification, analytical as well as eventual biological testing.[13] There are still few examples of SDL for drug discovery[13] in contrast to where this field has been accelerated by automation and computational approaches separately. These SDL for drug discovery could benefit from datasets to enable models with a much wider applicability domain as well as tools for the automated validation and benchmarking of such technologies in order to provide a firm foundation for these approaches.[14]

10.3 THE NEED FOR HIGH-QUALITY DATA

SDL is rapidly evolving as we fuse automation and AI to facilitate autonomous experimentation[15] and molecule synthesis and testing.[16–21] These laboratories fundamentally face a chicken-and-egg scenario because in order to generate machine learning models, experimental data is needed, and in order to decide upon future experimentation, AI predictions using previous data are required. Supply of such high-quality curated data for machine learning is therefore critical and likely a key factor in predicting success.

The NIH has such datasets that may be needed to train such machine learning (ML) models distributed across numerous databases, e.g. PubChem,[22,23] Tox21,[24] CEBS,[25]

TABLE 10.1
Selected Examples of Diverse SAR Databases and Datasets That Could Aid Drug Discovery via SDL

Database/ Dataset	Website	Data Types	Notes	Institute
National Institute of Allergy and Infectious Diseases ChemDB: Division of AIDS Therapeutics Database	https://chemdb.niaid.nih.gov	Contains small molecule data for HIV, TB, and other opportunistic infections	Requires CRADA to access it. Data cannot be readily extracted	NIAID
COMPARE	https://dtp.cancer.gov/databases_tools/compare.htm	Data for tens of thousands of molecules tested against 59 cell lines	Data is accessible in PubChem	NCI
PDSP	https://pdsp.unc.edu/databases/kidb.php	A database of K_i data for different GPCRs	Data is downloadable	NIMH
Tox21 toolbox	https://ntp.niehs.nih.gov/whatwestudy/tox21/toolbox/index.html	Screened >14,000 compounds against various toxicity targets (enzymes, receptors etc.)	Data is downloadable	NIEHS
Chemical effects in biological systems	https://manticore.niehs.nih.gov/cebssearch	Data for Ames, in vivo micronucleus, comet data, reproductive data etc.	Data is downloadable	NIEHS
Integrated chemical environment	https://ice.ntp.niehs.nih.gov/DATASETDESCRIPTION	Acute oral toxicity, dermal toxicity, inhalation toxicity, endocrine, eye, skin toxicity, physicochemical properties	Data is downloadable	NIEHS

(Continued)

TABLE 10.1 (*Continued*)
Selected Examples of Diverse SAR Databases and Datasets That Could Aid Drug Discovery via SDL

Database/ Dataset	Website	Data Types	Notes	Institute
PubChem	https://pubchem.ncbi.nlm.nih.gov	Data on assays, diseases, targets etc. Over 111 million compounds and 1 million bioassays	Data is downloadable	NLM
ChEMBL	https://www.ebi.ac.uk/chembl/	Manually curated database with over 13,000 targets, ~1.9M compounds, 16M activities	Data is downloadable	EMBL-EBI
ToxCast	https://www.epa.gov/chemical-research/exploring-toxcast-data-downloadable-data	821 assay endpoints, 1,800 chemicals	Data is downloadable	EPA

HIV ChemDB[26], and others (Table 10.1). We estimate there are likely on the order of 100 such databases representing millions of molecules and datapoints.[27] In particular, the ever-growing NIH datasets of small-molecule and bioactivity data (structure-activity relationship, SAR) has met with increased demand for access and analysis. With a large repertoire of ML software (either open source or commercial) now available, the bottleneck in obtaining useful knowledge from these datasets often lies with the extraction and curation of data. This data is often poorly curated in the databases or not in a format that is generally readily useable to output for machine learning models. We have seen this with databases like PubChem[22,23] which while a valuable repository, the data is suboptimally curated and not particularly accessible for generating such models. Contrast that with the ChEMBL database[28] in which the data is comparatively well curated, and has been widely extracted and used for ML by many groups.[29–38] Still, even the structure activity relationship (SAR) data in ChEMBL is not in an ideal format, and time-consuming manual curation is often required before it can be used for model building. Making these NIH ligand-based SAR datasets more accessible by providing the underlying datasets in a ready-to-model format would certainly be useful in the future. In doing so, this would eliminate the biggest challenge in data accessibility. Second, if these datasets were used to make readily available a significant number of trained and validated machine learning models that users could access and apply instantly in their laboratories that would also be beneficial. There is, therefore, an opportunity for linking and auto-curation of NIH public databases which use SAR data such as that described as IC_{50}, K_i, EC_{50}, MIC,

% inhibition sorted by target and /or disease enabled by a machine learning model ontology. The US in particular needs to maintain its position at the forefront of biomedical research, and leveraging the knowledge created through machine learning using already generated data (funded in large part by the NIH and possibly others) will be increasingly critical and likely also important for SDL.

10.4 LIMITATIONS OF SDL

The cost of setting up an SDL is very high currently so efforts to decrease this would increase their use and this could be facilitated by using low-cost, accessible tools rather than off-the-shelf equipment. To date there are also few examples were hardware and software for SDL have been made openly available.[39]

There also needs to be consideration of the safety and security measures if the AI is in control in order to prevent it from doing undesirable experiments or those that could be seen as unethical. If an SDL invents a molecule or material, understanding whether it is ultimately patentable is a valid concern. Certainly, it would be desirable to create something novel that could be patented, such as a molecule that is outside other companies' freedom to operate.

We may be far from seeing SDL in common use due to limited commercial tools and a lack of integration between vendors. The customer base is currently small due to the limited demand, and this may be holding vendors back as well. Integration of software, robotics, synthesis, liquid handling, purification, and analytical technology for multiple systems will be complex and may create opportunities for smaller companies. Alternatively, consortia could enable these interconnections by leveraging the SDL expertise in academia, industry, vendors, and elsewhere to spread the financial and scientific risk of developing SDL.

10.5 SDL IN THE FUTURE

SDL will likely be the future laboratory paradigm, but how long it will take is debatable. Laboratories have not really changed in over 100 years; while the equipment in them has developed dramatically, there is virtually always one or more scientists physically in there as well. The usual lab-coat-wearing scientist will be a different type in these SDL. For one, they will not need to be 'in' the lab. They may need a combination of computational, robotics, biology, and chemistry, or perhaps they will be engineers. They will likely be using generative algorithms at the core of their process and feeding data back until they meet design criteria. The human input may ultimately be limited to maintenance and benefitting only from the outputs of this technology. It will certainly be fascinating to see how quickly SDL develops, the scale of SDL that has become the norm, and whether it can become the dominant form of scientific laboratory. In SDL, the generative algorithm is but one important component that is integrated with the others to enable the function of the whole unit. Imagining other scenarios where generative algorithms may play a similar role is worth considering as they expand their scope beyond just being another 'de novo design' tool.

ACKNOWLEDGMENTS

The organizers, speakers, panelists, and fellow attendees at the Future Labs workshop are acknowledged for inspiring this chapter.

REFERENCES

1. Future Labs [cited 2024 Jan 16]. Available from: https://research.ncsu.edu/futurelabsworkshop/about.
2. SynFini 2024. Available from: https://www.sri.com/platform/synfini/.
3. Urbina F, Batra K, Luebke KJ, White JD, Matsiev D, Olson LL, Malerich JP, Hupcey MAZ, Madrid PB, Ekins S. UV-adVISor: Attention-based recurrent neural networks to predict UV-vis spectra. *Anal Chem.* 2021;93(48):16076–85. Epub 2021/11/24. doi: 10.1021/acs.analchem.1c03741. PubMed PMID: 34812602; PMCID: PMC9137254.
4. Scannell JW, Blanckley A, Boldon H, Warrington B. Diagnosing the decline in pharmaceutical R&D efficiency. *Nat Rev Drug Discov.* 2012;11(3):191–200. Epub 20120301. doi: 10.1038/nrd3681. PubMed PMID: 22378269.
5. Park M, Leahey E, Funk RJ. Papers and patents are becoming less disruptive over time. *Nature.* 2023;613(7942):138–44. Epub 20230104. doi: 10.1038/s41586-022-05543-x. PubMed PMID: 36600070.
6. Pacheco Gutierrez D, Folkmann LM, Tribukait H, Roch LM. How to accelerate R&D and optimize experiment planning with machine learning and data science. *Chimia (Aarau).* 2023;77(1–2):7–16. Epub 20230222. doi: 10.2533/chimia.2023.7. PubMed PMID: 38047848.
7. Epps RW, Bowen MS, Volk AA, Abdel-Latif K, Han S, Reyes KG, Amassian A, Abolhasani M. Artificial chemist: An autonomous quantum dot synthesis bot. *Adv Mater.* 2020;32(30):e2001626. Epub 20200604. doi: 10.1002/adma.202001626. PubMed PMID: 32495399.
8. Martin HG, Radivojevic T, Zucker J, Bouchard K, Sustarich J, Peisert S, Arnold D, Hillson N, Babnigg G, Marti JM, Mungall CJ, Beckham GT, Waldburger L, Carothers J, Sundaram S, Agarwal D, Simmons BA, Backman T, Banerjee D, Tanjore D, Ramakrishnan L, Singh A. Perspectives for self-driving labs in synthetic biology. *Curr Opin Biotechnol.* 2023;79:102881. Epub 20230103. doi: 10.1016/j.copbio.2022.102881. PubMed PMID: 36603501.
9. Koscher BA, Canty RB, McDonald MA, Greenman KP, McGill CJ, Bilodeau CL, Jin W, Wu H, Vermeire FH, Jin B, Hart T, Kulesza T, Li SC, Jaakkola TS, Barzilay R, Gomez-Bombarelli R, Green WH, Jensen KF. Autonomous, multiproperty-driven molecular discovery: From predictions to measurements and back. *Science.* 2023;382(6677):eadi1407. Epub 20231222. doi: 10.1126/science.adi1407. PubMed PMID: 38127734.
10. Angello NH, Rathore V, Beker W, Wolos A, Jira ER, Roszak R, Wu TC, Schroeder CM, Aspuru-Guzik A, Grzybowski BA, Burke MD. Closed-loop optimization of general reaction conditions for heteroaryl Suzuki-Miyaura coupling. *Science.* 2022;378(6618):399–405. Epub 20221027. doi: 10.1126/science.adc8743. PubMed PMID: 36302014.
11. Lehmann JW, Blair DJ, Burke MD. Towards the generalized iterative synthesis of small molecules. *Nat Rev Chem.* 2018;2(2):0115. doi: 10.1038/s41570-018-0115.
12. Trobe M, Burke MD. The Molecular Industrial Revolution: Automated Synthesis of Small Molecules. *Angew Chem Int Ed Engl.* 2018;57(16):4192–214. Epub 20180307. doi: 10.1002/anie.201710482. PubMed PMID: 29513400; PMCID: PMC5912692.

13. Coley CW, Eyke NS, Jensen KF. Autonomous discovery in the chemical sciences part I: Progress. *Angew Chem Int Ed Engl.* 2020;59(51):22858–93. Epub 20200608. doi: 10.1002/anie.201909987. PubMed PMID: 31553511.
14. Coley CW, Eyke NS, Jensen KF. Autonomous discovery in the chemical sciences part II: Outlook. *Angew Chem Int Ed Engl.* 2020;59(52):23414–36. Epub 20200611. doi: 10.1002/anie.201909989. PubMed PMID: 31553509.
15. Häse F, Roch LM, Aspuru-Guzik A. Next-generation experimentation with self-driving laboratories. *TRAC.* 2019;1(3):282–91. doi: 10.1016/j.trechm.2019.02.007.
16. Ozin G, Siler T. Autonomous chemical synthesis 2020. Available from: https://www.advancedsciencenews.com/autonomous-chemical-synthesis/.
17. Sanderson K. Automation: Chemistry shoots for the Moon. *Nature.* 2019;568(7753):577–79. Epub 2019/04/25. doi: 10.1038/d41586-019-01246-y. PubMed PMID: 31015690.
18. Porwol L, Kowalski DJ, Henson A, Long D-L, Bell NL, Cronin L. An autonomous chemical robot discovers the rules of inorganic coordination chemistry without prior knowledge. *Angew Chem Int Ed Engl.* 2020;59:11256–61.
19. Bedard AC, Adamo A, Aroh KC, Russell MG, Bedermann AA, Torosian J, Yue B, Jensen KF, Jamison TF. Reconfigurable system for automated optimization of diverse chemical reactions. *Science.* 2018;361(6408):1220–25. Epub 2018/09/22. doi: 10.1126/science.aat0650. PubMed PMID: 30237351.
20. Coley CW, Thomas DA, 3rd, Lummiss JAM, Jaworski JN, Breen CP, Schultz V, Hart T, Fishman JS, Rogers L, Gao H, Hicklin RW, Plehiers PP, Byington J, Piotti JS, Green WH, Hart AJ, Jamison TF, Jensen KF. A robotic platform for flow synthesis of organic compounds informed by AI planning. *Science.* 2019;365(6453):eaax1566. Epub 2019/08/10. doi: 10.1126/science.aax1566. PubMed PMID: 31395756.
21. Bettenhausen C. AI and robotics come together for synthesis. *C&E News.* 2020;98.
22. Kim S, Thiessen PA, Bolton EE, Chen J, Fu G, Gindulyte A, Han L, He J, He S, Shoemaker BA, Wang J, Yu B, Zhang J, Bryant SH. PubChem substance and compound databases. *Nucleic Acids Res.* 2016;44(D1):D1202–13. doi: 10.1093/nar/gkv951. PubMed PMID: 26400175; PMCID: PMC4702940.
23. Anon. The PubChem Database. Available from: http://pubchem.ncbi.nlm.nih.gov/.
24. Tice RR, Austin CP, Kavlock RJ, Bucher JR. Improving the human hazard characterization of chemicals: a Tox21 update. *Environ Health Perspect.* 2013;121(7):756–65. Epub 2013/04/23. doi: 10.1289/ehp.1205784. PubMed PMID: 23603828; PMCID: PMC3701992.
25. Waters M, Stasiewicz S, Merrick BA, Tomer K, Bushel P, Paules R, Stegman N, Nehls G, Yost KJ, Johnson CH, Gustafson SF, Xirasagar S, Xiao N, Huang CC, Boyer P, Chan DD, Pan Q, Gong H, Taylor J, Choi D, Rashid A, Ahmed A, Howle R, Selkirk J, Tennant R, Fostel J. CEBS--Chemical Effects in Biological Systems: a public data repository integrating study design and toxicity data with microarray and proteomics data. *Nucleic Acids Res.* 2008;36(Database issue):D892–900. Epub 2007/10/27. doi: 10.1093/nar/gkm755. PubMed PMID: 17962311; PMCID: PMC2238989.
26. Zorn KM, Lane TR, Russo DP, Clark AM, Makarov V, Ekins S. Multiple machine learning comparisons of HIV cell-based and reverse transcriptase data sets. *Mol Pharm.* 2019;16(4):1620–32. Epub 2019/02/20. doi: 10.1021/acs.molpharmaceut.8b01297. PubMed PMID: 30779585.
27. Lipinski CA, Litterman NK, Southan C, Williams AJ, Clark AM, Ekins S. Parallel worlds of public and commercial bioactive chemistry data. *J Med Chem.* 2015;58(5):2068–76. Epub 2014/11/22. doi: 10.1021/jm5011308. PubMed PMID: 25415348; PMCID: PMC4360371.

28. Gaulton A, Bellis LJ, Bento AP, Chambers J, Davies M, Hersey A, Light Y, McGlinchey S, Michalovich D, Al-Lazikani B, Overington JP. ChEMBL: a large-scale bioactivity database for drug discovery. *Nucleic Acids Res.* 2012;40(Database issue):D1100–7. PubMed PMID: 21948594.
29. Lenselink EB, Ten Dijke N, Bongers B, Papadatos G, van Vlijmen HWT, Kowalczyk W, AP IJ, van Westen GJP. Beyond the hype: Deep neural networks outperform established methods using a ChEMBL bioactivity benchmark set. *J Cheminform.* 2017;9(1):45. doi: 10.1186/s13321-017-0232-0. PubMed PMID: 29086168; PMCID: PMC5555960.
30. Mayr A, Klambauer G, Unterthiner T, Steijaert M, Wegner JK, Ceulemans H, Clevert DA, Hochreiter S. Large-scale comparison of machine learning methods for drug target prediction on ChEMBL. *Chem Sci.* 2018;9(24):5441–51. Epub 2018/08/30. doi: 10.1039/c8sc00148k. PubMed PMID: 30155234; PMCID: PMC6011237.
31. Lee K, Kim D. In-silico molecular binding prediction for human drug targets using deep neural multi-task learning. *Genes (Basel).* 2019;10(11). Epub 2019/11/11. doi: 10.3390/genes10110906. PubMed PMID: 31703452; PMCID: PMC6896155.
32. Tejera E, Carrera I, Jimenes-Vargas K, Armijos-Jaramillo V, Sanchez-Rodriguez A, Cruz-Monteagudo M, Perez-Castillo Y. Cell fishing: A similarity based approach and machine learning strategy for multiple cell lines-compound sensitivity prediction. *PLoS One.* 2019;14(10):e0223276. Epub 2019/10/08. doi: 10.1371/journal.pone.0223276. PubMed PMID: 31589649; PMCID: PMC6779297.
33. Awale M, Reymond JL. Polypharmacology browser PPB2: Target prediction combining nearest neighbors with machine learning. *J Chem Inf Model.* 2019;59(1):10–7. Epub 2018/12/19. doi: 10.1021/acs.jcim.8b00524. PubMed PMID: 30558418.
34. Škuta C, Cortés-Ciriano I, Dehaen W, Kříž P, van Westen GJP, Tetko IV, Bender A, Svozil D. QSAR-derived affinity fingerprints (part 1): fingerprint construction and modeling performance for similarity searching, bioactivity classification and scaffold hopping. *J. Cheminform.* 2020;12(1):39. doi: 10.1186/s13321-020-00443-6.
35. Wan F, Zhu Y, Hu H, Dai A, Cai X, Chen L, Gong H, Xia T, Yang D, Wang MW, Zeng J. DeepCPI: A deep learning-based framework for large-scale in silico drug screening. *GPB.* 2019;17(5):478–95. Epub 2020/02/09. doi: 10.1016/j.gpb.2019.04.003. PubMed PMID: 32035227; PMCID: PMC7056933.
36. Watson OP, Cortes-Ciriano I, Taylor AR, Watson JA. A decision-theoretic approach to the evaluation of machine learning algorithms in computational drug discovery. *Bioinformatics.* 2019;35(22):4656–63. Epub 2019/05/10. doi: 10.1093/bioinformatics/btz293. PubMed PMID: 31070704; PMCID: PMC6853675.
37. Robinson MC, Glen RC, Lee AA. Validating the validation: reanalyzing a large-scale comparison of deep learning and machine learning models for bioactivity prediction. *J Comput Aided Mol Des.* 2020;34(7):717–30. Epub 2020/01/22. doi: 10.1007/s10822-019-00274-0. PubMed PMID: 31960253; PMCID: PMC7292817.
38. Casciuc I, Horvath D, Gryniukova A, Tolmachova KA, Vasylchenko OV, Borysko P, Moroz YS, Bajorath J, Varnek A. Pros and cons of virtual screening based on public "Big Data": In silico mining for new bromodomain inhibitors. *Eur J Med Chem.* 2019;165:258–72. Epub 2019/01/28. doi: 10.1016/j.ejmech.2019.01.010. PubMed PMID: 30685526.
39. Baird SG, Sparks TD. Building a "Hello World" for self-driving labs: The closed-loop spectroscopy lab light-mixing demo. *STAR Protoc.* 2023;4(2):102329. Epub 20230531. doi: 10.1016/j.xpro.2023.102329. PubMed PMID: 37267112; PMCID: PMC10244891.

11 The Future of Generative Drug Discovery

Fabio Urbina, Joshua S. Harris, and Sean Ekins

11.1 INTRODUCTION

In recent years, the interest in generative AI for drug discovery (as described in the preceding chapters) has exploded. But what do we have to show for it? If we are to measure success by the number of molecules in the clinic to date derived from this technology, we are likely limited to a handful of molecules that can be genuinely attributed to generative AI versus docking or virtual screening with machine learning approaches. No drug discovered by generative AI has been approved by the FDA or any other regulator for that matter at this time. In eyes of many, this is an abysmal showing for the likely well over \$1–2B that has been invested in some of the biggest companies.[1] Many of the clinical candidates resulting from such investments have already failed. So where does that leave us? Obviously, this is just the "early days," and we need to put aside all the hype and iron out all the wrinkles in terms of whatever may be limiting the success of generative AI in drug discovery. This could be poor target selection or overall lack of target validation, noisy or inconsistent training data underlying the models, or even lack of consideration of enough molecular properties early in the discovery process etc. Certainly, if we give any technology long enough and invest enough money in it, then there will eventually be some success that can be attributed to it. Recent reviews have at least started to temper the enthusiasm for generative AI in drug discovery and highlight some of the challenges, although in general, these reviews also come back to the "transformative potential" of the technology.[1]

At this point, we should certainly look to the future and identify where generative AI may have its impact on drug discovery, as this may not be in the areas of the initial forays (namely, small molecule drug discovery, which is most of the focus of the earlier chapters). For example, generative biology is applying the same generative algorithms described in earlier chapters yet applying them to the design of proteins. One recent review focused specifically on the generative design of antibodies and detailed the challenges in protein drug discovery while also illustrating areas where machine learning was able to predict drug-like and developability properties (viscosity, *in vivo* behavior, pharmacokinetics, and immunogenicity).[2] This seems like a rather narrow perspective, as it excluded other types of biologics and did not include the potential for developing proteins for other applications outside human health.

A second potential application is structure-based *de novo* drug design. Whereas most of the earlier examples of generative drug discovery have focused on small molecule design in the absence of the protein, clearly adding some structural information

DOI: 10.1201/9781003399346-16

from the target may be important when there is no existing structure-activity relationship data with which to build machine learning models for scoring molecules during generative drug design. This may be just one potential scenario where 3D structural data could be valuable.[3] Of course, there are also additional complexities related to the 3D conformations of molecules, how they dock in the protein, and how they are scored such that a predicted "binding affinity" is obtained.[4] As with purely 2D methods, there are also issues around whether molecules are constructed from fragments or readily available building blocks to simplify synthesis and ensure synthetic accessibility. For both 2D and 3D methodologies, to date, there have been few prospective validation examples for these structure-based generative AI approaches[4] and most have relied on retrospective approaches.[3]

If we can apply the generative AI approaches to small molecules for drug discovery, there is also the potential to design molecules for other applications. For example, we could design materials that could be useful in aiding drug delivery; these could be non-bioactive elements of pharmaceutical formulations, new coatings, or other important components. And if we can design any "material", why stop at drug discovery? There is a whole universe of consumer products that are ripe for innovation. It has been acknowledged that research on materials may take as long as or longer than research on drugs (10–20 years or more), whether that is on batteries, fuel cells or other advanced materials.[5] Again, the types of algorithms used are identical to those that are used in generative drug discovery. Already there have been several applications in energy materials and structural materials.[5] As with all the other applications, there are few prospective validation examples for generative design in the area of materials discovery.[5]

We now highlight several additional areas where we think there may be value to using generative approaches, such as natural products, polypharmacology, bigger molecules, quantum machine learning and freedom to operate.

11.2 NATURAL PRODUCTS

The history of natural products as therapeutics is long and varied.[6] For example, of the 175 anticancer drugs approved between the 1940s and 2014, 49% were natural products or natural product derivatives.[7] The anti-infective drug discovery area is still highly dependent on natural products and their structures.[7] It has been suggested that approximately 50% of new chemical entities are based on natural products and derivatives.[8] From 1981 to 2010, 64% of FDA approved drugs were natural products or analogues.[9] More recent analyses of natural products as sources of new drugs suggest a figure of 33.5%, and this number increases to 64.9% when including natural product mimics and those made by total synthesis.[10] Natural products offer high potencies selected by evolution, and we have barely scratched the surface of what is out there.[8] For example, rapamycin and tetracycline have been important natural product drugs.[11,12] Marine natural products alone have led to eight drugs or cosmeceuticals (compounds that can be used in cosmetics or as drugs) approved by the FDA and EMA (e.g. FDA approved marine-derived drugs, namely cytarabine, depocyt, vidarabine, and ziconotide; at least 10 candidates in clinical trials[13]; and also a large number of marine chemicals in the preclinical pipeline[14]). Other classes of natural products, such as scents, represent a relatively untapped source of biologically active molecules[15] (e.g., menthol[16–23]).

Recently, there have been considerable efforts to use computational approaches for different aspects of natural product drug discovery; however, it was recently suggested that providing information on the bioactivity potential of natural products prior to their isolation is still lacking and is of key interest for identifying valuable natural products.[24] Other researchers have reviewed the role of *in silico* approaches to identify bioactives in natural products, and these methods include virtual screening and "target fishing".[25] There have been many individual quantitative structure activity relationship (QSAR) approaches used with natural products, such as prediction of antitumor or antibiotic activity using data from PubChem, chemical development kit (CDK) and quantum-chemical descriptors, and then testing on marine and microbial natural products.[26] Novartis researchers have proposed predicting a drug's biological function given just a structure by searching a library of compounds with known activities. They have also suggested that 2D methods outperform 3D methods in this regard for target prediction, although combining such descriptors is more effective than a single method.[27] Novartis have also used data from natural products screened against 100s of targets to build fingerprints that were then compared to a reference mechanism of action panel of activities and compounds, to predict targets. These fingerprints performed better than standard chemical descriptors, and 73.8% of predictions were confirmed *in vitro*.[28] There have been other approaches using natural language processing,[29] activity spectra,[30] Bayesian belief networks,[31] 3D pharmacophore approaches,[32–35] drug target networks and network pharmacology,[36,37] docking,[38–40] machine learning models,[41,42] combinations of machine learning and docking,[43] and other virtual screens.[44] These represent some of the many computational approaches applied to natural products and drug discovery. The growing number of databases of natural products from different organisms suggests a considerable need for computational efforts to mine them.[38,45,46] Most of the available target prediction tools do not focus on natural products but instead address synthetic compounds; for example, SwissTargetPrediction uses 2D or 3D similarity and molecules from ChEMBL.[47] These computational approaches fail to predict targets for natural products because they are generally different from the synthetic molecules which comprise the majority of the molecules in the public domain databases used to train these models.[48] There are also limitations in that only previously evaluated targets can be predicted (as there must be data available). The target rank order should also be considered as qualitative and only weakly correlates to potency; hence, their main value may be in prioritizing testing.[48] Recent target prediction methods have started to use transfer learning. One used a multitask neural network trained on CHEMBL and validated using several approaches with high AUC scores and target prediction for 62/139 approved drugs derived from natural products.[49] This approach was also superior to the recently reported stacked ensemble target fishing approach called STarFish.[50] Most machine learning studies propose modeling approaches and use internal testing but not prospective testing of methods.[51] Validation strategies for target prediction methods have been proposed with many recommendations but these have not been focused on natural product evaluations.[52] Overall, to date there has been relatively limited prediction of natural products and drug-target interactions[36,42,53–57] so there remains significant untapped potential for developing computational approaches to do this. Similarly, there is a great potential for using natural products as a starting point for generative design while using predictive models to focus their activity towards certain targets and away from others, as we have demonstrated recently by generating tabernanthalog, an ibogaine analogue with desirable properties, as had been previously demonstrated in the literature.[58] Other examples of computational approaches have applied Weighted Holistic Atom Localization and Entity Shape (WHALES) descriptors to natural products to enable scaffold hopping from hard-to-synthesize natural products to molecules with the same 3D structure or shape, resulting in simpler drug-like molecules with similar biological activity.[59] Natural product fragments can also be combined together to generate pseudo natural products with structures as well as biological activities that have not been reported before likely due to their shape and diversity.[60] These could be combined with generative approaches to aid in the creation of natural product like or pseudo natural products.

We could also use the biological data that is accumulating in the public domain, as we have shown with MacrolactoneDB[61], to use these as a starting point for the generative design of new macrolactones. Macrolactones are a broad, diverse structural class with various levels of complexity, and the database of macrolactones needs to be useful for different research project needs. For example, biosynthetic chemists who work closely with "classic" macrolides such as erythromycin, pikromycin, etc., may be interested in a specific set of twelve-to-sixteen-membered macrolides with sugars present. Additionally, the definition of "macrolides" has evolved in the past 50 years due to developments in medicinal research, such as the first, second, and third generation of macrolides, ketolides, etc. Thus, to accommodate researchers who focus on different areas of macrolactones, we constructed a web application with multiple filters to allow users to extract a highly specific subset of interest. MacrolactoneDB[61] is, therefore a new web application hosting ~13.7k macrolactones, including macrolides mined from public repositories such as NANPDB,[62] StreptomeDB,[63] unpd,[64] NuBBe,[64] ZINC15,[65] TIPdb,[66] AfroDB,[45] BindingDB,[67] AfroMalariaDB,[68] BIOFACQUIM,[69] ChEMBL[70] and PubChem[71] along with available biological information extracted from ChEMBL.[70] It consists of a database of macrolactones with bioactivities and a front-end web application that allows users to specify a subset of chemical space among molecules via multiple filters on chemical properties such as ring size, number of sugars, molecular weight, etc. This was developed using the *RDKit Molecule Substructure Filter* node and SMARTS patterns in Knime.[72] All filtered structures were curated using a similar protocol proposed by Fourches et al.[73]: (a) removal of mixtures, inorganics, (b) structural conversion, cleaning/removal of salts, (c) structural normalization, and (d) removal of structural duplicates. This resulted in 13,721 diverse macrolactones in MacrolactoneDB[61], which we have provided to the community.

Additionally, we conducted a cheminformatics analysis of MacrolactoneDB[61] to better understand the chemical diversity and scope of this structural class. We analyzed the chemical distribution in terms of several important molecular properties: molecular weight (MW), polar surface area (PSA), hydrophobicity (SlogP), hydrogen bond donors (HBA), hydrogen bond acceptors (HBA), rotatable bonds (NRB), and ring size (RS). We have also observed that contemporary chemical descriptors or fingerprints lack information to sufficiently account for large bioactive ring structures, such as frequency of ring sizes larger than12, sugars, etc. Thus, they may not fully characterize macrolactone molecules. Consequently, the lack of these important details can adversely affect Quantitative Structure-Activity Relationship (QSAR) studies, modeling, and Mechanism of Action (MoA) studies. Thus, we developed 91 new descriptors (which we called - mrc) to complement mordred descriptors, which account for smallest and largest ring sizes (≥12-membered), frequency of sugars, and occurrence of esters within the core rings, to better characterize macrolactones and macrolides. We mined this database for large datasets suitable for QSAR modeling and identified 3 for use as case studies to compare machine learning algorithms and descriptors. This involved QSAR modeling using a variety of machine-learning algorithms and molecular descriptor sets. We conducted tenfold cross-validation (CV) on our three case studies and examined the relevance and usefulness of different cheminformatics methods and tools on these highly complex, large ring molecules. Our overarching goal was to determine the optimal combination of machine learning algorithm and fingerprint set and to provide chemical insights into macrolactones. Our workflow then uses contemporary machine learning algorithms such as Random Forest (RF), Support Vector Regression (SVR), Naïve Bayes (NB), K Nearest Neighbor (KNN), Deep Neural Nets (DNN), Consensus (CSS, averaged prediction among all the aforementioned machine-learning algorithms), and Hybrid approaches from the two best algorithms (RF_KNN, averaged prediction from RF and KNN; and RF_DNN, averaged prediction from RF and DNN). Our workflow also incorporated explicit and implicit molecular descriptors, which include mordred, mrc (newly developed descriptors to address macrolide characteristics), mordred_mrc, MACCS, ECFP6, 2Drdkit, and "all" (which are a merger of unique, aforementioned descriptor sets).

We described three case studies which examined the distribution of pIC_{50} for *Plasmodium falciparum* (Malaria, CHEMBL364), pIC_{50}/pEC_{50} for Hepatitis C targets (CHEMBL379), and pIC_{50} for T-cells (CHEMBL614309). Malaria had 223 macrolactone ligands with an almost normal distribution of pIC_{50}s ranging from 4.67 to 8.61 with a mean of 6.59 ± 0.65. Hepatitis C had 129 macrolactone ligands with a slightly left-skewed distribution of pIC_{50}/pEC_{50}s ranging from 4.48 to 9.59 with a mean of 7.29 ± 1.04. T-cells had 103 macrolactone ligands with a non-normal distribution of pIC_{50}s ranging from 4.93 to 9.74 with a mean of 8.24 ± 1.07. Overall, all the datasets had a good range of activities suitable for QSAR regression models. We compared the performance of molecular descriptors and machine learning models from tuned methods for all three case studies. In the *Plasmodium falciparum* dataset, "all" descriptors provided the best tenfold cross-validation prediction results consistently across seven machine learning models based on R^2, and MAE. In Hepatitis C, the descriptor sets had very similar R^2 and MAE across eight machine learning models, with "all" descriptors slightly better with R^2_{max} 0.76 and MAE_{min} 0.37. T-cells results showed a significant difference in the performance between explicit and implicit descriptors. Explicit descriptors (mordred, mordred_mrc, and merger "all") had R^2_{max} 0.78 and MAE_{min} 0.39 across machine learning models. On the other hand, implicit fingerprints, namely ECFP6 ($R^2_{max} = 0.56$, $MAE_{min} = 0.47$) and MACCS ($R^2_{max} = 0.17$,

$MAE_{min} = 0.62$), yielded very poor performance.[61] Overall, the prediction results from the case studies agreed with our hypothesis that explicit descriptors (mordred, mordred_mrc) would perform better than implicit chemical fingerprints (MACCS or ECFP6), especially in the Malaria and T-cells case studies. Of note, "all" descriptors performed best among others, closely followed by either mordred or mordred_mrc in all cases. When consensus and hybrid modeling approaches were applied, we noticed an increase in R^2 across our case studies, especially for *Plasmodium falciparum* and Hepatitis C. We further validated and eliminated the possibility of chance correlation in our QSAR models by conducting y-randomization with a ten-fold CV for the three case studies, demonstrating significant differences. The highest y-randomized R^2 for the combination of machine learning algorithms and descriptor sets were 0.11 ($<<$ 0.64 from actual QSAR tenfold CV R^2) for Malaria, 0.14 ($<<$ 0.76 from actual QSAR tenfold CV R^2) for Hepatitis C virus, and 0.18 ($\ll$0.78 from actual QSAR tenfold CV R^2) for T-cells. The poor cross-validation statistics of the y-randomized model rule out the possibility of chance correlation for our QSAR models. Of note, our machine learning workflow was built with only 2D fingerprints/descriptors; hence, the information characterizing these macrolactones likely does not capture conformational information such as intra-hydrogen bonding properties. Yet, the predictive power of models built with 2D descriptors alone was rather impressive ($R^2 = 0.64$ for Plasmodium falciparum, $R^2 = 0.76$ for Hepatitis C Virus, $R^2 = 0.78$ for T-cells). Conformational analysis of macrocycles still remains a complex, challenging problem wherein a small structural modification can result in the conformational reorganization of remote regions of a macrocyclic backbone.[74] Our three case studies showed that RF was the best predictor among individual machine learning algorithms across six descriptor sets. These combined efforts[61] have led us to further develop these technologies so we can license them to other companies or use them in our fee-for-service consulting.

Databases of natural product molecules like Canvass[75] have been screened primarily against cytotoxicity endpoints and not human targets. Other natural product databases have been compiled using natural product data for assays from public databases such as ChEMBL, so we are unlikely to find much additional data to validate our models that are built with ChEMBL data alone. A second challenge is that virtually all the machine learning models developed use small drug-like molecules (or pesticides, agrochemicals, etc.), and this means there is very rarely much overlap between natural products and model training sets. The tools that are publicly available will all have this limitation. Using 3D descriptors may help to improve the predictions from such models. There are also likely to be issues in the model applicability domain with limited overlap between compounds being predicted and the model training sets. Certainly there are plenty of areas to develop so we could apply generative approaches to natural products for drug discovery.

11.3 POLYPHARMACOLOGY

Many drugs interact with or inhibit several different human proteins, and these are described as having polypharmacology. This goes beyond the classic paradigm of a drug hitting a single target, which would usually be ideal to avoid undesirable or off-target effects. Drugs that display polypharmacology may be desirable in some instances, as they could hit several targets in a pathway that may be important to the bioactivity and have additive or synergistic effects. This has been observed with kinase inhibitors, where selective inhibitors may be less effective than molecules hitting several kinases. The challenge with designing molecules that hit several targets is that there are potentially conflicting requirements for each target (binding site size, molecule property requirements, differences in pharmacophores, differences in tissue expression or localization, etc.). With the curation of datasets for various biological targets from sources such as ChEMBL[70], PubChem,[71],[76] Tox21,[77] CEBS,[78] HIV ChemDB[79], and other similar databases, large datasets can be used to train machine learning models and generative AI to enable the prediction and design of molecules that inhibit multiple targets of interest. One recent example is a tool called POLYGON based on generative reinforcement learning trained on data from ChEMBL to design molecules targeting MEK1 and mTOR. After synthesizing a small number of generated molecules, several demonstrated inhibition at low μM concentrations to illustrate the potential for designing polypharmacology of molecules.[80]

In recent years, graph-based models have emerged,[81] capable of learning relationships between a large number of targets and molecules in a knowledge graph containing information for multiple targets and multiple activities. At least one graph-based model, GraphSAGE, exists, which allows inference on new targets and new molecules not present during the training of the initial model.[81] GraphSAGE is capable of learning SAR between molecules and targets, as well as being capable of generalizing to targets and molecules that it has never been seen before with sufficient accuracy. In addition, new graph-based models including graph convolutional networks (GCNs), graph attention networks (GATs), and message passing neural networks (MPNNs) have shown state-of-the-art predictive capabilities in benchmark molecular datasets.[82–84] In addition to graph-based networks, multi-task learning has been shown to increase the predictive capabilities of ML models.[85] These results suggest that GraphSAGE and other multi-task graph-based models are capable of sharing information across targets and molecules, learning a more robust underlying relationship between targets, and are particularly promising for datasets with lower amounts of data or restricted chemical space. GraphSAGE merges SAR data with target-related 3D data. We have used a GraphSAGE[81] implementation as a link-prediction heterogeneous graph, in which compounds and targets are used as nodes, and edges have attributes of 1/0 for binary activity predictions or -logM values for predicting EC_{50}/IC_{50} activity values. The only edges constructed between nodes are those with known activity. All compound nodes have their fingerprints (ECFP6) as attributes, and all target protein nodes have a 147-dimensional float vector representing computed composition, transition, and distribution (CTD) descriptors based on the different properties of amino acid descriptors. The key feature is that predictions can be made on new compound-target pairs that the model has not seen before, including targets that may have no known activity data. By combining all targets of a given type into one model, our GCN, GAT, and MPNN multi-task networks will allow the cross-sharing of information between different datasets and, when combined with Bayesian optimization for hyperparameter picking, can comprise robust

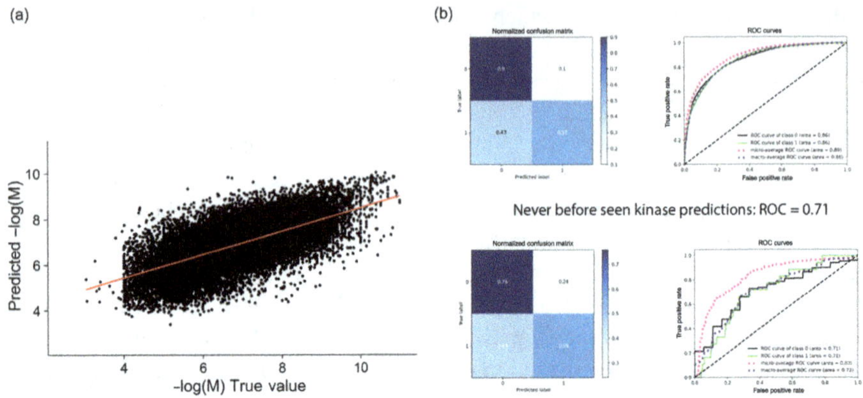

FIGURE 11.1 (a) GraphSAGE model is built using primarily kinase datasets from ChEMBL (474) and incorporates 20 more targets of various proteins to facilitate transfer learning. The ROC of the full model on a 20% test set is 0.86 (predicting a heterogeneous mix of activities on each of the ~474 targets). (b) We next queried the model against PFKB3, a kinase that was not in the original training set, and made predictions without any more training. ROC on PFKB3 was 0.71.

predictive models for a compound's activity. We have used this approach recently to generate models from a set of 24,700 compound activities for 475 kinase targets. GraphSAGE is robust to dataset size, as these datasets range from ~100 molecule activities to over 4,000, yet there is little bias in predictions (that is, our model does not abandon learning smaller dataset representations in lieu of predicting only large datasets correctly (Figure 11.1).

Another alternative machine learning approach we can use is *convolutional-long short-term memory* (ConvLSTM),[86] which we have recently used as end-to-end models in order to rapidly generate computational predictions for a billion molecules in a DNA-encoded library (Table 11.1). The final model developed was a neural network based in Pytorch comprised of ConvLSTM layers that act on SMILES strings, which outputs a prediction score between 0 and 1. Each unique character in the SMILES vocabulary was represented as a separate integer, except for Br and any closed-bracket notation, which were given their own separate integers. Each SMILES string was thus tokenized by converting into an integer representation, which was then used as the input sequence for the model. The test column is the binary activity value to be predicted. The model was trained using a randomized 70:15:15 (train:test: validation) split. Hyperparameter optimization was performed using the validation set, and final model statistics were calculated for the test set. All training data was converted into binary activity data, where a cut-off is chosen based on generally accepted cutoffs for such activity assays or based on reasonable model performance and reasonable expectation of activity. Based on the F1 scores (Table 11.1), this ML approach compares favorably to individual ML models generated using ECFP6 descriptors alone for several datasets.[87,88]

As an additional example of using LSTM, we have curated datasets from ChEMBL[70] on 42 targets used in the SafetyScreen44 *in vitro* screen and built a

TABLE 11.1
Comparison of Different Machine Learning Approaches to ADME/Tox Models Using F1 Scores after Fivefold Cross Validation and Highlighting the Conv-LSTM Method

Model Datasets	Actives/Total	Adaboost	Bayes	XGboost	K-NN	Linear Regression	Random Forest	SVC	Conv-LSTM
Water solubility	502/17,443	0.24	0.38	0.48	0.48	0.25	0.27	0.30	**0.49**
Blood-brain barrier	1,777/2,291	0.93	0.93	0.95	0.91	0.91	0.95	0.96	0.93
CHO cytotoxicity	367/822	0.68	0.71	0.70	0.70	0.66	0.72	0.69	**0.74**
CYP3A4 inhibition	2,546/3,756	0.84	0.83	0.85	0.82	0.80	0.83	0.85	0.80
Plasma protein binding	682/990	0.85	0.84	0.87	0.86	0.85	0.87	0.88	0.82

Bold values indicate where conv-LSTM is the best.

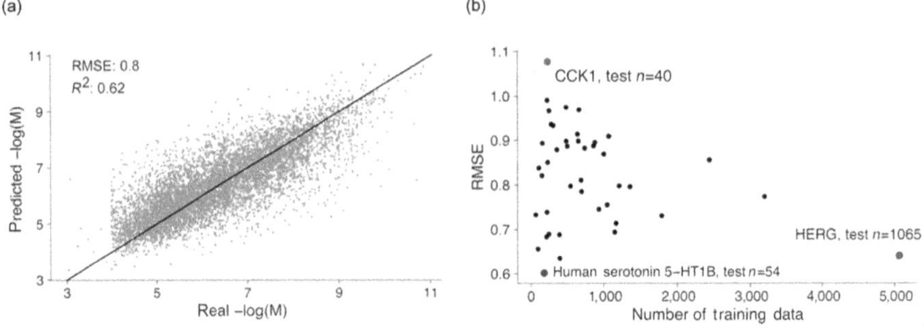

FIGURE 11.2 ConvLSTM model was built to predict 42 toxicity endpoints (IC_{50} values) based on *in vitro* data. (a) Predictions for 42 mixed targets, predicted vs. actual -log(Molar) values for a test-set of compounds, with at least 10 data points for each of the 42 toxicity targets. RMSE and R^2 are shown for the combined predictions. (b) RMSE vs. size of the training data for each target. The highest RMSE (red, CCK1) and lowest RMSE (Serotonin 5HT1B, blue) are highlighted, along with the toxicity target with the largest training set (hERG, pink).

multi-task neural network that predicts compound -logM binding affinity to the targets (Figure 11.2). The embedding layer in the model takes tokenized SMILES strings directly as inputs, which allows parallelizing training and inference on GPUs in an end-to-end manner. We used a stratified random splitting strategy to ensure all targets had representation in the training and test sets for downstream analysis. The model had an excellent performance on a hold-out test set of compounds (Figure 11.2a). We also trained a similar LSTM model with ECFP6 as the input, which showed that the SMILES-based model achieves near-identical results. The size of the training data for each target had no correlation with the test root-mean-squared error (RMSE, Figure 11.2b), indicating the model was not overfitting on targets with the most training points and that it was leveraging the multi-task architecture to learn to generalize across endpoints.

Both graphSAGE and ConvLSTM could be used effectively for multitarget prediction capabilities alone or as an ensemble machine learning model approach, perhaps integrating few shot learning or other available machine learning approaches.[87,88] These approaches could be integrated in to generative approaches for molecule design in order to predict molecules with selectivity or promiscuity towards different targets like kinases or avoiding targets that are part of the SafetyScreen44.

11.4 LARGE MOLECULES

11.4.1 PROTACS

The design and optimization of large molecules such as proteolysis targeting chimeras (PROTACS, composed of warhead, linker, and E3 ligase) as well as other molecules that are beyond the rule of 5 (bRo5, and generally considered non-drug-like which will likely impact ADME properties) has been rarely considered for design with generative AI. A few studies have used small sets of PROTACS to develop approaches to score molecules or describe the optimal chemical space for bioavailability and permeability of PROTACS as follows. One early study used simple descriptors (MW, nC, NAR, PHI, nhDon, NHAcc, and TPSA) to describe permeable PROTACS that occupied a particular region of chemical space.[89] Similarly, measured solubilities for 21 PROTACS correlated with LogD and LogP.[90] Machine learning models to predict solubility for PROTACS have also been built, but no external validation was performed. Interestingly, the observation that TPSA > 289.31 led to high solubility was noted.

There are a few examples of generative approaches used with PROTACS. One study described GraphINVENT, which was trained to produce PROTACs using 4120 molecules from protac.db then fine-tuned with a protein degradation model. This was applied to IRAK3 degradation, and 82% of the final sampled molecules were predicted as active, but no experimental validation was performed.[91] We have explored using our MegaSyn generative approach[58] (see Chapter 6) to produce PROTAC structures. The MegaSyn model was pre-trained on ~2.6 million ChEMBL dataset molecules. We modified the training approach for PROTACS generation by curating a dataset of 1100 known linkers for PROTACS structures (derived from protac.db[5]) and then fine-tuned MegaSyn by training on this until it learned to generate PROTACS linkers. We then used an algorithm which accepted a Warhead and E3 ligase SMILES structure with specific attachment points, and generated potential linkers from MegaSyn. Ultimately we combined the generated molecule as a linker with the Warhead and E3 Ligase to form a PROTACS structure, and finally scored valid molecules against ADME machine learning models. Starting with naive generation (essentially, generating small molecules), we were able to fine-tune training on the linkers dataset until it began generating PROTACS linkers almost exclusively, which required a scoring function defined by a low-weighted contribution from quantitative estimate of drug-likeness (QED) scores as well as contributions from heavily weighted scores based on ADME properties (solubility and hERG). Only PROTACS fulfilling the design criteria were kept for analysis. It will be important to ultimately demonstrate that generative approaches like this can identify synthesizable and active PROTACs in the future.

11.4.2 Polypeptides

We have previously also described how our MegaSyn algorithm could be trained with a set of 1554 antimicrobial peptides in order to learn how to build polypeptides that were scored with a model for glucagon-like peptide-1 (GLP-1) agonist activity using data from ChEMBL.[92] We then used dimensionality reduction using a t-SNE plot and nearest neighbor distance of generated proposed GLP-1 agonists to visualize *de novo* generated GLP-1 agonists alongside commercial GLP-1 drugs.[92] This demonstrated that the proposed GLP-1 agonists were close in terms of structural and predicted bioactivity to commercial GLP-1 agonists. We did not synthesize or test any of the designed molecules, but our analysis suggested that these generative approaches could be readily applied to larger biologically active molecules and could be applicable to different targets, other diseases, or even structural scaffolds of molecular entities in order to prioritize what to make in the future.[92]

11.4.3 Polymers

We have also used MegaSyn to generate polymers that maximize predicted properties of interest within other property constraints.[1] We built custom fingerprints for polymers into MegaSyn and custom scoring models for handling these types of fingerprints. The polymer fingerprints represent the structural features of polymers constructed from one or more repeat units that can be chained together (including branching structures). The first step involves creating a structural fingerprint vector based on the repeat unit structures and the relative ratios of repeat units. The second step involves appending metadata about the polymer (molecular weight, polydispersion) to the fingerprint vector, yielding the final fingerprint. These polymer fingerprints are then used as input for machine learning models (e.g. support vector regression). Before training the MegaSyn model to optimize a particular polymer property, we primed the model by training it on randomized realistic structures of interest; therefore, before training begins, the MegaSyn model has already learned to generate randomized structures of the molecule of interest. To achieve this, we decomposed the entire ChEMBL library into BRICS fragments[2] (RDKit implementation), keeping all fragments with two attachment points. We randomly selected fragments to attach between the molecular groups of interest, using a filtering process to select more realistic molecules. While MegaSyn learned to generate the molecules of interest, occasionally, there were also irrelevant features, such as a phosphorus atom or a C-C triple bond. By "irrelevant features," we mean features that the scoring models have not been trained on. Features such as these will not contribute positively or negatively to the model prediction, so they can occur by random chance during MegaSyn structure optimization. The generative software is clearly only as good as the predictive models that it trains against. If we can build predictive models based on a more diverse set of the molecules of interest in the training data in the future, then the generative design software will likely be able to discover even more interesting structures with good, predicted properties.

11.5 QUANTUM MACHINE LEARNING

Quantum computers are a powerful technology that uses the principles of quantum mechanics to solve problems that classical computers cannot solve in a reasonable timeframe and may have the potential to help in machine learning applications.[93,94] This technology is still in its earliest stages, and companies have generally not applied it to drug discovery applications such as cheminformatics. There is, therefore, a considerable opportunity to develop the software technologies needed to leverage it for challenging problems such as the identification of inhibitors of various drug discovery targets or the accurate prediction of toxicity. Utilizing quantum computers for machine learning for small molecules has potentially much broader applications in the design of new efficacious and safe small molecule drugs. Our extensive machine learning experience[95–112] has focused heavily in the last decade on machine learning and generative models for ADME/Tox properties.[95,100,113–126] This has led to models with good receiver-operator characteristic scores (>0.7).[95] Open-source implementation of the ECFP6/FCFP6 fingerprints[127] and Bayesian model building module[95,128] has enabled their use in new software implementations. We initially developed our proprietary Assay Central software,[95,128] which is a framework for curating high-quality datasets and generating machine-learning models for prospective drug discovery and toxicology predictions.[79,95,123,129–138] As these datasets increase in size, they will lead to challenges for methods such as SVM and deep learning, which are generally more compute-intensive (GPUs can help with the latter). Most recently we have used several of our drug discovery and toxicology datasets for evaluating preliminary quantum computing technologies accessed via the IBM Qhub and NC State University.[139] ECFP6 descriptors are usually generated as 2048 bits. Classical computers can deal with this easily, but state-of-the-art quantum computers have lower limits on the number of qubits, so we have had to develop a fingerprint compression algorithm. To date, we have implementations of SVM, DNN, and several other algorithms which can run on quantum computers. We found similar levels of accuracy on cross-validation with these methods, whether we used classical or quantum computers for a large Tuberculosis dataset.[139] However, initial testing on a quantum computer simulator outperformed classical computers with the SVM algorithm in terms of time. For example, simulations for the quantum computer ran in the range of 1–3 seconds and for classical computers the range was 4–5 minutes.[139] Running a computation on an actual quantum computer takes longer, as the job is segmented and run over the cloud. There is a need to build and validate quantum machine learning (QML) models for drug discovery, but few, if any, commercial tools exist that can develop, deploy, and validate QML models for drug discovery and toxicology. Though the use of quantum computing for generative design has been recently demonstrated using quantum simulations,[140] we still await the use of a quantum computer to design a molecule, which is then subsequently synthesized, tested, and shown to have the desired activity and properties. This approach is still in the earliest stages of research, but we should be exploring the potential of quantum computers for machine learning and generative drug discovery approaches.

11.6 FREEDOM TO OPERATE

The future of molecule design across different industries will increasingly require machine learning models for the design and optimization of molecules. An important feature will be to teach the AI what is novel and how to create intellectual property (IP). Understanding the freedom to operate (FTO) for a new molecule will be important not only from the point of view of molecular structure but also whether it is for a new use or application (e.g. drug repurposing). While there have been significant efforts in the areas of *de novo* design and autonomous synthesis, we are not aware of other solutions or tools to assist in FTO for generative drug discovery. One of the most significant challenges not addressed is whether new IP is created when new molecules are generated by such AI. Exhaustively testing to see if generated molecules already exist would be one approach to assess FTO, e.g. by comparing similarity to existing molecules in databases or patent databases. Still, this approach would not capture the entire space of patents as often covered by Markush structures, and the context of the patents the molecules are involved in would have to be investigated to understand if the patent is also relevant for the desirable use case. This can take significant human hours to investigate even a single molecule, let alone a whole library of novel structures. We suggest there needs to be more effort to develop tools for FTO. For example, one could integrate various datasets such as the United States Patent and Trademark Office (USPTO) and SureChEMBL[141,142] datasets in order to check whether a molecule is novel and is likely to have FTO, which clarifies whether a product or its potential commercialization infringes on other existing IP rights. Providing patent lawyers and scientists with a score of likely FTO would assist them in their efforts. The corpus of US patents is available at the USPTO. While interpretation of patents is often a manual task, two recent developments have provided new tools to distill patent information: (a) recent advances in NLP, particularly text classification and context prediction, and (b) the advent of semi-supervised machine learning models, which require only a small subset of data to be labeled. We would propose scraping this data to extract information on small molecules and their uses, organized by distinct disease and target ontologies. Similarly, there are several other datasets that could be also helpful such as SureChEMBL[141,142] and PubChem.[143,144] The structure-patent association is not enough; often, the context is the most critical missing knowledge when investigating the patent molecular space, such as whether a molecular structure is merely part of a chemical synthesis route or has a specific disease use-case spelled out. When investigating an already-patented molecule, often the use case can be interpreted as strong or weak, depending on the specificity of the language used. To aid in this decision process, we could use machine learning to perform context and sentiment analysis, predicting the structure's use case in each compound-patent link as well as the specificity of the use cases in a semi-supervised manner. To perform this, we would classify a small number of documents manually based on synthesis routes or use cases using a disease or target ontology, and then use semi-supervised learning to classify most of the documents. Critically, the use of semi-supervised learning reduces the manual classification significantly, and these model predictions will give a quantitative score to patent language, informing novel drug discovery decisions.

We have recently prototyped an approach that uses the combination of Murcko scaffolds and ECFP6 similarity along with *t*-distributed stochastic neighbor embedding (t-SNE) and clustering algorithms to capture the chemical space and quantify the overlap of a molecule of interest and the available chemistry space for small molecules and patents, based on full molecular structures or the common structural motifs adapted from the recently described Drug Discovery Maps.[145] Our approach is as follows: first, ECFP6 fingerprints are generated for the set of molecules. A t-SNE algorithm is applied with two components and a perplexity based on the dataset size and is run for at least 1,000 iterations. This embeds the chemical space of the patent data into a 2D latent representation. Query compounds can be embedded into the lower dimensional t-SNE space by fixing the patent t-SNE chemical coordinates and performing the t-SNE embedding allowing only the query molecules to stochastically move (Figure 11.3). Once embedded, the closeness of test compounds can be visualized to determine if they fall within a representative region of chemical space covered by the patent set. Density-Based Spatial Clustering (DBSCAN) is applied with an epsilon radius of 0.9 as a decision rule as to whether the query molecule(s) are covered; DBSCAN groups data into their labeled clusters and, importantly, generates

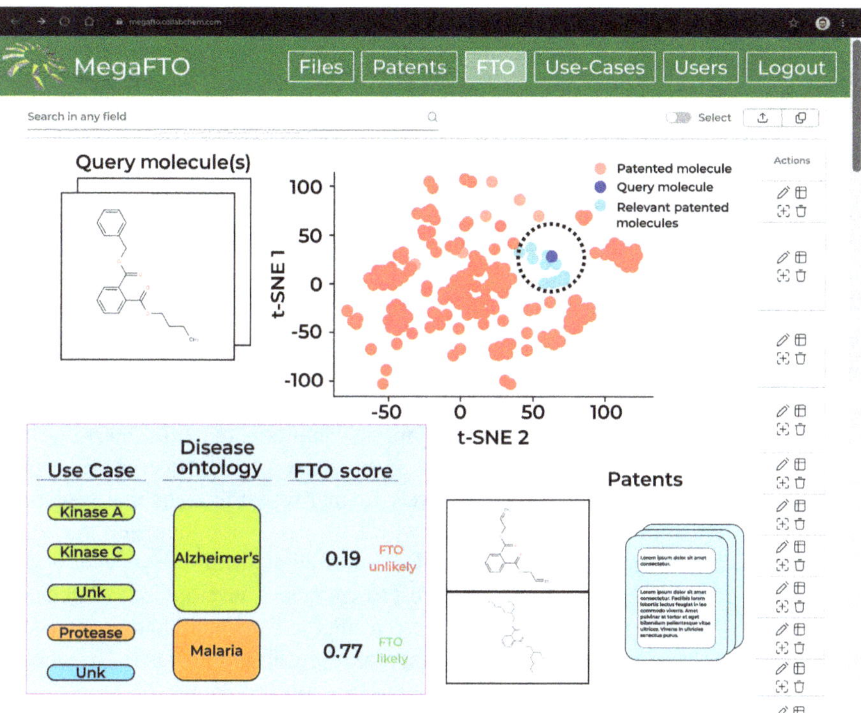

FIGURE 11.3 Schematic of MegaFTO user interface, showing approaches to understanding the overlap of a molecule and known compounds and patents.

a separate cluster label for data that does not belong to any group and is considered noise. If query compounds are assigned a group, a score of 1 is granted. The closest patented compound in the grouped space is queried, and patent space is then enumerated and summarized. Critically, Markush structures in patents will also be enumerated. If any query compounds are relegated to the noise class of DBSCAN, those compounds are determined to be insufficiently close to the patent set and a score of 0 is assigned, suggesting novel chemical space. This algorithm is applied a second time to the Murcko-scaffold decomposition of the datasets. This then allows a comparison of distinct scaffold representations and a more discrete view of the molecular space (Figure 11.3). Finally, similarity maps based on model predictions are generated for each compound in the query set.

These approaches can be used to visualize the user's specific compound with all available molecules and patents assisting in decision-making. In addition to t-SNE based on ECFP6 fingerprints alone, we can also use a combination of features, including use-case and language context scores in addition to ECFP6, to embed patent knowledge and determine if the representation is more robust than that of chemical fingerprints alone. As the previously described GraphSAGE algorithm is capable of learning structure-activity relationships between molecules and targets, we can use this approach to learn the relationships between small molecules and their target uses and patents. By using our annotated patent database, we can then build prediction models to infer the likely use of a molecule based on patent data alone.

11.7 SUMMARY

We anticipate that interest in generative AI for drug discovery will certainly continue in the future based on the considerable funding and investments (many billions of dollars) made by industry and governments to date. In this chapter, we have provided some selected examples of where we think there might be other opportunities to expand its application further, primarily driven by our own interests as a small pharmaceutical company. We have highlighted several potential applications of generative approaches to areas including natural products, polypharmacology, larger molecules (PROTACS, polypeptides, polymers), quantum machine learning, and freedom to operate around patents. In some of these areas, we or others have already provided examples. Certainly, there are likely further research areas that generative AI for drug discovery could be applied to which we have not anticipated due to the current direction of the industry. We are also admittedly still in the very early days of this field, and it will certainly be of interest to see how it develops and what can be delivered for the sums invested. In time, these results will dictate whether generative drug discovery truly becomes the prevailing paradigm for the industry, or whether we must continue the search for the next tool to develop and apply.

ACKNOWLEDGMENTS

We kindly acknowledge Dr. Phyo Phyo Kyaw Zin and Dr. Gavin J Williams for collaborations on MacrolactoneDB which are described in this chapter.

FUNDING

We kindly acknowledge NIH funding from R44GM122196-02A1 from NIGMS and 1R44ES031038-01 and 1R43ES033855-01 from NIEHS for our machine learning software development and applications. "Research reported in this publication was supported by the National Institute of Environmental Health Sciences of the National Institutes of Health under Award Number R44ES031038 and 1R43ES033855-01. We also acknowledge 1R43DA055419-01 from NIDA and 1R43AT010585-01 from NCCIH. The content is solely the responsibility of the authors and does not necessarily represent the official views of the National Institutes of Health."

REFERENCES

1. Gangwal A, Lavecchia A. Unleashing the power of generative AI in drug discovery. *Drug Discov Today*. 2024;29(6):103992. Epub 20240423. doi: 10.1016/j.drudis.2024.103992. PubMed PMID: 38663579.
2. Mock M, Langmead CJ, Grandsard P, Edavettal S, Russell A. Recent advances in generative biology for biotherapeutic discovery. *Trends Pharmacol Sci*. 2024;45(3):255–67. Epub 20240219. doi:10.1016/j.tips.2024.01.003. PubMed PMID: 38378385.

3. Bleicher LS, van Daelen T, Honeycutt JD, Hassan M, Chandrasekhar J, Shirley W, Tsui V, Schmitz U. Enhanced utility of AI/ML methods during lead optimization by inclusion of 3D ligand information. *Front Drug Discov.* 2022;2. doi:10.3389/fddsv.2022.1074797.
4. Tang Y, Moretti R, Meiler J. Recent advances in automated structure-based de novo drug design. *J Chem Inf Model.* 2024;64(6):1794–805. Epub 20240314. doi:10.1021/acs.jcim.4c00247. PubMed PMID: 38485516; PMCID: PMC10966644.
5. Menon D, Ranganathan R. A generative approach to materials discovery, design, and optimization. *ACS Omega.* 2022;7(30):25958–73. Epub 20220724. doi:10.1021/acsomega.2c03264. PubMed PMID: 35936396; PMCID: PMC9352221.
6. Spainhour CB. Naturla products. In: Gad SC, editor. *Drug Discovery Handbook.* Hoboken, NJ: John Wiley & Sons; 2005, pp. 11–72.
7. Newman DJ, Cragg GM. Natural products as sources of new drugs from 1981 to 2014. *J Nat Prod.* 2016;79(3):629–61. doi:10.1021/acs.jnatprod.5b01055. PubMed PMID: 26852623.
8. Paterson I, Anderson EA. Chemistry. The renaissance of natural products as drug candidates. *Science.* 2005;310(5747):451–3. Epub 2005/10/22. doi:10.1126/science.1116364. PubMed PMID: 16239465.
9. Newman DJ, Cragg GM. Natural products as sources of new drugs over the 30 years from 1981 to 2010. *J Nat Prod.* 2012;75(3):311–35. doi:10.1021/np200906s. PubMed PMID: 22316239; PMCID: 3721181.
10. Newman DJ, Cragg GM. Natural products as sources of new drugs over the nearly four decades from 01/1981 to 09/2019. *J Nat Prod.* 2020;83(3):770–803. Epub 2020/03/13. doi:10.1021/acs.jnatprod.9b01285. PubMed PMID: 32162523.
11. Vezina C, Kudelski A, Sehgal SN. Rapamycin (AY-22,989), a new antifungal antibiotic. I. Taxonomy of the producing streptomycete and isolation of the active principle. *J Antibiot (Tokyo).* 1975;28(10):721–6. PubMed PMID: 1102508.
12. Chopra I, Roberts M. Tetracycline antibiotics: mode of action, applications, molecular biology, and epidemiology of bacterial resistance. *Microbiol Mol Biol Rev.* 2001;65(2):232–60; second page, table of contents. doi:10.1128/MMBR.65.2.232-260.2001. PubMed PMID: 11381101; PMCID: 99026.
13. Li R. Marinopyrroles: Unique drug discoveries based on marine natural products. *Med Res Rev.* 2016;36(1):169–89. doi:10.1002/med.21359. PubMed PMID: 26332654.
14. Mayer AM, Glaser KB, Cuevas C, Jacobs RS, Kem W, Little RD, McIntosh JM, Newman DJ, Potts BC, Shuster DE. The odyssey of marine pharmaceuticals: A current pipeline perspective. *Trends Pharmacol Sci.* 2010;31(6):255–65. doi:10.1016/j.tips.2010.02.005. PubMed PMID: 20363514.
15. Kaiser R. *Meaningful Scents around the World.* Zurich: Wiley, VCH; 2006.
16. Tokunaga T, Sugawara H, Tadano C, Muro M. Effect of stimulation of cold receptors with menthol on EMG activity of quadriceps muscle during low load contraction. *Somatosens Mot Res.* 2017;34(2):85–91. doi:10.1080/08990220.2017.1299004. PubMed PMID: 28325123.
17. Suchodolski J, Feder-Kubis J, Krasowska A. Antifungal activity of ionic liquids based on (-)-menthol: A mechanism study. *Microbiol Res.* 2017;197:56–64. doi:10.1016/j.micres.2016.12.008. PubMed PMID: 28219526.
18. Wondergem R, Bartley JW. Menthol increases human glioblastoma intracellular Ca2+, BK channel activity and cell migration. *J Biomed Sci.* 2009;16:90. doi:10.1186/1423-0127-16-90. PubMed PMID: 19778436; PMCID: 2758849.
19. Park EJ, Kim SH, Kim BJ, Kim SY, So I, Jeon JH. Menthol enhances an antiproliferative activity of 1alpha,25-dihydroxyvitamin D(3) in LNCaP cells. *J Clin Biochem Nutr.* 2009;44(2):125–30. doi:10.3164/jcbn.08-201. PubMed PMID: 19308266; PMCID: 2654468.

20. Watt EE, Betts BA, Kotey FO, Humbert DJ, Griffith TN, Kelly EW, Veneskey KC, Gill N, Rowan KC, Jenkins A, Hall AC. Menthol shares general anesthetic activity and sites of action on the GABA(A) receptor with the intravenous agent, propofol. *Eur J Pharmacol.* 2008;590(1–3):120–6. doi:10.1016/j.ejphar.2008.06.003. PubMed PMID: 18593637.
21. Shahverdi AR, Fazeli MR, Rafii F, Kakavand M, Jamalifar H, Hamedi J. Inhibition of nitrofurantoin reduction by menthol leads to enhanced antimicrobial activity. *J Chemother.* 2003;15(5):449–53. doi:10.1179/joc.2003.15.5.449. PubMed PMID: 14598936.
22. Juergens UR, Stober M, Vetter H. The anti-inflammatory activity of L-menthol compared to mint oil in human monocytes in vitro: a novel perspective for its therapeutic use in inflammatory diseases. *Eur J Med Res.* 1998;3(12):539–45. PubMed PMID: 9889172.
23. Zimmermann M, Preac-Mursic V. In vitro activity of taurolidine, chlorophenol-camphor-menthol and chlorhexidine against oral pathogenic microorganisms. *Arzneimittelforschung.* 1992;42(9):1157–9. PubMed PMID: 1445486.
24. Olivon F, Allard PM, Koval A, Righi D, Genta-Jouve G, Neyts J, Apel C, Pannecouque C, Nothias LF, Cachet X, Marcourt L, Roussi F, Katanaev VL, Touboul D, Wolfender JL, Litaudon M. Bioactive natural products prioritization using massive multi-informational molecular networks. *ACS Chem Biol.* 2017;12(10):2644–51. doi:10.1021/acschembio.7b00413. PubMed PMID: 28829118.
25. Olgac A, Orhan IE, Banoglu E. The potential role of in silico approaches to identify novel bioactive molecules from natural resources. *Future Med Chem.* 2017;9(14):1663–84. doi:10.4155/fmc-2017-0124. PubMed PMID: 28841048.
26. Pereira F, Latino DA, Gaudencio SP. QSAR-assisted virtual screening of lead-like molecules from marine and microbial natural sources for antitumor and antibiotic drug discovery. *Molecules.* 2015;20(3):4848–73. doi:10.3390/molecules20034848. PubMed PMID: 25789820.
27. Nettles JH, Jenkins JL, Bender A, Deng Z, Davies JW, Glick M. Bridging chemical and biological space: "target fishing" using 2D and 3D molecular descriptors. *J Med Chem.* 2006;49(23):6802–10. doi:10.1021/jm060902w. PubMed PMID: 17154510.
28. Wassermann AM, Lounkine E, Urban L, Whitebread S, Chen S, Hughes K, Guo H, Kutlina E, Fekete A, Klumpp M, Glick M. A screening pattern recognition method finds new and divergent targets for drugs and natural products. *ACS Chem Biol.* 2014;9(7):1622–31. doi:10.1021/cb5001839. PubMed PMID: 24802392.
29. Percha B, Altman RB. Learning the structure of biomedical relationships from unstructured text. *PLoS Comput Biol.* 2015;11(7):e1004216. doi:10.1371/journal.pcbi.1004216. PubMed PMID: 26219079; PMCID: 4517797.
30. Lagunin A, Filimonov D, Poroikov V. Multi-targeted natural products evaluation based on biological activity prediction with PASS. *Curr Pharm Des.* 2010;16(15):1703–17. PubMed PMID: 20222853.
31. Abdo A, Leclere V, Jacques P, Salim N, Pupin M. Prediction of new bioactive molecules using a Bayesian belief network. *J Chem Inf Model.* 2014;54(1):30–6. doi:10.1021/ci4004909. PubMed PMID: 24392938.
32. Schuster D, Waltenberger B, Kirchmair J, Distinto S, Markt P, Stuppner H, Rollinger JM, Wolber G. Predicting cyclooxygenase inhibition by three-dimensional pharmacophoric profiling. Part I: model generation, validation and applicability in ethnopharmacology. *Mol Inform.* 2010;29(1–2):75–86. doi:10.1002/minf.200900071. PubMed PMID: 27463850.
33. Rollinger JM, Haupt S, Stuppner H, Langer T. Combining ethnopharmacology and virtual screening for lead structure discovery: COX-inhibitors as application example. *J Chem Inf Comput Sci.* 2004;44(2):480–8. doi:10.1021/ci030031o. PubMed PMID: 15032527.

34. Hochleitner J, Akram M, Ueberall M, Davis RA, Waltenberger B, Stuppner H, Sturm S, Ueberall F, Gostner JM, Schuster D. A combinatorial approach for the discovery of cytochrome P450 2D6 inhibitors from nature. *Sci Rep.* 2017;7(1):8071. doi:10.1038/s41598-017-08404-0. PubMed PMID: 28808272; PMCID: 5556109.
35. Rollinger JM, Schuster D, Danzl B, Schwaiger S, Markt P, Schmidtke M, Gertsch J, Raduner S, Wolber G, Langer T, Stuppner H. In silico target fishing for rationalized ligand discovery exemplified on constituents of Ruta graveolens. *Planta Med.* 2009;75(3):195–204. doi:10.1055/s-0028-1088397. PubMed PMID: 19096995; PMCID: 3525952.
36. Fang J, Wu Z, Cai C, Wang Q, Tang Y, Cheng F. Quantitative and systems pharmacology. 1. In silico prediction of drug-target interactions of natural products enables new targeted cancer therapy. *J Chem Inform Model.* 2017;57(11):2657–71. doi:10.1021/acs.jcim.7b00216. PubMed PMID: 28956927.
37. Ding W, Gu J, Cao L, Li N, Ding G, Wang Z, Chen L, Xu X, Xiao W. Traditional Chinese herbs as chemical resource library for drug discovery of anti-infective and anti-inflammatory. *J Ethnopharmacol.* 2014;155(1):589–98. doi:10.1016/j.jep.2014.05.066. PubMed PMID: 24928828.
38. Gu J, Gui Y, Chen L, Yuan G, Lu HZ, Xu X. Use of natural products as chemical library for drug discovery and network pharmacology. *PloS One.* 2013;8(4):e62839. doi:10.1371/journal.pone.0062839. PubMed PMID: 23638153; PMCID: 3636197.
39. Bhatti HA, Tehseen Y, Maryam K, Uroos M, Siddiqui BS, Hameed A, Iqbal J. Identification of new potent inhibitor of aldose reductase from Ocimum basilicum. *Bioorg Chem.* 2017;75:62–70. doi:10.1016/j.bioorg.2017.08.011. PubMed PMID: 28917123.
40. Chen YZ, Ung CY. Computer automated prediction of potential therapeutic and toxicity protein targets of bioactive compounds from Chinese medicinal plants. *Am J Chin Med.* 2002;30(1):139–54. doi:10.1142/S0192415X02000156. PubMed PMID: 12067089.
41. Chagas-Paula DA, Oliveira TB, Zhang T, Edrada-Ebel R, Da Costa FB. Prediction of anti-inflammatory plants and discovery of their biomarkers by machine learning algorithms and metabolomic studies. *Planta Med.* 2015;81(6):450–8. doi:10.1055/s-0034–1396206. PubMed PMID: 25615275.
42. Keum J, Yoo S, Lee D, Nam H. Prediction of compound-target interactions of natural products using large-scale drug and protein information. *BMC Bioinf.* 2016;17 (Suppl 6):219. doi:10.1186/s12859-016-1081-y. PubMed PMID: 27490208; PMCID: 4965709.
43. Lorenzo VP, Alves MF, Scotti L, Dos Santos SG, de Fatima Formiga Melo Diniz M, Scotti MT. Computational chemistry study of natural alkaloids and homemade databank to predict inhibitory potential against key enzymes in neurodegenerative diseases. *Curr Top Med Chem.* 2017;17(26):2926–34. doi:10.2174/1568026617666170821150538. PubMed PMID: 28828994.
44. Luo H, Liang DF, Bao MY, Sun R, Li YY, Li JZ, Wang X, Lu KM, Bao JK. In silico identification of potential inhibitors targeting Streptococcus mutans sortase A. *Int J Oral Sci.* 2017;9(1):53–62. doi:10.1038/ijos.2016.58. PubMed PMID: 28358034; PMCID: 5379162.
45. Ntie-Kang F, Zofou D, Babiaka SB, Meudom R, Scharfe M, Lifongo LL, Mbah JA, Mbaze LM, Sippl W, Efange SM. AfroDb: A select highly potent and diverse natural product library from African medicinal plants. *PLoS One.* 2013;8(10):e78085. Epub 2013/11/10. doi:10.1371/journal.pone.0078085. PubMed PMID: 24205103; PMCID: PMC3813505.
46. Onguene PA, Simoben CV, Fotso GW, Andrae-Marobela K, Khalid SA, Ngadjui BT, Mbaze LM, Ntie-Kang F. In silico toxicity profiling of natural product compound libraries from African flora with anti-malarial and anti-HIV properties. *Comput Biol Chem.* 2017;72:136–149. doi:10.1016/j.compbiolchem.2017.12.002. PubMed PMID: 29277258.

47. Daina A, Michielin O, Zoete V. SwissTargetPrediction: Updated data and new features for efficient prediction of protein targets of small molecules. *Nucleic Acids Res.* 2019;47(W1):W357–W64. Epub 2019/05/21. doi:10.1093/nar/gkz382. PubMed PMID: 31106366; PMCID: PMC6602486.
48. Rodrigues T, Reker D, Schneider P, Schneider G. Counting on natural products for drug design. *Nat Chem.* 2016;8(6):531–41. Epub 2016/05/25. doi:10.1038/nchem.2479. PubMed PMID: 27219696.
49. Qiang B, Lai J, Jin H, Zhang L, Liu Z. Target prediction model for natural products using transfer learning. *Int J Mol Sci.* 2021;22(9):4632. Epub 2021/05/01. doi:10.3390/ijms22094632. PubMed PMID: 33924898; PMCID: PMC8124298.
50. Cockroft NT, Cheng X, Fuchs JR. STarFish: A stacked ensemble target fishing approach and its application to natural products. *J Chem Inf Model.* 2019;59(11):4906–20. Epub 2019/10/08. doi:10.1021/acs.jcim.9b00489. PubMed PMID: 31589422; PMCID: PMC7291623.
51. Rayan A, Raiyn J, Falah M. Nature is the best source of anticancer drugs: Indexing natural products for their anticancer bioactivity. *PLoS One.* 2017;12(11):e0187925. doi:10.1371/journal.pone.0187925. PubMed PMID: 29121120; PMCID: 5679595.
52. Mathai N, Chen Y, Kirchmair J. Validation strategies for target prediction methods. *Brief Bioinform.* 2020;21(3):791–802. Epub 2019/06/21. doi:10.1093/bib/bbz026. PubMed PMID: 31220208; PMCID: PMC7299289.
53. Fang H, Wang K, Zhang J. Transcriptome and proteome analyses of drug interactions with natural products. *Curr Drug Metab.* 2008;9(10):1038–48. PubMed PMID: 19075620.
54. Fricker G. Drug interactions with natural products at the blood brain barrier. *Curr Drug Metab.* 2008;9(10):1019–26. PubMed PMID: 19075618.
55. Goldman RD, Rogovik AL, Lai D, Vohra S. Potential interactions of drug-natural health products and natural health products-natural health products among children. *J Pediatr.* 2008;152(4):521–6, 6 e1–4. doi:10.1016/j.jpeds.2007.09.026. PubMed PMID: 18346508.
56. Staudinger JL, Ding X, Lichti K. Pregnane X receptor and natural products: beyond drug-drug interactions. *Expert Opin Drug Metab Toxicol.* 2006;2(6):847–57. PubMed PMID: 17125405; PMCID: 2978027.
57. Bailey DG, Dresser GK. Natural products and adverse drug interactions. *CMAJ.* 2004;170(10):1531–2. PubMed PMID: 15136542; PMCID: 400713.
58. Urbina F, Lowden CT, Culberson JC, Ekins S. MegaSyn: Integrating generative molecular design, automated analog designer, and synthetic viability prediction. *ACS Omega.* 2022;7(22):18699–713. Epub 2022/06/14. doi:10.1021/acsomega.2c01404. PubMed PMID: 35694522; PMCID: PMC9178760.
59. Grisoni F, Merk D, Consonni V, Hiss JA, Tagliabue SG, Todeschini R, Schneider G. Scaffold hopping from natural products to synthetic mimetics by holistic molecular similarity. *Commun Chem.* 2018;1(1):44. doi:10.1038/s42004-018-0043-x.
60. Karageorgis G, Foley DJ, Laraia L, Waldmann H. Principle and design of pseudo-natural products. *Nat Chem.* 2020;12(3):227–35. doi:10.1038/s41557-019-0411-x.
61. Zin PPK, Williams GJ, Ekins S. Cheminformatics analysis and modeling with MacrolactoneDB. *Sci Rep.* 2020;10(1):6284. Epub 2020/04/15. doi:10.1038/s41598-020-63192-4. PubMed PMID: 32286395; PMCID: PMC7156526.
62. Ntie-Kang F, Telukunta KK, Doring K, Simoben CV, Moumbock AFA, Malange YI, Njume LE, Yong JN, Sippl W, Gunther S. NANPDB: A resource for natural products from northern african sources. *J Nat Prod.* 2017;80(7):2067–76. Epub 2017/06/24. doi:10.1021/acs.jnatprod.7b00283. PubMed PMID: 28641017.
63. Klementz D, Doring K, Lucas X, Telukunta KK, Erxleben A, Deubel D, Erber A, Santillana I, Thomas OS, Bechthold A, Gunther S. StreptomeDB 2.0--an extended resource of natural products produced by streptomycetes. *Nucleic Acids Res.* 2016;44(D1):D509–14. Epub 2015/11/29. doi:10.1093/nar/gkv1319. PubMed PMID: 26615197; PMCID: PMC4702922.

64. Zani CL, Carroll AR. Database for rapid dereplication of known natural products using data from MS and fast NMR experiments. *J Nat Prod.* 2017;80(6):1758–66. Epub 2017/06/16. doi:10.1021/acs.jnatprod.6b01093. PubMed PMID: 28616931.
65. Sterling T, Irwin JJ. ZINC 15--ligand discovery for everyone. *J Chem Inf Model.* 2015;55(11):2324–37. Epub 2015/10/20. doi:10.1021/acs.jcim.5b00559. PubMed PMID: 26479676; PMCID: PMC4658288.
66. Lin YC, Wang CC, Chen IS, Jheng JL, Li JH, Tung CW. TIPdb: a database of anticancer, antiplatelet, and antituberculosis phytochemicals from indigenous plants in Taiwan. *Sci World J.* 2013;2013:736386. Epub 2013/06/15. doi:10.1155/2013/736386. PubMed PMID: 23766708; PMCID: PMC3666282.
67. Gilson MK, Liu T, Baitaluk M, Nicola G, Hwang L, Chong J. BindingDB in 2015: A public database for medicinal chemistry, computational chemistry and systems pharmacology. *Nucleic Acids Res.* 2016;44(D1):D1045–53. doi:10.1093/nar/gkv1072. PubMed PMID: 26481362; PMCID: PMC4702793.
68. Onguene PA, Ntie-Kang F, Mbah JA, Lifongo LL, Ndom JC, Sippl W, Mbaze LM. The potential of anti-malarial compounds derived from African medicinal plants, part III: An in silico evaluation of drug metabolism and pharmacokinetics profiling. *Org Med Chem Lett.* 2014;4(1):6. Epub 2015/11/10. doi:10.1186/s13588-014-0006-x. PubMed PMID: 26548985; PMCID: PMC4970435.
69. Pilon-Jimenez BA, Saldivar-Gonzalez FI, Diaz-Eufracio BI, Medina-Franco JL. BIOFACQUIM: A Mexican compound database of natural products. *Biomolecules.* 2019;9(1):31. Epub 2019/01/20. doi:10.3390/biom9010031. PubMed PMID: 30658522; PMCID: PMC6358837.
70. Gaulton A, Bellis LJ, Bento AP, Chambers J, Davies M, Hersey A, Light Y, McGlinchey S, Michalovich D, Al-Lazikani B, Overington JP. ChEMBL: A large-scale bioactivity database for drug discovery. *Nucleic Acids Res.* 2012;40(Database issue):D1100–7. PubMed PMID: 21948594.
71. Kim S, Thiessen PA, Bolton EE, Chen J, Fu G, Gindulyte A, Han L, He J, He S, Shoemaker BA, Wang J, Yu B, Zhang J, Bryant SH. PubChem substance and compound databases. *Nucleic Acids Res.* 2016;44(D1):D1202–13. doi:10.1093/nar/gkv951. PubMed PMID: 26400175; PMCID: PMC4702940.
72. Fillbrunn A, Dietz C, Pfeuffer J, Rahn R, Landrum GA, Berthold MR. KNIME for reproducible cross-domain analysis of life science data. *J Biotechnol.* 2017;261:149–56. Epub 2017/08/02. doi:10.1016/j.jbiotec.2017.07.028. PubMed PMID: 28757290.
73. Cherkasov A, Muratov EN, Fourches D, Varnek A, Baskin, II, Cronin M, Dearden J, Gramatica P, Martin YC, Todeschini R, Consonni V, Kuz'min VE, Cramer R, Benigni R, Yang C, Rathman J, Terfloth L, Gasteiger J, Richard A, Tropsha A. QSAR modeling: Where have you been? Where are you going to? *J Med Chem.* 2014;57(12):4977–5010. Epub 2013/12/20. doi:10.1021/jm4004285. PubMed PMID: 24351051; PMCID: PMC4074254.
74. Appavoo SD, Huh S, Diaz DB, Yudin AK. Conformational control of macrocycles by remote structural modification. *Chem Rev.* 2019;119(17):9724–52. Epub 2019/08/15. doi:10.1021/acs.chemrev.8b00742. PubMed PMID: 31411458.
75. Kearney SE, Zahoranszky-Kohalmi G, Brimacombe KR, Henderson MJ, Lynch C, Zhao T, Wan KK, Itkin Z, Dillon C, Shen M, Cheff DM, Lee TD, Bougie D, Cheng K, Coussens NP, Dorjsuren D, Eastman RT, Huang R, Iannotti MJ, Karavadhi S, Klumpp-Thomas C, Roth JS, Sakamuru S, Sun W, Titus SA, Yasgar A, Zhang YQ, Zhao J, Andrade RB, Brown MK, Burns NZ, Cha JK, Mevers EE, Clardy J, Clement JA, Crooks PA, Cuny GD, Ganor J, Moreno J, Morrill LA, Picazo E, Susick RB, Garg NK, Goess BC, Grossman RB, Hughes CC, Johnston JN, Joullie MM, Kinghorn AD, Kingston DGI, Krische MJ, Kwon O, Maimone TJ, Majumdar S, Maloney KN, Mohamed E, Murphy BT, Nagorny P, Olson DE, Overman LE, Brown LE, Snyder JK, Porco JA, Jr., Rivas F, Ross SA, Sarpong R, Sharma I, Shaw JT, Xu Z, Shen B, Shi

W, Stephenson CRJ, Verano AL, Tan DS, Tang Y, Taylor RE, Thomson RJ, Vosburg DA, Wu J, Wuest WM, Zakarian A, Zhang Y, Ren T, Zuo Z, Inglese J, Michael S, Simeonov A, Zheng W, Shinn P, Jadhav A, Boxer MB, Hall MD, Xia M, Guha R, Rohde JM. Canvass: A crowd-sourced, natural-product screening library for exploring biological space. *ACS Cent Sci.* 2018;4(12):1727–41. Epub 2019/01/17. doi:10.1021/acscentsci.8b00747. PubMed PMID: 30648156; PMCID: PMC6311695.

76. Anon. The PubChem Database. Available from: https://pubchem.ncbi.nlm.nih.gov/.
77. Tice RR, Austin CP, Kavlock RJ, Bucher JR. Improving the human hazard characterization of chemicals: A Tox21 update. *Environ Health Perspect.* 2013;121(7):756–65. Epub 2013/04/23. doi:10.1289/ehp.1205784. PubMed PMID: 23603828; PMCID: PMC3701992.
78. Waters M, Stasiewicz S, Merrick BA, Tomer K, Bushel P, Paules R, Stegman N, Nehls G, Yost KJ, Johnson CH, Gustafson SF, Xirasagar S, Xiao N, Huang CC, Boyer P, Chan DD, Pan Q, Gong H, Taylor J, Choi D, Rashid A, Ahmed A, Howle R, Selkirk J, Tennant R, Fostel J. CEBS--Chemical effects in biological systems: A public data repository integrating study design and toxicity data with microarray and proteomics data. *Nucleic Acids Res.* 2008;36(Database issue):D892–900. Epub 2007/10/27. doi:10.1093/nar/gkm755. PubMed PMID: 17962311; PMCID: PMC2238989.
79. Zorn KM, Lane TR, Russo DP, Clark AM, Makarov V, Ekins S. Multiple machine learning comparisons of HIV cell-based and reverse transcriptase data sets. *Mol Pharm.* 2019;16(4):1620–32. Epub 2019/02/20. doi:10.1021/acs.molpharmaceut.8b01297. PubMed PMID: 30779585.
80. Munson BP, Chen M, Bogosian A, Kreisberg JF, Licon K, Abagyan R, Kuenzi BM, Ideker T. De novo generation of multi-target compounds using deep generative chemistry. *Nat Commun.* 2024;15(1):3636. Epub 20240506. doi:10.1038/s41467-024-47120-y. PubMed PMID: 38710699; PMCID: PMC11074339.
81. Hamilton WL, Ying R, Leskovec J. Inductive representation learning on large graphs. *arXiv* 2017; 1706.02216.
82. Kipf TN, Welling M. Semi-supervised classification with graph convolutional networks. *arXiv* 2016; 1609.02907.
83. Veličković P, Cucurull G, Casanova A, Romero A, Liò P, Bengio Y. Graph attention networks. *arXiv* 2017; 1710.10903.
84. Gilmer J, Schoelholz SS, Riley PF, Vinyals O, Dahl GE. Neural message passing for quantum chemistry. *arXiv* 2017; 1704.01212.
85. Cichońska A, Ravikumar B, Allaway RJ, Wan F, Park S, Isayev O, Li S, Mason M, Lamb A, Tanoli Z, Jeon M, Kim S, Popova M, Capuzzi S, Zeng J, Dang K, Koytiger G, Kang J, Wells CI, Willson TM, Tan M, Huang C-H, Shih ESC, Chen T-M, Wu C-H, Fang W-Q, Chen J-Y, Hwang M-J, Wang X, Ben Guebila M, Shamsaei B, Singh S, Nguyen T, Karimi M, Wu D, Wang Z, Shen Y, Öztürk H, Ozkirimli E, Özgür A, Lim H, Xie L, Kanev GK, Kooistra AJ, Westerman BA, Terzopoulos P, Ntagiantas K, Fotis C, Alexopoulos L, Boeckaerts D, Stock M, De Baets B, Briers Y, Luo Y, Hu H, Peng J, Dogan T, Rifaioglu AS, Atas H, Atalay RC, Atalay V, Martin MJ, Jeon M, Lee J, Yun S, Kim B, Chang B, Turu G, Misák Á, Szalai B, Hunyady L, Lienhard M, Prasse P, Bachmann I, Ganzlin J, Barel G, Herwig R, Oršolić D, Lučić B, Stepanić V, Šmuc T, Oprea TI, Schlessinger A, Drewry DH, Stolovitzky G, Wennerberg K, Guinney J, Aittokallio T. Crowdsourced mapping of unexplored target space of kinase inhibitors. *Nat Commun.* 2021;12(1):3307. doi:10.1038/s41467-021-23165-1.
86. Shi X, Chen Z, Wang H, Yeung D-Y, Wong W, Woo W. Convolutional LSTM network: A machine learning approach for precipitation nowcasting. *arXiv* 2015; 1506.04214.
87. Finn C, Abbeel P, Levine S. Model-agnostic meta-learning for fast adaptation of deep networks. *arXiv* 2017; 1703.03400.
88. Wang Y, Yao Q, Kwok J, Ni LM. Generalizing from a few examples: A survey on few-shot learning. *arXiv* 2019; 1904.05046.

89. Jimenez DG, Sebastiano MR, Caron G, Ermondi G. Are we ready to design oral PROTACs(R)? *ADMET DMPK.* 2021;9(4):243–54. Epub 2022/03/19. doi:10.5599/admet.1037. PubMed PMID: 35300370; PMCID: PMC8920102.
90. Garcia Jimenez D, Rossi Sebastiano M, Vallaro M, Mileo V, Pizzirani D, Moretti E, Ermondi G, Caron G. Designing soluble PROTACs: Strategies and preliminary guidelines. *J Med Chem.* 2022;65:12639–12649. Epub 2022/04/27. doi:10.1021/acs.jmedchem.2c00201. PubMed PMID: 35469399.
91. Nori D, Coley CW, Mercado R. De novo PROTAC design using graph-based deep generative models2022, November 01, 2022:[arXiv:2211.02660 p.]. Available from: https://ui.adsabs.harvard.edu/abs/2022arXiv221102660N.
92. Urbina F, Ekins S. The commoditization of AI for molecule design. *Artif Intell Life Sci.* 2022;2:100031. Epub 2022/10/11. doi:10.1016/j.ailsci.2022.100031. PubMed PMID: 36211981; PMCID: PMC9541920.
93. Havlicek V, Corcoles AD, Temme K, Harrow AW, Kandala A, Chow JM, Gambetta JM. Supervised learning with quantum-enhanced feature spaces. *Nature.* 2019;567(7747):209–12. Epub 2019/03/15. doi:10.1038/s41586-019-0980-2. PubMed PMID: 30867609.
94. Schuld M. Machine learning in quantum spaces. *Nature.* 2019;567(7747):179–81. Epub 2019/03/15. doi:10.1038/d41586-019-00771-0. PubMed PMID: 30867605.
95. Clark AM, Dole K, Coulon-Spector A, McNutt A, Grass G, Freundlich JS, Reynolds RC, Ekins S. Open source Bayesian models: 1. Application to ADME/Tox and drug discovery datasets. *J Chem Inf Model.* 2015;55:1231–45. doi:10.1021/acs.jcim.5b00143.
96. Kortagere S, Ekins S. Troubleshooting computational methods in drug discovery. *J Pharmacol Toxicol Methods.* 2010;61(2):67–75. PubMed PMID: 20176118.
97. Gupta RR, Gifford EM, Liston T, Waller CL, Bunin B, Ekins S. Using open source computational tools for predicting human metabolic stability and additional ADME/TOX properties. *Drug Metab Dispos.* 2010;38:2083–90.
98. Ekins S, Williams AJ. Precompetitive preclinical ADME/Tox data: Set it free on the web to facilitate computational model building to assist drug development. *Lab Chip.* 2010;10:13–22.
99. Ekins S, Honeycutt JD, Metz JT. Evolving molecules using multi-objective optimization: Applying to ADME. *Drug Discov Today.* 2010;15:451–60. PubMed PMID: 20438859.
100. Bahadduri PM, Polli JE, Swaan PW, Ekins S. Targeting drug transporters - Combining in silico and in vitro approaches to predict in vivo. *Methods Mol Biol.* 2010;637:65–103. PubMed PMID: 20419430.
101. Ekins S, Bugrim A, Brovold L, Kirillov E, Nikolsky Y, Rakhmatulin E, Sorokina S, Ryabov A, Serebryiskaya T, Melnikov A, Metz J, Nikolskaya T. Algorithms for network analysis in systems-ADME/Tox using the MetaCore and MetaDrug platforms. *Xenobiotica.* 2006;36(10–11):877–901. Epub 2006/11/23. doi:10.1080/00498250600861660. PubMed PMID: 17118913.
102. Ekins S, Andreyev S, Ryabov A, Kirillov E, Rakhmatulin EA, Sorokina S, Bugrim A, Nikolskaya T. A combined approach to drug metabolism and toxicity assessment. *Drug Metab Dispos.* 2006;34:495–503. PubMed PMID: 16381662.
103. Ekins S. Systems-ADME/Tox: Resources and network approaches. *J Pharmacol Toxicol Methods.* 2006;53(1):38–66. Epub 2005/08/02. doi:10.1016/j.vascn.2005.05.005. PubMed PMID: 16054403.
104. Chang C, Ekins S. Pharmacophores for human ADME/Tox-related proteins. In: Langer T, Hoffman RD, editors. *Pharmacophores and Pharmacophore Searches.* Weinheim: Wiley-VCH; 2006, pp. 299–324.
105. Ekins S, Nikolsky Y, Nikolskaya T. Techniques: application of systems biology to absorption, distribution, metabolism, excretion and toxicity. *Trends Pharmacol Sci.* 2005;26(4):202–9. Epub 2005/04/06. doi:10.1016/j.tips.2005.02.006. PubMed PMID: 15808345.

106. Ekins S, Andreyev S, Ryabov A, Kirillov E, Rakhmatulin EA, Bugrim A, Nikolskaya T. Computational prediction of human drug metabolism. *Expert Opin Drug Metab Toxicol.* 2005;1(2):303–24. Epub 2006/08/23. doi:10.1517/17425255.1.2.303. PubMed PMID: 16922645.
107. Balakin KV, Ivanenkov YA, Savchuk NP, Ivaschenko AA, Ekins S. Comprehensive computational assessment of ADME properties using mapping techniques. *Curr Drug Disc Tech.* 2005;2:99–113.
108. Ekins S, Swaan PW. Computational models for enzymes, transporters, channels and receptors relevant to ADME/TOX. *Rev Comp Chem.* 2004;20:333–415.
109. Ekins S, Boulanger B, Swaan PW, Hupcey MA. Towards a new age of virtual ADME/TOX and multidimensional drug discovery. *Mol Divers.* 2002;5(4):255–75. Epub 2003/01/29. PubMed PMID: 12549676.
110. Ekins S, Wrighton SA. Application of in silico approaches to predicting drug--drug interactions. *J Pharmacol Toxicol Methods.* 2001;45(1):65–9. Epub 2001/08/08. doi:S1056–8719(01)00119-8 [pii]. PubMed PMID: 11489666.
111. Ekins S, Waller CL, Swaan PW, Cruciani G, Wrighton SA, Wikel JH. Progress in predicting human ADME parameters in silico. *J Pharmacol Toxicol Methods.* 2000;44(1):251–72. Epub 2001/03/29. doi:S1056–8719(00)00109-X [pii]. PubMed PMID: 11274894.
112. Ekins S, Ring BJ, Grace J, McRobie-Belle DJ, Wrighton SA. Present and future in vitro approaches for drug metabolism. *J Pharmacol Toxicol Methods.* 2000;44(1):313–24. Epub 2001/03/29. doi:S1056–8719(00)00110-6 [pii]. PubMed PMID: 11274898.
113. Perryman AL, Stratton TP, Ekins S, Freundlich JS. Predicting mouse liver microsomal stability with "pruned" machine learning models and public data. *Pharm Res.* 2015;33:433–49. doi:10.1007/s11095-015-1800-5.
114. Ekins S. Progress in computational toxicology. *J Pharmacol Toxicol Methods.* 2014;69(2):115–40. doi:10.1016/j.vascn.2013.12.003. PubMed PMID: 24361690.
115. Dong Z, Ekins S, Polli JE. Structure-activity relationship for FDA approved drugs as inhibitors of the human sodium taurocholate cotransporting polypeptide (NTCP). *Mol Pharm.* 2013;10(3):1008–19. PubMed PMID: 23339484.
116. Astorga B, Ekins S, Morales M, Wright SH. Molecular determinants of ligand selectivity for the human multidrug and toxin extrusion proteins, MATE1 and MATE-2K. *J Pharmacol Exp Ther.* 2012;341(3):743–55. PubMed PMID: 22419765.
117. Pan Y, Li L, Kim G, Ekins S, Wang H, Swaan PW. Identification and validation of novel hPXR activators amongst prescribed drugs via ligand-based virtual screening. *Drug Metab Dispos.* 2011;39:337–44. PubMed PMID: 21068194.
118. Zientek M, Stoner C, Ayscue R, Klug-McLeod J, Jiang Y, West M, Collins C, Ekins S. Integrated in silico-in vitro strategy for addressing cytochrome P450 3A4 time-dependent inhibition. *Chem Res Toxicol.* 2010;23(3):664–76. PubMed PMID: 20151638.
119. Ekins S, Williams AJ, Xu JJ. A predictive ligand-based bayesian model for human drug induced liver injury. *Drug Metab Dispos.* 2010;38:2302–8. PubMed PMID: 20843939.
120. Diao L, Ekins S, Polli JE. Quantitative structure activity relationship for inhibition of human organic cation/carnitine transporter. *Mol Pharm.* 2010;7:2120–30. PubMed PMID: 20831193.
121. Zheng X, Ekins S, Raufman JP, Polli JE. Computational models for drug inhibition of the human apical sodium-dependent bile acid transporter. *Mol Pharm.* 2009;6(5):1591–603. Epub 2009/08/14. doi:10.1021/mp900163d. PubMed PMID: 19673539; PMCID: 2757534.
122. Ekins S, Kortagere S, Iyer M, Reschly EJ, Lill MA, Redinbo MR, Krasowski MD. Challenges predicting ligand-receptor interactions of promiscuous proteins: the nuclear receptor PXR. *PLoS Comput Biol.* 2009;5(12):e1000594. Epub 2009/12/17. doi:10.1371/journal.pcbi.1000594. PubMed PMID: 20011107; PMCID: 2781111.

123. Minerali E, Foil DH, Zorn KM, Lane TR, Ekins S. Comparing machine learning algorithms for predicting drug-induced liver injury (DILI). *Mol Pharm.* 2020;17:2628–2637. Epub 2020/05/19. doi:10.1021/acs.molpharmaceut.0c00326. PubMed PMID: 32422053.
124. Dong Z, Ekins S, Polli JE. Quantitative NTCP pharmacophore and lack of association between DILI and NTCP inhibition. *Eur J Pharm Sci.* 2014;66C:1–9. doi:10.1016/j.ejps.2014.09.005. PubMed PMID: 25220493; PMCID: PMC4362924.
125. Ekins S, Diao L, Polli JE. A substrate pharmacophore for the human organic cation/carnitine transporter identifies compounds associated with rhabdomyolysis. *Mol Pharm.* 2012;9:905–13. PubMed PMID: 22339151.
126. Diao L, Ekins S, Polli JE. Novel inhibitors of human organic cation/carnitine transporter (hOCTN2) via computational modeling and in vitro testing. *Pharm Res.* 2009;26:1890–900. PubMed PMID: 19437106.
127. Clark AM, Sarker M, Ekins S. New target predictions and visualization tools incorporating open source molecular fingerprints for TB Mobile 2.0. *J Cheminform.* 2014;6:38.
128. Clark AM, Ekins S. Open source Bayesian models: 2. Mining a "big dataset" to create and validate models with ChEMBL. *J Chem Inf Model.* 2015;55:1246–60. doi:10.1021/acs.jcim.5b00144.
129. Lane T, Russo DP, Zorn KM, Clark AM, Korotcov A, Tkachenko V, Reynolds RC, Perryman AL, Freundlich JS, Ekins S. Comparing and validating machine learning models for Mycobacterium tuberculosis drug discovery. *Mol Pharm.* 2018;15(10):4346–60. Epub 2018/04/20. doi:10.1021/acs.molpharmaceut.8b00083. PubMed PMID: 29672063; PMCID: PMC6167198.
130. Russo DP, Zorn KM, Clark AM, Zhu H, Ekins S. Comparing multiple machine learning algorithms and metrics for estrogen receptor binding prediction. *Mol Pharm.* 2018;15(10):4361–70. Epub 2018/08/18. doi:10.1021/acs.molpharmaceut.8b00546. PubMed PMID: 30114914; PMCID: PMC6181119.
131. Wang PF, Neiner A, Lane TR, Zorn KM, Ekins S, Kharasch ED. Halogen substitution influences ketamine metabolism by cytochrome P450 2B6: In vitro and computational approaches. *Mol Pharm.* 2019;16(2):898–906. Epub 2018/12/28. doi:10.1021/acs.molpharmaceut.8b01214. PubMed PMID: 30589555.
132. Sandoval PJ, Zorn KM, Clark AM, Ekins S, Wright SH. Assessment of substrate-dependent ligand interactions at the organic cation transporter OCT2 using six model substrates. *Mol Pharmacol.* 2018;94(3):1057–68. Epub 2018/06/10. doi:10.1124/mol.117.111443. PubMed PMID: 29884691; PMCID: PMC6070079.
133. Hernandez HW, Soeung M, Zorn KM, Ashoura N, Mottin M, Andrade CH, Caffrey CR, de Siqueira-Neto JL, Ekins S. High throughput and computational repurposing for neglected diseases. *Pharm Res.* 2018;36(2):27. Epub 2018/12/19. doi:10.1007/s11095-018-2558-3. PubMed PMID: 30560386; PMCID: PMC6792295.
134. Ekins S, Puhl AC, Zorn KM, Lane TR, Russo DP, Klein JJ, Hickey AJ, Clark AM. Exploiting machine learning for end-to-end drug discovery and development. *Nat Mater.* 2019;18(5):435–41. Epub 2019/04/20. doi:10.1038/s41563-019-0338-z. PubMed PMID: 31000803; PMCID: PMC6594828.
135. Ekins S, Gerlach J, Zorn KM, Antonio BM, Lin Z, Gerlach A. Repurposing approved drugs as inhibitors of Kv7.1 and Nav1.8 to treat pitt Hopkins syndrome. *Pharm Res.* 2019;36(9):137. Epub 2019/07/25. doi:10.1007/s11095-019-2671-y. PubMed PMID: 31332533; PMCID: PMC6814258.
136. Dalecki AG, Zorn KM, Clark AM, Ekins S, Narmore WT, Tower N, Rasmussen L, Bostwick R, Kutsch O, Wolschendorf F. High-throughput screening and Bayesian machine learning for copper-dependent inhibitors of Staphylococcus aureus. *Metallomics.* 2019;11(3):696–706. Epub 2019/03/07. doi:10.1039/c8mt00342d. PubMed PMID: 30839007; PMCID: PMC6467072.

137. Anantpadma M, Lane T, Zorn KM, Lingerfelt MA, Clark AM, Freundlich JS, Davey RA, Madrid PB, Ekins S. Ebola virus Bayesian machine learning models enable new in vitro leads. *ACS Omega*. 2019;4(1):2353–61. Epub 2019/02/08. doi:10.1021/acsomega.8b02948. PubMed PMID: 30729228; PMCID: PMC6356859.
138. Korotcov A, Tkachenko V, Russo DP, Ekins S. Comparison of deep learning with multiple machine learning methods and metrics using diverse drug discovery datasets. *Mol Pharm*. 2018;14:4462–75.
139. Batra K, Zorn KM, Foil DH, Minerali E, Gawriljuk VO, Lane TR, Ekins S. Quantum machine learning algorithms for drug discovery applications. *J Chem Inf Model*. 2021;61(6):2641–7. Epub 2021/05/26. doi:10.1021/acs.jcim.1c00166. PubMed PMID: 34032436; PMCID: PMC8254374.
140. Kao PY, Yang YC, Chiang WY, Hsiao JY, Cao Y, Aliper A, Ren F, Aspuru-Guzik A, Zhavoronkov A, Hsieh MH, Lin YC. Exploring the advantages of quantum generative adversarial networks in generative chemistry. *J Chem Inf Model*. 2023;63(11):3307–18. Epub 20230512. doi:10.1021/acs.jcim.3c00562. PubMed PMID: 37171372; PMCID: PMC10268960.
141. Papadatos G, Davies M, Dedman N, Chambers J, Gaulton A, Siddle J, Koks R, Irvine SA, Pettersson J, Goncharoff N, Hersey A, Overington JP. SureChEMBL: A large-scale, chemically annotated patent document database. *Nucleic Acids Res*. 2016;44(D1):D1220–8. Epub 2015/11/20. doi:10.1093/nar/gkv1253. PubMed PMID: 26582922; PMCID: PMC4702887.
142. Falaguera MJ, Mestres J. Identification of the core chemical structure in SureChEMBL patents. *J Chem Inf Model*. 2021;61(5):2241–7. Epub 2021/05/01. doi:10.1021/acs.jcim.1c00151. PubMed PMID: 33929850.
143. Wang Y, Cheng T, Bryant SH. PubChem BioAssay: A decade's development toward open high-throughput screening data sharing. *SLAS Discov*. 2017;22(6):655–66. Epub 2017/03/28. doi:10.1177/2472555216685069. PubMed PMID: 28346087; PMCID: PMC5480605.
144. Anon. PubChem 2020. Available from: https://pubchem.ncbi.nlm.nih.gov/.
145. Janssen APA, Grimm SH, Wijdeven RHM, Lenselink EB, Neefjes J, van Boeckel CAA, van Westen GJP, van der Stelt M. Drug discovery maps, a machine learning model that visualizes and predicts kinome-inhibitor interaction landscapes. *J Chem Inf Model*. 2019;59(3):1221–9. Epub 2018/10/30. doi:10.1021/acs.jcim.8b00640. PubMed PMID: 30372617; PMCID: PMC6437696.

Index

For Product Safety Concerns and Information please contact our EU representative GPSR@taylorandfrancis.com
Taylor & Francis Verlag GmbH, Kaufingerstraße 24, 80331 München, Germany

www.ingramcontent.com/pod-product-compliance
Lightning Source LLC
LaVergne TN
LVHW010558110826
845149LV00003B/691

* 9 7 8 1 0 3 2 5 0 6 2 5 8 *